Never Satisfied

Never Satisfied

A Cultural History of Diets,
Fantasies and Fat

Hillel Schwartz

THE FREE PRESS
A Division of Macmillan, Inc.
NEW YORK

Collier Macmillan Publishers
LONDON

The Free Press
A Division of Macmillan, Inc.
866 Third Avenue, New York, N.Y. 10022

Collier Macmillan Canada, Inc.

Printed in the United States of America

printing number
1   2   3   4   5   6   7   8   9   10

Library of Congress Cataloging-in-Publication Data

Schwartz, Hillel
    Never satisfied.

    Bibliography: p.
    1. Reducing—Social aspects—United States—History.
2. Body image. 3. Obesity—Social aspects—United
States—History. 4. Body, Human—Social aspects—
United States. I. Title.
RM222.2.S357   1986   391′.62′0973   86-19552
ISBN 0-02-929250-6

For my parents,
at whose table I was first satisfied

Contents

CHAPTER ONE

Prologue: Ritual and Romance

It would be interesting if some student of manners would trace with precision the process whereby what finicking people call "embonpoint" came into general discredit. Fat is now regarded as an indiscretion, and almost as a crime.

—*Living Age* (Feb. 28, 1914) 573.

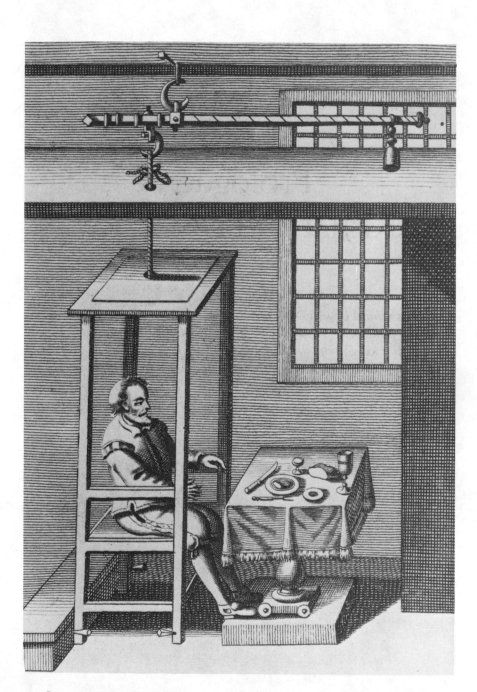

Santorio Santorio in his hanging chair, from an English edition of his Aphorisms *(1712).* Courtesy of the National Library of Medicine

Fantasies of the Body

E LLA MAE STEPPED on the bathroom scale. She played with it, lifting one foot off, on, off, sending the numbers whirling. "This was weight, this was all weight was, this is what one could do with weight. . . . She knew this machine well; it could purr or hiss or spit like a cat. She knew there was no trusting it, that the number it finally put there had nothing to do with her, told nothing about who she was."[1]

This is a book about the experience of weight, how it has changed in the United States over the last 150 years, and what it tells about us now.

This is also a book about fat and fatness, which we have commonly confused with weight.

A history of the American experience of weight and of fatness must willy-nilly be a history of dieting. Slimming. Reducing. That this should be so is already a curiosity, something that entreats explanation. In other parts of the world, fatness does not bear immediate reference to pounds put on or calories consumed; in other times, personal weight has not been finely calibrated to age or height or worth.

Weight is a cultural condition. A scale does not make it more or less real. Fatness too is a cultural condition. Calipers are a pretext and pretense. There can be no timelessly perfect diet because the act of losing weight or shedding fat, like the desire itself, is culturally bounded.

The desire to be slim is not simply a result of fashion. It must be understood in terms of a confluence of movements in the sciences and in dance, in home economics and political economy, in medical technology and food marketing, in evangelical religion and life insurance. Our sense of the body, of its heft and momentum, is shaped more by the theater of our lives than by our costume. Our furniture, our toys, our architecture, our etiquette are designed for, or impel us toward, a certain kind of body and a certain feeling of weight.

Each epoch has had different tolerances for weight and for fatness. Since the 1880s, those tolerances have grown especially narrow, especially demanding. We take for granted now a constant personal vigil against overweight and obesity. Who among us cannot tell our weight within, say, 5 lbs? Who does not feel cheated if the birth announcement fails to give the baby's weight to the exact ounce?

What we most take for granted often seems least susceptible to history, as if only our crises require a chronicle. Indeed, aside from some hasty reviews in medical journals and a few passages in works by fashion historians, slimming has been left entirely without context: People liked being fat a century ago; now they like being thin.[2] The absence of an analytical tradition is almost startling, given more than a century of failed diets. After so many disappointments, people might have looked back and taken stock.

Slimming, however, has to do with fantasies. It has always been a sort of science fiction, extrapolating into the best and lightest of futures. The culture of slimming is uncomfortable with retrospect. Dieters cannot make peace with the past because each diet carries forward fantasies of a body released and transformed. As slow miracle or instant metamorphosis, diets deal in possibility. The fantasy of a body newly buoyant or balanced is far more appealing than the conscientious rehearsal of failed promises.

Why people choose to diet, when they diet, how they go about dieting—these are determined by prevailing fantasies about the body, its weight and its fat. Where, for example, fat is imagined to be inert, local and anonymous, dieters may hope to dissolve it away or pound it out in sporadic gestures of remorse. Where fat is imagined (as it is now) to be active, itinerant, and individual, dieters must fight against it tooth and nail, thoroughly, systematically, day and night.

This book, then, deals as much with shared fictions as with physiological fact. It will be inhabited by ghosts, cannibals, boa constrictors, mechanical horses, and tapeworms. Shifting perceptions of how the body should move and how it should feel while in motion—the kinaesthetics of our lives—will make people aware of and uneasy with their bodies. Shifting fantasies about weight and fat will accommodate new wonder drugs and eight-day diets. Shifting theories about metabolism and appetite will entail new therapies for reducing.

Each successive chapter in this book is devoted to explaining the cultural fit between shared fictions about the body and the reducing methods of the era. Since these fictions come to be shared only through the lively interplay of high culture (the sciences, the fine arts, philosophy, political economy) and popular culture (folk medicine, county fairs, cookery, comic strips), we must range widely in order to make sense of the national drive toward a lighter, thinner body. The scientific urge to weigh and measure the human body must be hinged to a popular faith in that body as a reliable index to the self within: How do Americans become convinced that weight reveals something desperately true about the person beneath the pounds? The statistical, businesslike disposition to calculate longevity on the basis of height, weight and age must be hinged to less exact, more common experiences of lightness and vitality: How do Americans become convinced that the streamlined body is the perfect body, the streamlined diet the perfect diet?

Diets have come and gone, but the passion for slimming has mounted steadily. Weight-watching and dieting have become part of the customary fabric of American society, from the nightclub to the nursery. Slimming, I shall argue, is the modern expression of an industrial society confused by its own desires and therefore never satisfied. On the one hand we seem to want more of everything; on the other hand we are suspicious of surplus. Increasingly perplexed or intimidated by abundance, Americans have taken the protocols of slimming as the protocols for social and spiritual renewal. This has been as true of Horace Fletcher's 1899 campaign for slow chewing and intestinal asepsis as it is now of Jane Fonda's Workout and buttock tucks. Each program for reducing has harbored an implicit program for coping with abundance and excess in the body politic. The hostility toward fat extends far beyond physiology.

Our language itself is laden with metaphors of fatness and heaviness. If we cannot speak or write without images of fat and weight entering our discourse, then the culture of slimming may have deep roots in those parts of our lives which seem entirely separate and distant from it. I have not shied away from those analogies which seem on their surfaces to be *only* matters of language, *only* figures of speech. Nor have I shied away from the inherent theatricality of that language. Diets arise in settings so much like those of folk tales or gothic romances that it would be foolish to abandon their drama for the sake of a dull scholasticism. In fact, it has been just this dramatic, mythic quality which has sustained many diets so that they may be reincarnated from epoch to epoch.

This book must therefore seem at times to be in suspense. It is structured as much by the demands of drama as by the demands of chronicle. Social historian, dancer and playwright must collude in plotting the paths and forces by which so many ostensibly disparate parts of American life have been caught up in the culture of slimming. As in dance and theater, the method of this book is inductive and cumulative, moving from the particular (the image, the gesture, the sensation, the event) toward the more universal.

Dieting and History

History drags. It is a weight on us. Most diet book authors and most dieters are as impatient with that weight as with their own extra pounds. When dieters look back, as often they must, it is through the agency of nostalgia for the body that once was, or through the gothic tale of unremitting horror. The culture of slimming is not without an historical conscience, but it is without much sense of process. Diets seem to appear out of nowhere, in no time at all, like barbarians or wandering saints, and they seem to disappear as easily and as swiftly as they come. Because of this, the typical chronicle of slimming is a discrete set of flashing points, enlightenment to dark age to enlightenment, discontinuous and disappointing. Even at its most sophisticated, the dieter's sense of history tends to be catastrophic, a cycle of disasters and victories. The more obvious the vicious circle, the more extreme the next diet. As Judith Thurman reviewed her own life in 1977, she recalled that she had seen she was fat at twelve, had fasted and become thin but was fat again by the end of high school, and on and on: "Perhaps my feelings themselves actually became obese—fuel I couldn't turn into energy. I began crazily to desire some extremity of experience—a catastrophe, a fever, a 'real' deprivation, by which I meant an exotic one—that would burn them up."[3] The move toward—the desire for—extremes becomes part of the vicious circle of the culture of slimming itself.

The dieter is therefore little disturbed by the apparent contradictions between one diet and the next. It is not as if a dieter follows a logical program or steps progressively from a worse diet to a better diet. It is hard to know exactly where the extremes lie or how to measure them.

Diets and diet experts can thus make the most surprising blue-smoke-and-trap-door entrances and exits, change their costumes, reappear as new and miraculous. John T. Andreadis in 1946 sold the Glamour Mold Self-Massage Kit for spot reducing; in 1948 he sold the Hollywood Two-Way Plan for weight loss; in the early 1950s he sold Propex appetite suppressants; soon enough, while patenting a rubber balloon doll with cardboard feet that could walk down an inclined plane, he established the Wonder Drug Company and sold Regimen. Regimen's green, pink and yellow pills were for "No-diet reducing." Andreadis marketed them with special intensity in 1959: 218,000 one-minute TV spots, 1,064,000 lines of newspaper advertising, and housewives testing the diet week after week on the scales of the "Today Show." The clinical reports on Regimen were invented, the housewives were hired actresses who lost weight on their own diets of coffee and phenobarbital, but Andreadis had sold $16 million worth of Regimen by 1965.[4]

A box of Regimen pills cost thirty cents to manufacture and sold for five dollars. The pills contained benzocaine, ammonium chloride and phenylpropanolamine hydrochloride (PPA or PPH). The FDA pursued Andreadis for fraud in the 1960s, but twenty years later an FDA panel has reviewed benzocaine and PPA and found both to be safe and mildly effective as over-the-counter appetite suppressants. PPA has returned in force with Anorexine, Appedrine, Ayds, Coffee Tea & A New Me, Dexatrim, Diet-Trim, Prolamine, Spantrol. With such twists and turns even of the officially approved repertoire of weight-control drugs, a long memory can only handicap.[5]

The same holds for the high-fat, low-carbohydrate diet proposed in Germany in the 1880s, then in this country by Vilhjalmur Stefansson in 1946, then in the 1950s as the Du Pont Diet, again in the first best-selling diet of the 1960s, Herman Taller's *Calories Don't Count*, again as Sidney Petrie's *Martinis & Whipped Cream* (1966), and once more as *The New Drinking Man's Diet and Cookbook* (1974).[6] Each time the diet has reappeared, it has been impervious to its past. The rejuvenation of diets is as much a part of the culture of slimming as the rejuvenation of the dieter.

Dieters are discouraged by and dissuaded from the long prospect. History as a disjunct collection of points is far more congenial to hope. Without continuity and context, any diet, drug or device may seem startlingly new and promising.

This book offers a different sense of history, one less advantageous to the culture of slimming. Insofar as I give historical momentum and social context to the process of dieting and the choices of dieters, I must come across as a critic of that culture. But I shall not rate the many diets we encounter,[7] nor shall I take a stand on whether slimming of itself is good or bad, fatness healthy or unhealthy. Rather, I go to some lengths to make momentarily attractive or reasonable even the most unusual of diets and devices. It is better that we appreciate the allure of each diet or device as it slides out from the historical wings than that we leap to judgment.

I cannot say whether an historically informed dieter will be a better (healthier, more successful) dieter. Certainly, this book cannot make the act of reducing any easier to maintain or the state of fatness any easier to endure within American life.

If, however, the active cognizance of our bodies requires a sense of proportion, then we should be equally obliged to a sense of social proportions. The culture of slimming is tending now toward such weightlessness that it is difficult to acknowledge those social proportions: the relationship between economic abundance and personal appetite; the relationship between the truth told by the body and the truth told by the self; the relationship between our longings and our fears.

Should someone insist upon a moral to this book, it is that fatness is so obstinate a problem in our society precisely because it is so richly situated at its center.

That has not always been so.

Ritual and Romance

In late medieval morality plays, Gluttony misled men to banquets in hell, where sauces were seasoned with sulfur and devils stuffed gluttons with toads from stinking rivers. Such banquets stood in sorry contrast to the paradises for gluttons, the Land of Cockaigne (Pieter Brueghel's "Luylekkerland") and Hans Sachs's Schlaraffenland with its pork porches, sausage fences, wine wells. A 1606 map of the Land of Cake (Paese di Chucagna) showed lakes of fresh butter, ravioli trees, clouds of fried fowl. There were as well the awestruck tales of legendary gluttons—the tyrant Denys of Heraclea, Cornish King Grallon, Flemish King Gambrinus—not to mention Gargantua himself, who as an infant required the milk from 17,913 cows.[8]

During centuries of European image-making about gluttons and gluttony, the aesthetic and theological emphases were on the act itself, the overeating, and not on the weight or shape of the glutton. Manuals of penance never mentioned corpulence, and stiffer penalties held for the arrogance of excessive fasting than for the sensuality of the feast. A carnal sin, gluttony implied disordered appetite, the refusal to take the true measure of one's human needs. Penance was heaviest when gluttony became theft or sacrilege, lightest when merely a sociable overindulgence at meals.[9]

In the early modern period, medical epitaphs were slowly substituted for moral warnings. The punishment for Gargantua's indulgence was neither spiritual distress nor the pain of obesity but eighteen chins and a phlegmatic temperament. The fat Falstaff must know "the grave doth gape / For thee thrice wider than for other men."

"O wretched, miserable Italy!" wrote octogenarian Luigi Cornaro. "Dost not thou plainly see, that Gluttony deprives thee of more Souls yearly, than either a War, or the Plague itself could have done?" Himself a victim of gout and stomach disorders, Cornaro at forty had abandoned all medicines for a temperate life of 12 oz of food and 14 oz of drink each day. He became a new man, spry, free of disease, quickly healed of broken bones. Writing in 1558 from Venice, home of a phalanx of esteemed doctors, Cornaro was nonetheless sure that "every Man . . . might become his own Physician" if only he would keep a strict watch over his appetite, "which indeed ought to be every one's Chief Business and Concern."[10]

Santorio Santorio was just a child when Cornaro died in 1566 at the age of ninety-one, but Santorio it was who undertook most diligently that strict watch upon which Cornaro insisted. Around the age of forty, accustomed as a physician to close measurement and patient experiment, Santorio fastened a chair to the beam of an enormous steelyard scale so that the chair hung a finger's breadth from the floor of his room. For the next three decades he would weigh himself often and regularly, with practiced attention to the nature of his meals, his exercise, his sexual activity and his evacuations.[11]

The good doctor of Padua was in methodical if static pursuit of something arithmetical—"the mean proportion of the latitude of healthy ponderation"—and of something invisible. This last he called "insensible perspiration," the secret yet telltale index of health: "He only who knows, to what quantity, and when, the secret perspiration of a man's body amounts to more or less, shall find out how much, and when, any thing ought to be added, or subtracted in order to the preservation, or recovery of his Health." Such perspiration amounted to 50 oz as a man lay asleep at night, to 5 lbs daily on a diet of 8 lbs of food and drink. The numbers varied according to the seasons, one's age and the weight of one's clothes. They varied also according to one's state of mind: grief inhibited insensible perspiration, happiness opened the pores and passages. In general, steadiness was the best sign, and the subtler the insensible perspiration, the healthier one was likely to be.[12]

Neither Cornaro nor Santorio was much concerned with corpulence *per se*. Had they been consulted, they would have given mildly opposed advice, Cornaro inclining toward leanness, Santorio toward ponderosity. But both would have agreed that absolute weight, all else being equal, was of less import than steady weight. The problem was not poundage but flux. So may be dated, almost too neatly, the origins of obsessive weight-watching in the modern West.

Cornaro's strictures on appetite have since been translated and reprinted more widely than any similar aphorisms of Hippocrates.[13] Etchings of Santorio in his hanging chair have taken pride of place in the iconography of dieting. The two men have become the prototypes for the two fundamental modes of dieting, romance and ritual. Those modes will remain virtually constant throughout this book, conditioning not only the form but also the spirit of most of the diets we shall encounter. We must understand their implications before we can proceed from the Old World to the New.

For Cornaro, dietetic restraint began with an inner change which was outwardly rewarded and permanently blessed. His cure was painless and thoroughgoing. From the relatively simple decision to lead a temperate life came the magnificent gifts of rejuvenation and longevity.[14]

This romance of dieting works in a way that other medical fantasies do not. The dieter's battle against gluttony is a magical battle; every step taken against the glutton doubles the hero's strength, gives him at once more youth and more power. Lighter, he is more agile and more alert. The longer the battle lasts, the more vigor he has.

Cornaro in his valetudinarian pride became the model for a victory over gluttony which was also a return to youth and to beauty. As in the typical 16th-century romance, the hero changes himself and so changes the world. Personal renovation has cosmic consequences. It may reverse time, restore justice, establish order.

Santorio would seem to have been working that vein of 17th-century self-examination that had as its initial image not the dark wood of the romance but the dark night of the soul. The weighing of the body as a metaphor for the weighing of the soul is an ancient figure, and the image of the balance has long accompanied the rhetoric of moderation.[15] But the portraits of Santorio do not show the second pan of the classical equal-arm balance. His steelyard scale has only one obviously weight-bearing arm, from which Santorio hangs in his dependable chair; the counterpoise on the other longer arm is simply not credible. Such a scale is scarcely appropriate, visually or dramatically, for the weighing of good against bad. Rather, the steelyard demonstrates the measurement of the visible by the invisible, Santorio's bulk by an abstract set of calculated ratios. Santorio's scrutiny of the self was a ritual scrutiny of the body, on the premise that the body is in constant if sometimes invisible commerce with the world. Hellenistic Stoics and medieval Christian philosophers had assumed such an intercourse, but Santorio was after something more measurable than a world fluid (pneuma) or an imponderable fog (miasma). Like his Italian contemporaries studying air pressure and specific gravity, Santorio directed his thirty-year experiment toward the discovery of laws about the changes in natural bodies.[16] The fineness and stamina of his observations were akin to the newly styled manners of autobiography, which made public the warts, weals and woes of unheroic man.

Dieting ritual, like autobiography, begins with the critical acknowledgment of disproportion. Call this disproportion ugliness, awkwardness or fatness, it must be named and measured. The measurement is the warrant of honest intent; as Santorio explained, "'tis no unseemly thing to weigh the excrements."[17] So the ritual scrutiny commences with a bald look in the mirrors which Venetian glassmakers were just then improving, and it moves on through Santorio's meticulous accounts to such familiarity with scales that weight-watching is established as an unimpeachable habit. Between the mirror and the scale lie acts of confession and repentance.

The dieting romance is impatient, working from the inside out, explosive. The dieting ritual is patient, working from outside in, implosive.

Clearly, the impatience of romance and the patience of ritual may not be compatible, as the famous Dr. Cheyne learned for himself half a century after the death of Santorio. George Cheyne was born in Scotland in 1673 to parents healthy but disposed to corpulence. As a child his glands were lax, his solid parts feeble. In his youth he migrated to London, where he gamboled with a free-living crowd and grew "excessively fat, short-breath'd, lethargick and listless." Cured of an autumnal intermittent fever by quinine, he remained in a "jumbled and turbid" humor for a year, then suffered a "vertiginous Paroxysm close to Apoplexy." Deserted by his festive companions, he withdrew to the countryside for a simpler, more vegetarian life. There he took vomits, volatile salts, bitters, chalybeat (iron) waters. Still he was pursued by headaches and melancholy. He tried laudanum (opium) and mercurial medicines such as calomel (a powerful cathartic), acquiring in the process liver and gall bladder problems. As a side effect of his diseases, his medications and their diseases, his body was "melting away like a Snowball in Summer," but he felt otherwise so dreary that he set himself to meditate on religion. From the fountain of divinity he turned to the faucets of Bath, at whose spas he was much relieved. He began again to indulge his appetite for animal foods—too fast and too much, so thence to the waters of Bristol and gentle vomits. Not yet to up snuff, he met a clergyman who jogged his memory of a wonderful milk cure that worked for epileptics. On the milk diet for half a year, Cheyne was considerably revived and much thinner, having become "Lank, Fleet and Nimble, but still, upon any Error even in this Low Diet, I found more or less Oppression and Lowness." He mistook a pain in the pit of his stomach for lung disease and was frightened into a furious abstemiousness, 10 miles of horseback riding each day, and a bitter purgative every fortnight. Chewing more quinine, he felt miraculously changed and heartier of appetite. He indulged once again in animal food and incurred, alas, a depuratory fever which prepared the way for his exhausted body to suck up the juices of food "like a Sponge, and thereby suddenly grew *plump, fat* and *hale* to a Wonder; but indeed too fast." He swelled to nearly 450 lbs and was assailed by asthma, scorbutic ulcers and erysipelas before he returned to a milk and white meat diet, then to a milk and vegetable diet. He was in his forties.[18]

Some ten years later, after further indiscretions of appetite and eructations of the body, Cheyne had settled on a vegetarian diet with milk, tea and coffee. "The thinner my diet is," he wrote in 1733, "the easier, more cheerful and lightsome I find myself."[19] This "lightsome" had three avenues of reference—to light (the glow of health), to lightness (buoyancy), and to light-headedness (a mind undisturbed, a soul unoppressed). The "English Malady" which Cheyne himself so named had to do with the weight of the body and the weight of the soul bearing directly upon one another. Cheyne had been caught between them just as he had been caught between the ritual and romance of dieting.

I have lingered over Cheyne's afflictions because it was he who best demonstrated to later generations the delicate relationship between ritual and romance. His intermittent but feverish desires for an instant cure made prescriptions difficult to follow, while the formal comforts of ritual made his bursts of heroic abstinence seem quirky and insincere.

We can see him struggling between Cornaro and Santorio in his popular and influential book, *An Essay of Health and Long Life*:

> Since then our Appetites are deceitful and Weight and Measure troublesome and singular; we must have Recourse to a Rule independent of our Sensations. . . . I know nothing but Eating and Drinking by our Eye: that is, determining first of all either by Weight or Measure, or by particular Observation or Experiment, the Bulk, or Number of Mouthful of Flesh Meat, and the Number of Glasses of strong Liquors, *under* which we are best; and then by our eye determining an equal Quantity at all times for the future. . . . For we are so wisely contrived, that our Food need not be adjusted to *mathematical* Points: A little over or under will make no Difference in our Health.[20]

Here was the 18th-century virtuoso aching at once for precision and conviviality, the rule of reason and the rule of thumb. Here was the eminent physician trying at once to be exact and good-natured, sharp-eyed and mild-mannered. After decades, he managed a persuasive reconciliation. For that reason among others, his advice on diet would be frequently quoted across the waters in the English colonies of North America.

The colonists had their local Cornaro and Santorio. Their Cornaro was Benjamin Franklin, who died at the advanced age of eighty-four after living a life somewhat more profligate than the one he preached. "Wouldst thou enjoy a long life, a healthy Body, and a Vigorous Mind, and be acquainted also with the wonderful works of God?" he asked readers of his *Poor Richard's Almanack*. "Labour in the first place to bring thy Appetite into Subjection to Reason." Like Cheyne, Franklin weaseled on dietetic arithmetic, deciding that "The Difficulty lies, in finding out an exact Measure; but eat for Necessity, not Pleasure, for Lust knows not where Necessity ends." Daily exercise, an occasional fast, and gastronomic rectitude would bring on the cheerful life of one such as Cornaro, whom Franklin had dying at the age of one hundred twenty.[21]

Franklin was a poorer imitation of his Italian master than Dr. John Lining was of his. Lining meant to repeat in South Carolina's climate the observations of Santorio in Padua. He began in March 1740 to weigh himself, his food, his drink, his urine and stools. He correlated this data with the weather, the room temperature, the time of day and the local air pressure, making "these tedious Calculations" for more than a year. His observations were as scrupulous as the contemporary confessions of revival converts were expansive; on July 3, 1740, for example, "being cloathed in a Holland Jacket and Chince Gown, was exposed betwixt 12¾ and 2¾, to the Third Degree of the Wind's Force; eat 10⅝ Ounces of roasted Lamb, Bread and Shallots, drank 40 Ounces of Punch, and used no Exercise; in these Two Hours made 3⅜ Ounces of Urine and, being exposed to the Wind, perspired only 12 Ounces, though I sweated a little all the Time." During the summer he weighed himself once every three hours, sometimes every hour, hoping to determine some correspondence between his perspiration and the sultry, dangerous summer climate of the South.[22]

Lining was worried about the applicability of Old World measurement to the New World. Did the same laws of the body or of diet appertain here? Could he locate through the body the physical laws appropriate to this different world? His ritual was devoted to weight less as a personal issue than as a continental calendar.

The dieting romance—Cornaro's text, Franklin's sayings—presumes universality. The same changes in life or appetite entail the same results; the battle against gluttony is a generically human battle. Such is the promise of the cure-all, the elixir, the miracle reducing belt. In our common humanity, one regimen must be good for all.

The dieting ritual is in theory universal, but in practice it discriminates, localizes. No two people share the same numbers. Precise measurement distinguishes us one from the other, sets Charleston apart from Padua, England from New England. The closer the scrutiny, the less reliable any pat prescription or received wisdom. Dieting ritual celebrates separateness even as it claims to confirm a covering law.

We must therefore make peace with a tricky paradox, one that will haunt the rest of this book. The backwoods healers, those ornery, cantankerous eclectics, will not hesitate to proclaim a universal panacea, while the more socialized scientists and orthodox physicians will divagate, treating each set of symptoms as probably unique. The jack-of-all-tirades comes to seem most convincing and empirical; he will give practical, down-to-earth advice instantly, even by mail. And those who would on the face of things appear to be most at ease with clear hypothesis, careful experiment and thoughtful conclusion will seem popularly the most confused and unhelpful when it comes to questions of food and fat. If natural philosophers rail against gluttony, they have nothing on the more expert oratory of roadside evangelists. If doctors pronounce on the virtues of moderation, they appear old-hat and terribly vague. If physiologists propose a forcefully calculated system of feeding, they must be parodying themselves, as Dr. Cheyne well understood and as Dr. Thomas Moffett realized centuries before when he scorned the "inch diet." To "eat by drams, and drink by spoonfuls more perplexeth the mind then cureth the body, engendring a jealousie over every meat, suspition on every quantity, dread, fear, and terrour over every proportion (bereaving the head of quietness, the heart of security, and the stomack consequently of good concoction)."[23]

The stomach is always the leading casualty of the tensions between ritual and romance. For millennia, the stomach has been full when it ought to have been empty or empty when it ought to have been full. Anatomists have described it as if it were surrounded and besieged. Thus Thomas Vicary in 1548: The stomach "hath the liver on the right side chasing and beating him with his lobes or figures; and the spleen on the left side, with his fatness and veins, sending to him melancholy, to exercise his appetites; and about him is the heart, quickening him with his arteries . . . ."[24]

The siege mentality is particularly characteristic of the dieting romance, which makes of the stomach a kind of muscular architecture, the intestines a maze. Gluttony has overstocked the keep. The bowels are heavy with undigested matter, the entire belly a Castle of Indolence.

Lifting the siege requires an inner transformation: a change in one's desires or appetites; a catharsis; a redirection of one's forces. The transformation may be as plain as Cornaro's new resolve. It may be as fancy as those appetite suppressants which date back to the third century B.C. and Philon the Byzantine's "hunger and thirst checking pill" composed of sesame, honey, oil, almonds and sea onion.[25] It may be as lush as the laxatives and purgatives whose recipes return us to Old Kingdom Egypt.[26] It may be as Spartan as running and leaping.

Dieting ritual envisions the stomach as a holy vessel and the body as a "system of pipes, through which fluids are perpetually circulating." Although there is talk (as in the romance) of repletion and sluggishness, the stress is upon flood control and canal work. Not solids but fluids. The stomach is rather bloated than stuffed.[27]

Dieting ritual entails Santorio's unhurried attention to the pores and passages of the body. Relief arrives by the ounce: that pinching, bleeding and sweating which can draw out foul fluids from the bloated body. The cure begins from the outside, invoking a force separate from the victim. This is the ancient tradition of massage, mineral baths, sweathouses and their modern analogs: vibrating tables, jacuzzis, plastic sweatsuits. It is the tradition of the jockey and the middleweight boxer. It is the mechanics' tradition, first of cups and leeches, then of gleaming apparatus that introduce electricity or magnetism into the body to revive the internal fluids and set them flowing again: the galvanic reducing belt, the magnetic corset. It is the tradition of the liquid diet—Cheyne's milk, the Metrecal for Lunch Bunch, liquid protein.

Men, Women and Fat

It may seem strange, in all this discussion of ritual and romance, that no woman has appeared and that all the pronouns have been masculine. Although we now associate dieting most immediately with women, the classical texts of dieting until the 20th century were written by men who had made a drastic change in their habits in midlife. The archetypal public dieters were more often male until late in the 19th century, despite that stoutness so praiseworthy in Victorian rhetoric about men. Even during the 1760s, when there was a European vogue for weighing oneself at shops with large hanging scales, those who returned regularly—at least to Number 3 St. James's Street in London—were men. The records of Messrs. Berry Brothers & Rudd, winedealers, show that the Earl of Salisbury weighed 15 stone 9 (219 lbs) in 1787, 19 stone 4 (276) in 1798; Lord Guilford in 1801 was at 14 stone and ten years later at 18 stone 11. The rest of the amused peerage seem to have been equally heavy, but Lord Byron was obviously upset about his weight, 13 stone 12 in 1806. On a vinegar diet he got himself down under 9 stone by 1811. Beau Brummell, the dandy who weighed himself more than forty times, must also have been reducing, or was it age and disappointment which took him from 12 stone 10½ in 1815 to 10 stone 13 in 1822?[28]

I parade these figures as much for their specious precision as for their literary novelty. Sometimes the men were in boots, sometimes in shoes; some wore heavy clothes one time, light clothes the next, according to the weather and the season. Santorio would have thought them laughable. Some men, however, were weighed accurately and professionally. These were the jockeys, who tried every imaginable scheme to "waste" themselves before races. Perhaps they did not put on half a dozen waistcoats, run two or three miles, strip and immerse themselves in a hot dunghill, as one aspiring stableboy was conned into doing circa 1747, but their loyalty to sweating remains. As does that of the pugilists whose trainers were to be widely cited for their dieting strategies.[29]

Even with the sweating, the middle-aged men presented dieting as a muscular, willful act. It was, when men undertook it, a romance, an unburdening, a freeing up, a moral athleticism. The act of chewing could itself be athletic, with its own training motto, "Masticate, Denticate, Chump, Grind, and Swallow."[30]

Yet when men turned their eyes on overweight women, they made of women's dieting a fulsome and patent ritual. Since women's weights seemed to jump at puberty, marriage, pregnancy and menopause, women's reducing had to be spoken of in terms of fluids, internal secretions and sexual ichor, as if womb and stomach were identical twins. Hence the centuries of anecdote about male physicians mistaking a fat belly for maternity, gluttony for pregnancy. And since it seemed that a woman's fluids were not completely under her control, women were to be cured of corpulence by intervention, by an imposed order and extrinsic technique. Hence the male insistence (today still) that women dieters are exasperatingly uncooperative and cannot will their own transformation.

It follows that very fat men in Western society have been represented most often as gluttons or monsters, very fat women as patients or freaks. The glutton's temperament is sanguine, the monster's choleric, but both are fat by an act of will; the glutton is highly sensual, the monster without affections, but both are vivid and vital; the glutton is engagingly social, the monster isolated, but both are invested with a peculiar sort of power: the man who devours, the man who destroys.

Patients and freaks are objects of charity rather than subjects of awe. Their temperaments, bilious or lymphatic, make them irritable and yet unaware, overly sensitive but slothful. Where fat men inspire or terrify, fat women draw the camphor of sympathy and disgust—sympathy, because they cannot help themselves; disgust, because they are sexually ambiguous, emotionally sloppy.

These representations have become part of the popular medical landscape. Fat men contract diseases of the stomach and joints (as gluttons) or diseases of the heart (as monsters). Fat women endure glandular disturbances (as patients) and the misfortunes of heredity (as freaks). Men suffer from solidity and largeness: the paunch, the swollen heart. Women suffer from fluidity and smallness: the hormones, the chromosomes. The condition of fat men is reparable because more tangible and accessible; women's fat is intransigent because constitutional, deep and ultimately historical.

Reducing programs and propaganda have been fitted to this landscape. Campaigns directed at men have been framed as adventures, romances that will provoke an immediate change in the world: physical prowess, political action, business success. Campaigns directed at women have been framed as rituals of watchfulness in response to external threats. Domestic economy, nutrition education, public nursing have encouraged slimming as a strategic defense against the mounting-up of waste, fat and fatigue in an imposing world.

Since men abandoned form-fitting clothes in the 1860s, misshapen men have been publicly less conspicuous and privately less constrained than misshapen women. In this way, fashion has consistently upheld the sexual distinction between romance and ritual. Men have appeared not to need artificial bulwarks; they walk unassisted by secret devices. Women in their stays or in their elastic girdles have appeared to invoke external support. There have been curiously retrograde movements here, for while many men and most physicians deplored corsets as machines which crushed women's maternal organs, the same corsets confirmed men in their belief that the weaker sex was always in need of foreign aid. Similarly, while feminists might argue for unrestrictive clothing, other women equally self-assured could advocate tight-lacing as a sign of independence from middle-class male prudery or a drab masculine aesthetic.[31]

Fashion is a small part of that world of appearances which we are about to enter. It has to do with shape and texture, posture and quality of skin, not with weight. Our century's unique confusion of dimension, proportion, mass and weight has been compounded by fashion and fashion writing, but styles in clothing and cosmetics do not of themselves have causal priority. They cannot be enlisted to explain the thrust of scientific research or the popularity of bathroom scales.[32]

The body itself must stand at the center of this book—what it is, what it seems to be, what it could turn out to be. Ritual and romance underlie the patterns of dieting, and fashion reinforces those patterns, but it is the larger, more various experience of our bodies and our shared fictions about weight and fat that determine this history, its turns, its twists, its forward motion.

We move on now to the man who edited a new translation of Cornaro's *Discourses* in 1832, and we shall come to a halt some steps beyond the Datatrim electronic talking scale, more voluble and more perceptive than any device the venerable Santorio Santorio might have dreamed of.

CHAPTER TWO

The Thin Body
and the Jacksonians

The first American weight watchers were disciples of
Sylvester Graham, a health reformer whose dietary
program was meant to restore wholesome appetite to
a nation of gluttons. At issue, however, was neither
fatness nor overweight but indigestion and overex-
citement. Grahamites watched their weight not because they wanted to be thin but because they
needed to prove to a skeptical society that a simple,
abstinent diet could make them resilient and robust.
Jacksonians themselves were highly ambivalent
about thin bodies. In political terms, leanness bespoke vigor and honesty; in social terms, leanness bespoke lack of charity and the denial of a rightful
American abundance. Leanness might be acceptable
as a style, but not as a way of life.

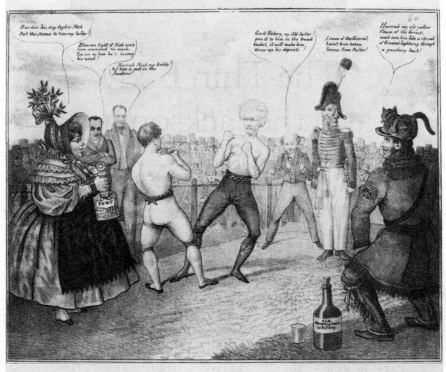

"The celebrated fight took place at Washington in 1834, Hickory was sec-onded by Little Van and Major Jack Downing, with Joe Tammany for bot-tle holder; Long Harry and Black Dan were Nick's seconds, and Old Mother Bank bottle holder. Several long and severe rounds were fought, and from the immense sums bet, many of the fancy were losers to a large amount. Old Mother B is said to have backed her champion to the tune of more than $150,000. Nick's weight of metal was superior as well as his sci-ence, but neither were sufficient for the pluck and wind of Hickory, who shewed through his training and sound condition so effectually that in the last round Nick was unable to come to time and gave in."

Set-to between Old Hickory and Bully Nick, lithograph c. 1834.
Courtesy of the Print Department, Boston Public Library

The First Weight Watchers

COMMUNION SERVICE, Portland, Maine, spring 1834. A man in a gown of black muslin stands over an immense loaf of bread made of bran and chopped straw. He pronounces a sermon in doggerel verse, then breaks the loaf into pieces, which are tossed around the room from man to laughing man. That night, carried away by the spirit of their burlesque, some thirty of the celebrants gather noisily outside the crowded hall in which the real Reverend Sylvester Graham is holding forth. Graham that week has completed four special lectures for mothers; now he is speaking on the evils of tea, coffee, tobacco and opium. He believes in a plain, abstinent diet: whole grains, vegetables, pure water. Spices and stimulants invite gluttony, which leads to indigestion, illness, sexual excess, social disruption and, ultimately, civic disorder. Graham's logic seems all too prophetic. The men outside become rowdier, police try to disperse them, they throw stones, and the nervous assembly elects to adjourn shortly after 9:30 P.M. The Reverend Graham, unharmed, escorts a lady home. On the following day there is a riot.[1]

That riot, Graham insisted, had nothing to do with his talks for mothers, talks which he had given without public murmur in Phila-

23

delphia, New York and Providence. But cause and effect were as cloudy in Sylvester Graham's life as they were in his *Lectures on the Science of Human Life*. When he came to speak in Boston during the winter of 1837, the Portland commotion lay heavily on the minds of such as Dr. John Bartlett, who had issued an appeal to "every husband, father, and brother who hears me, if he would not as willingly see his wife, daughter or sister issue from a brothel, as from the secret lectures of this infamous man."[2]

At his first Boston lecture for ladies on February 23, Graham was heckled by two reputed nightwalkers. At his third lecture, one woman grew faint and another walked out. By the date appointed for his fourth and final lecture, Graham had seen handbills urging that he be tarred and feathered, and nearly a thousand men were waiting to holler down "this most obscene, filthy and infamous scoundrel."[3]

Perhaps three hundred women braved the hooting of the mob to enter Amory Hall that Thursday, March 2. Some had weathered an earlier riot against abolitionist George Thompson and were hardly cowed by this new ruckus. They did, however, take the precaution of removing from the stage Graham's one visual aid, an anatomical transparency so designed for mixed company that it did not show even in outline any improper organs. Graham indeed had protested that his talks for mothers were open to men and were conducted with "religious solemnity," but the excitable editor of the *Daily Herald* knew otherwise. In Graham's absence (was he hiding in a side room?), Henry F. Harrington took to the podium and harangued the women, accusing them of harboring whores in their midst. Outside, the mob was hissing. "If they are going to hiss, I for one won't move an inch," declared a matron in the hall, but the city marshal begged them all to retire. As they left, the women hissed back at the men.[4]

"All the complicated interests of vice, —all the indulgencies of gross and degrading sensuality, —all the depravities of human nature, are put in jeopardy by my operations," proclaimed Graham a fortnight later.[5] But this was too smug an explanation for such sharp explosions in Graham's wake. A black and bandied communion, hooting mobs outside lecture halls *cum* brothels—how was it that a thin man with a slightly aquiline nose, a stoop to his shoulders and a pallid countenance drew such fire?[6]

From the moment he began as a lecturer on the Philadelphia Temperance Circuit in 1830, Graham had been on the trail of something larger than mere intemperance. He happened first on masturbation, then cholera, then gluttony. None was an original discovery, least of all gluttony. Prof. Charles Caldwell, veteran of Western lecture circuits, had figured in 1832 that "for every reeling drunkard that disgraces our country, it contains one hundred gluttons." Extrapolated by the health reformer William A. Alcott to an 1842 American population of 18,000,000, this meant a country of 30,000 disgraceful reeling drunkards and 3,000,000 gluttons. "GLUTTONY," wrote Graham in 1838, "and *not starvation* is the greatest of all causes of evil. . . . Excessive alimentation is the greatest dietetic error in the United States—and probably in the whole civilized world."[7]

Unlike alcoholism, presented most often as a man's curse (and a wife's travail), gluttony was universal. And unlike drunkenness, whose cure had to be effected as much by social changes as by personal conversion from spirits to the Spirit, gluttony could be cut to the quick by actions within the home, at table, by Woman. So, almost naturally, Graham arrived at an especial concern for mothers. And bread.

There was a fierce connection between the two. Good mothers baked their own bread; good bread was baked exclusively by good mothers. "The best bread-makers I have ever known," wrote Graham, "watch over their bread troughs while their dough is rising, and over their ovens while it is baking, with about as much care and attention as a mother watches over the cradle of her sick child." Only the mother who loved her children, Graham repeated, could bake perfect bread. The metaphorical resonance of bread and babe, of rising loaves and childrearing, was not inadvertent. Graham's theory of diet was also a theory of domestic relations and a social program.[8]

In simplest terms, this was the theory: Gluttony, arch sin, was born of civilization, which seduced the natural appetite and played digestion false. The spices and ferments of hectic commerce insinuated themselves into the kitchen of the innocent wife, wreaking havoc with her sacred duties as wife and mother. Fed too often because too often tempted, fed too ignorantly and therefore never satisfied, children grew weak, anxious and dyspeptic. The same children, appetites corrupted by the salt and pepper, the tea and coffee of an overly rich diet, became so accustomed to sensual excitements that self-pollution was the awful but common sequel. Habituated to public gluttony and thus to private lust, young husband and young wife would fall prey to the perils of sexual excess, which entailed most of the ills that flesh is heir to. Unhealthy parents in turn would spawn unhealthy children.[9]

And this was the cure, the social program: If a woman, a mother, truly understood the workings of her own body, she would appreciate the value of a simple diet. Her hearth and her table would be havens from the noxious excitements of an increasingly commercial world, her bran bread a reminder of the virgin soil from which, originally, we arose. The best bread would be coarse, honest and unleavened, free of that artificial excitement called yeast which, in the course of baking, turned sugar into alcohol. A light, sweet, unintoxicating bread was possible only with unbolted ripe wheat, lovingly washed and roughly milled. The dough would be kneaded with pure milk at blood heat, as New England mothers had done at the dawn of the Republic.[10]

Good bread would heal as it satisfied. With unadorned vegetables, a few fruits, pure cold water and deep breaths of clear air, bran bread would be the centerpiece of a stark but flavorful life, neither provocative nor indulgent. Children would grow into "the simple economy of the gospel," able to withstand the defilements of urban life. Soon the public world of mob violence, false pride and civic masturbation (the "wanton bestowment of civic honors") would be transformed in much the same way that vegetable foods could calm the vainglorious martial impulses of meat-eaters.[11]

Not intended as a weight-reducing regimen, the Graham system was spare enough in practice to make personal weight an important issue. The general absence of beef, pork and ale from the Graham system made for a widespread skepticism about the power of his diet to keep healthy flesh on human bones. Graham believed himself a martyr to the natural, to the restoration of wholesome appetite, harmonious relations between the internal organs, and integrity in civil life, but his enemies thought him perverse and unnatural, a man who wanted to upend civilization and drive abundance from the young temple of democracy. Graham seemed to be denying the bounties of this New World and the joys of a full American life. His disciples constantly appeared in a ghostly light, half alive, half dead. One critic, imagining a Grahamite boardinghouse at dinnertime, saw rather a mortuary feast. Around a table spread without linen were seated "some thirty lean-visaged, cadaverous disciples, eyeing each other askance—their looks lit up with a certain cannibal spirit, which, if there were any chance of making a full meal off each other's bones, might perhaps break into dangerous practice." Cold water to the right of them, bran bread to the left, and ahead of them "the corpses of potatoes," the Grahamite men sat like "busts in chalk," the women like "mummies preserved in saffron."[12]

Again and again, Grahamites tottered through contemporary accounts to the rattle of bones. "I once travelled all through the State of Maine with one of them" wrote Sam Slick (satirist Thomas C. Haliburton). "He was as thin as a whippin post. . . . He put me in mind of a pair of kitchen tongs, all legs, shaft, and head, and no belly; a real gander lookin critter, holler as a bamboo walkin cane, and twice as yeller."[13]

The disciples protested: They were neither cannibals nor rambling skeletons. They testified that they had gained both weight and resilience on a diet of vegetables and fruit, unbolted wheat bread, rice, sago, pure water and a bit of fresh cream. They had eaten slowly, chewed well, avoided condiments, gravies, tea, coffee, tobacco, butter and pastries. They took meals two or three times a day, six hours apart, and they never snacked. Now their health had been restored, their appetite regained, their spirits invigorated, their strength magnified—and their weight properly adjusted.[14]

From their letters and testimonials comes the first evidence of a coherent group of Americans conscious of exact personal weight, the first evidence of ordinary Americans weighing themselves with some regularity, and the first evidence of adult Americans occasionally weighing their food on a daily basis. Mr. Metcalf at first lost weight on the Graham diet but recovered 15 lbs within a year and left behind a history of ulcerated bowels to become a new man at forty-five. M. H. gained 10 lbs and was no longer weighing his food. Anna Maria Primrose had endured rheumatism, nosebleeds and asthma until she found Graham and a new body. S. from Dedham fell from 193 to 170 lbs but then rose to a comfortable 175, "which is sufficient bulk for any one to carry about." John Kilton reduced from 161 to 127, then reappeared at 146, with "a solidity in my system that never existed there before."[15]

Settling at a solid weight was a good sign that one was neither monster nor ghost. While P. T. Barnum hunted up fat boys and human skeletons for his American Museum in New York,[16] the Grahamites would not be freaks. Like Graham, his disciples were eager to lay claim to both spirit and substance. Their comparatively slender diet was meant to yield handsome, robust bodies. Thinness was never the goal; wholesome appetite was.

These first American weight watchers were much less concerned with fatness than they were with gluttony. They yearned not for leanness but for a "natural" weight, a tempered and temperate life.

If bits and pieces of Grahamism reappear in most present slimming diets (the whole wheat toast, the bias toward vegetables, the careful chewing, the exile of butter, gravies and pastry), it is because we have been led to confuse gluttony with fatness, fatness with heaviness, and heaviness with overweight. Those are modern confusions, confusions that I will be at pains to trace in the next several chapters as we watch the culture of slimming emerge in the midst of a new desire for a thin body.

First, however, we must confront a society highly ambivalent about thinness and not yet squared to any notion of abstinence. We must go back behind Sylvester Graham's discourses "poetical and rhetorical, mathematical and metaphorical, botanical and ornithological,"[17] to appreciate how deeply Graham's system was embedded within his own era and how at the same time it could seem so mean, so spiteful of appetite, and so unnatural.

The Stomach and the Polemics of Appetite

At the vital center of Graham's discourses lay the stomach. It was, to begin with, Graham's own stomach, aching and upset. It was, next, the model stomach, the stomach as contemplated by physiologists and philosophers. It was, last, the Jacksonian stomach, the underbelly of national politics.

Near the end of his life, Graham wrote in one of his typically sentimental poems:

> In gloom, in sadness, and in tears,
>   Through childhood's period thou did'st languish;
> And up through manhood's early years,
>   Thy every pulse was beat in anguish.

His friend, Dr. Russell T. Trall, took this stanza as partial explanation for Graham's early, severe and protracted case of indigestion or dyspepsia. An unhappy childhood had as it were fixed itself in Graham's stomach. "When in his best bodily condition, he was always subject to what he called 'gastric irritation,'" a morbid appetite which when indulged would bring on rheumatism and neuralgia. At his end, during the summer of 1851, trundled in a wheelbarrow like a sack of grain, Graham attributed his decline to that morbid appetite, which had distended his stomach and spent his vital forces.[18]

Graham was the seventeenth and last child of a spent man, the Reverend John Graham, Jr., who would die at the age of seventy-four two years after Sylvester's birth. In 1796 Ruth Graham, second wife of John and for the second time in her life a widow, was forty-one. She inherited one-third of a house, the right to bake in the oven, and the burden of caring for at least three small children. She was not up to all these numbers, and the children were soon parceled out to neighbors or kin. By the age of five, Sylvester was being raised by strangers, among them a tavernkeeper, and when he was seven his mother was declared "deranged." He would live with her off and on during the next years, but he too was in a fragile condition, rarely able to sustain either a job or an education. He worked in a paper mill, traveled with a horse dealer, clerked in a store, taught school and prepared for the ministry, his own body interrupting him with the anguish of dyspepsia, consumption, exhaustion and finally a total breakdown. He married the woman who nursed him through his convalescence and whose small dowry would finance his studies for the Presbyterian ministry. Ordained in 1826 at the age of thirty-four, he had scarcely a year in a regular pulpit before he entered upon a decade of itinerant lecturing. A baby son died in 1829, his mother died in a New Jersey sanatorium in 1834 and by 1838 he had withdrawn from public life with his wife Sarah and three children to live out an obstreperous retirement devoted to two thorough searches—one for the prooftexts on diet in the Bible, the other for remote illustrious ancestors of the Graham clan.[19]

Always an imperious man, often sharp-tongued, he was not on good terms with many of his living kin. In 1844 he would write a conciliatory letter from his house in Northampton, Massachusetts, to one of his three surviving brothers, apologizing for the tone of a previous letter whose causticity was that of an "intense and concentrated love which would tear out a fatal cancer from a brother's soul." His little daughter Caroline had just died, and he seemed to want the "little remnant of our father's household" to return to a hearth which, really, he had never shared. "Is not the all devouring grave," he asked, "hungering for us with a keen and earnest appetite?"[20]

For Graham the "devouring grave" was less a commonplace figure of speech than the coda of his life and his life's work. He who penned detailed, defensive letters to newspapers on the causes of his own ill health (due, he explained, to an extreme asceticism while under the pressure of preparing books and lectures against gluttony) would not be above assigning a literal and liberal appetite to death.[21]

"Life consists in the sum of the functions, by which death is resisted," wrote French physiologist Xavier Bichat (1771–1802). "The measure, then, of life in general, is the difference which exists between the effect of exterior powers, and that of interior resistance." We do not know whether Graham read this—a translation appeared in Boston in 1827—but he did own a book by Bichat's successor, François J. V. Broussais (1772–1838), who argued for a similar vitalism. Predictably, Graham was reluctant to acknowledge his sources. His ideas had to be his own, even when he borrowed them. Yet he was a vitalist; that is to say, true to his religious training, true also to his years of struggle with a frail constitution, he resisted a mechanical or chemical explanation for the workings of the body. There was something more to life, as Bichat wrote, than hydraulics.[22]

Graham simplified what was in Europe a complex philosophical and biological controversy.[23] The controversy revolved around questions of digestion, for if one could determine how dead matter (that is, food, animal *or* vegetable) could nourish living tissue, then one had discovered the secret of life itself. The locus of debate was the stomach, which seemed immediately responsible for the conversion of dead matter into nutriment. What exactly went on in the stomach? Through experiments with snakes, ducks and dogs, Continental scientists had followed some of the steps by which the digestive tract stripped food particles down to basic nutritive elements, though there was much debate whether the process was essentially mechanical (grinding and churning) or chemical (dissolving or fermenting the food). Then, in 1822, by the best of bad fortunes, a young Canadian trapper named Alexis St. Martin had an accident which left a permanent hole or fistula in his stomach. Through this aperture his American surgeon, William Beaumont, explored the action of the human stomach, extracting the gastric juices, dangling bits of food on strings, measuring the volume of fluids. With St. Martin's grudging help, Beaumont was able to confirm that the gastric juices were acidic, not alkaline, and that these juices did indeed dissolve many foods. He prepared a chart of the time it took the stomach to digest various meats and vegetables, raw or cooked. His chart would be widely used and then widely imitated for the next century by physiologists, cookbook authors, home economists and reducing experts.[24]

Was the stomach no more than an organic mixing bowl? Was digestion no more than a pitiful chemistry? What Sylvester Graham wanted to believe, and therefore did believe, was that life was alchemical. What one ate was not simply dissolved to basic elements; it was transformed. The vital economy of the body, Graham wrote, "can triumph over the chemical affinities and ordinary laws of inorganic matter, and bend them to its purposes at pleasure;—generating and transmuting from one form to another, with utmost ease, the substances which human science calls elements."[25]

Graham was most outraged by what Beaumont had to say about hunger. Beaumont wrote that "the sense of hunger resides in the stomach, and is as well allayed by putting the food directly into the stomach" as by starting at the mouth. Graham wanted to keep hunger within the realm of the moral and spiritual; he could not abide the removal of hunger from the control of the will. Already, in a footnote to his 1832 edition of the treatise of Luigi Cornaro, Graham had dared to correct that saintly Italian, who had supposed that if one listened to one's stomach, one could not go wrong with one's appetite. Graham disagreed: "The whole system of governing the head by the stomach, instead of governing the stomach by the head, is utterly wrong. Make your stomach the healthful minister of the body, and not the whole body the mere locomotive appendage of your stomach. Treat your stomach like a well governed child; carefully find out what is best for it, as the digestive organ of your body, and then teach it to conform to your regimen, and soon its habitude will become what is commonly called *nature*." The stomach, like the child, must be part of a larger and wiser community. If, as Beaumont had written, "the stomach is a creature of habit," it was as subject to a moral education as the child.[26]

The simile of course was biographical, and yet it was also neurological. As the health of the child was the measure of the moral well-being of a family, so the stomach was "the common index of the whole system" of the body. The stomach lay just below, and in intimate contact with, the solar plexus, which constituted "a kind of common centre of action and sympathy, to the whole system of organic nerves." The body was one "general web of nervous texture, . . . a community of life and energy." The stomach was its sensorium and could not (should not?) suffer alone. Since the mucous membranes of the alimentary canal were alive with nerve-endings, that inner surface was "most peculiarly the centre of sympathy to the whole organic system."[27]

The more the nerves were stimulated, the more sensitive and fragile they became. Gluttony wound through the body from bowels to brain like a convulsing snake, exhausting the system. This neurology Graham lifted from Broussais, whose theory of irritation and exhaustion fitted Graham's sense of life as a series of dead-earnest skirmishes against foul-mouthed rioters and personal frailty. The snake, an anaconda, had appeared in the pages of the *Boston Daily Advertiser*, swallowing whole a live fowl "and not being satisfied with its supper, had the conscience to swallow his bed also." The anaconda appeared again in the *Graham Journal of Health and Longevity* as a dyspeptic, devouring whatever fell his way.[28]

Plainly, people did not stop eating when the hunger in their stomachs was allayed. Just as plainly, such overindulgence led to overstimulation, exhaustion and disease. Graham used this rhetoric in his tract against masturbation, in his lectures on the treatment of cholera during the 1832 epidemic, and in his campaign against gluttony. In each case, the remedy was a naturally regulated appetite, exercise, cold baths, fresh air and pure water. Not that Americans should return to the state of savages: savages led chancy, dyspeptic lives of feasting and fasting. Graham was too little the Leatherstocking and too much the Presbyterian to embrace the primeval. He proposed rather a civilized rejection of civilization, a return not to the tribal primitive but to primitive Christianity, that apostolic community of covenant, *Brith*, which his grandfather had chosen to translate as "to Chuse and to Eat." Friends were drawn to loving communion, spake John Graham in 1734, by "Eating and Drinking, freely, lovingly and cheerfully, with the Persons, with whom the Covenant is made."[29]

Sylvester Graham stood on tricky ground here, one foot in a nostalgic New England, the other in a visionary New England, both of which were indebted to impossibly good women. But he had been born into a tricky world, his father the age of an old grandfather, his mother off kilter, his boyhood off track. And he became a man in Jacksonian America in among a hugger-mugger of reformers and utopians who spoke loudly of the Millennium and inaugurated their own new worlds at Brook Farm, Fruitlands, Oneida, New Lebanon, Nauvoo and New Harmony. Meanwhile, masses of young people were leaving the depleted soils of New England and the Carolinas for the Eastern metropolises or the settlements of the Ohio Valley, and they were coming unchaperoned, by stage and canal, into frontier and commercial worlds of tricksters, hucksters and confidence men.[30]

That oldest of confidence men, time, lay in wait for them. "It is the nature of vital properties to exhaust themselves," wrote Xavier Bichat; "time wastes them." Sylvester Graham the vitalist placed himself staunchly in time's way. His system was meant to keep time at bay, so much so that naysayers and yeasayers alike were never quite sure whether he had actually promised his audiences lives of a hundred years. Lecturing for hours with frequent asides, prescribing a method of breadmaking thrice as long as usual, and searching for ancient ancestors, Graham was slowing life down. That rejuvenation which Luigi Cornaro had experienced and which diet books would bespeak ever and anon was for Graham a temporary release from the erosion of time. When they wanted to make clear how very well they felt, Grahamites spoke of their "buoyancy," a floating above time.[31]

The opposite of buoyancy was petrifaction. As Graham clipped an article about the Petrified Forest from the *New York Tribune* in 1844, he must have been impressed by the fact that the "old theory of slow decay . . . is now exploded. Matter, vegetable and animal, is found turned to stone in the air." He must surely have remarked the somatic parallel to this instant paralysis of the natural world, for he had discoursed at length on the ills of constipation, with which "It is true, probably, speaking within bounds, to say that nine tenths of the adults, and nearly as large a proportion of youth in civic life, are more or less afflicted." Constipation was the result of being taken in by superfine flour, pastries, and other sensuous deceits of civilization. Gluttony, hurrying appetite ahead of hunger, desire ahead of need, could bring the vital body to an untimely, motionless end.[32]

Out of Graham's fears for his own body came a nervous, bony defense of vitalism and a spirited theory of appetite that subordinated the stomach to mind and soul. Graham's campaign against gluttony was the crusade of a romantic who was desperately apprehensive of the ravages of time. It was not that gluttony made one fat but that it exhausted the mortal body, paralyzed its organs, cut life short. And if such were the penalties for a personal abandon, what would happen when a nation's appetites ran loose?

The Politics of Appetite

In no other era have references to gluttony and the luxuries of the table been so prevalent and effective on the national political stage. From the contest over the Bank of the United States before and after Andrew Jackson's reelection in 1832, through the Panic of 1837, to the 1840 battle for the presidency between William Henry Harrison and Martin Van Buren, fatness and repletion were the recurrent images.

Chartered in 1816 in response to local bank failures after the liquidation of the first Bank of the United States and a subsequent business recession, the Second Bank of the United States had been granted a twenty-year term. By 1828 and Jackson's election, the Bank was a solvent, well-managed institution or a devouring hydra-headed monster. For Whigs, the Bank facilitated the deposit and short-term transfer of funds from branch to branch in an expanding commercial market. For Democrats, the Bank was the classic confidence man, encouraging speculation, seducing people with credit, making money out of air as thin as fine flour. The Bank's success, which meant to the Whigs a healthy seacoast economy, meant to Jackson and his Democrats demonic monopoly and the disappearance of hard money from the inland frontier.[33]

Grown fat on its deposits and aristocratic on its exclusive privileges, the Bank in this Democratic fable was now challenged by that champion of the lean frontier, Andrew Jackson. As a young man, Jackson had suffered the springs and furrows of land speculation and bankruptcy; he intended to let the monster expire during his second term. The Whig director of the Bank, Nicholas Biddle, an efficient financier but an edgy politician, put the charter up for renewal four years early. Hoping to convert the Bank's fiscal strength into political capital, he made the Bank *the* issue in Jackson's 1832 bid for relection.[34]

So Old Hickory, 6 feet, 1 inch, thin and grizzled, squared off against Bully Nick, 5 feet, 7 inches, round and fair. We have an illustration of this boxing match. There is Biddle, seconded by fat Old Mother Bank holding a large bottle of port. "Blow me tight," says a spectator, "if Nick ain't been crammed too much—You see as how he's losing his wind!" Another cheers on Jackson: "Go it Hickory, my old buffer! give it to him in the bread basket, it will make him throw up his deposits!" No matter that Jackson was thin because subject to nephritis and chronic dysentery; no matter that Biddle was not especially round or self-indulgent. The fable required that the thin be fit and the fat be fought. The cartoon itself was drawn in 1834, when the "pluck and wind" of asthmatic, dropsical Jackson had indeed overcome natty Nick's "weight of metal." In the summer of 1833, the public deposits were withdrawn from the Bank.[35]

In 1837, with the once-opulent Bank reduced to a state charter in Pennsylvania, Jackson's heir, Martin Van Buren, faced a financial panic. Nearly half the banks established after 1830 would fail between 1837 and 1843. The vital economy seemed to have lost its vitality. Van Buren explained the situation to Congress in a message whose grammar of stimulation and excess Sylvester Graham could have claimed as his own: "[O]ur present condition is chiefly to be attributed to overaction in all the departments of business—an overaction . . . stimulated to its destructive consequences by excessive issues of bank papers and by other facilities for the acquisition and enlargement of credit." Once again, the physiological had become the political; gluttony, hurry and the false confidences of time were making a nervous wreck of the national body.[36]

The metaphors worked both ways. Critics saw Graham's system as a kind of ultra-republicanism. The satirist Richard Selden in 1839 assumed the voice of one of these levelers: "I am not certain in my own mind as yet, that the true stopping place in the glorious temperance reformation is at bran and water, because I do not know but some chemical discovery may yet show us that stone puddings are wholesomer for breakfast, and a little dirt and water better for supper than genuine coarse bran." Then he drew his bead: "When we consider the awful and unrelenting tyranny of appetite, when once it has the mastery over man, we should be as jealous of pampering it in the least as of tolerating aristocracy. I am certain, in a political point of view, that there is no way of effecting a complete equality in this happy country, until all men are levelled up to the standard of true Grahamites."[37]

On April 14, 1840, politics overtook parody. Charles Ogle, a Whig congressman from Pennsylvania, moved to amend the appropriations bill before the House. He wished to strike $3,665 meant for work on the White House, its furniture and grounds. A niggling matter, one would suppose, but Ogle was digging up more than shrubs and compost. He accused President Van Buren of violating the "plain, simple and frugal notions of our republican People." If the Jacksonians had denounced John Quincy Adams's 1825 purchase of a billiard table, cues and balls at a cost of $61, how much more legitimate was a Whig protest now against Van Buren's extravagance of $11,191.32 for White House table settings. And what settings: "massive gold plate and French sterling silver services, blue and gold French tambours, compotiers on feet, stands for bonbons with three stages, gilded French plateaus, garnished with mirrors and garlands, and gaudy artificial flowers." This luxury was scarcely intended for those "old and unfashionable dishes, '*hog and hominy*,' '*fried meat and gravy*,' '*schnitz, knep,* and *sourcrout*,' with a mug of 'hard cider.' No, sir, no. All these substantial preparations are looked upon by *gourmands, French cooks* and *locofoco Presidents* as exceedingly vulgar." Upon what did Van Buren condescend to dine? Ogle printed a sample menu in the *Congressional Record*: a soup course (turtle, pea or Julienne); a fish course (salmon, bass); a meat course (including filet of beef in champagne); an entremets (salad, filet mignon, calves brains, pigeon); fowl (wild duck, guinea fowl); pastries; desserts and liqueurs. It was time the people knew that "their money goes to buy for their plain hard-handed democratic President, knives, forks, and spoons of gold, that he may dine in the style of the monarchs of Europe."[38]

When Van Buren read Ogle's speech (said the Whigs), he was "in such a rage . . . that he actually *burst his corset*." Ogle and his friends had framed the entire election as a question of bodies, menus and habits of dining. It was William Henry Harrison's log cabin cider against Van Buren's chateau wine. The tall, slender Tippecanoe, plain eater, was set opposite the short Little Magician, Van the epicure. No matter that Harrison's wealthy father had been a Virginian gourmet or that Harrison's own abstinence was due to chronic indigestion; no matter that Van Buren had risen from the humbler family of a tavernkeeper or that the gold tableware was silver gilt and had been purchased years before by President Monroe. Although now the Whigs had staked out the lean frontier and cast the Democrats as sumptuous urban aristocrats, the fable was the same. The simple, the home-grown, the coarse and blunt must triumph over the elegant, the manufactured, the refined and diplomatic. If there were to be spoons, they must be like those of the frontiersman Hawkeye, the Pathfinder, measuring his skill across the rapids by the spoonfuls of white water in his canoe.[39]

Graham would have squirmed in that canoe—and squirmed mightily against any praise of hog and hominy, fried meat and gravy, sauerkraut or hard cider. But his system did fit within the

Jacksonian fable that so consistently put democracy to its test within the "national kitchen." Wrote one of Graham's defter critics, "Green peas, cabbage, and spinet [spinach] are enrolled in a new catalogue. They are no longer culinary and botanical. They take rank above that. They are become metaphysical."[40]

When Old Tippecanoe died after one month in office, a national fast was proclaimed. Benjamin Labaree, president of Middlebury College, in a sermon delivered on that occasion, took the country to task for the tragedy. Americans had an inordinate desire of gain, he said. The country was an immense mart swept by a national passion for buying and selling. The frenzy of speculation and the mania for profit had led to broken promises and, he implied, to the first death of a President in office.[41] For such a miserable state of affairs the traditional anodynes were repentance, piety, sobriety and devotion. Given the Jacksonian penchant toward gastronomic metaphor, the national fast might just as well have been taken literally, as prescribed by Sylvester Graham: natural appetite (against greed), slow eating (against frantic commerce), plain unspiced food (against speculation), few fats (against profit mania), honest bread (against broken promises). The outcome would be endurance, resilience, regularity, buoyancy, integrity and longevity.

Those diet policies and their promises recur often over the next 150 years, more and more closely allied to programs for losing weight. No diet comes without a larger social agenda. Every diet program is both conservative and prophetic: conservative, because its strategies and rationale are deeply embedded in the era in which it first appears; prophetic, because its agenda is invariably visionary, a picture of the world as it must be when we are less gluttonous, less dyspeptic, less constipated—or thinner, sleeker, lighter. Graham and the Jacksonians thought there was much wrong with their society, and they took the ailing human body as its totem. The theory of the cure followed upon the diagnosis of the disease. But how accurate was the diagnosis? Were people so very gluttonous? Were they eating too much? Were they thinner or fatter than they had been or than they should have been?

The Jacksonian Experience of the Body

Art and fashion between 1820 and 1850 showed women with tapered arms and "prune and prism" mouths, their waists drawn in and their ankles impractical. The "steel-engraving" woman, at first romantic and then (in the 1840s) sentimental, skipped then glided on the arm of her consort, a slender, elegant man in close-fitting trousers and coat. Both might wear corsets, not because they were fat but because they required a certain erect posture and a certain inverted shape that would lead the eye to a center so magical it could not seem to hold. Whether sleeves and collars billowed out above or skirts and tails billowed out below, between lay a spiritualized stomach, pivotal yet invisible.[42]

This was the stomach imagined by the fashionably romantic and anorectic poet Byron, who by 1822 had "starved himself into an unnatural thinness." If he himself dieted on hard biscuits and soda water, or on potatoes flattened and drenched in vinegar, his diet for women was at once more fanciful and more severe. "A woman," he wrote, "should never be seen eating or drinking, unless it be *lobster salad* and *champagne*, the only truly feminine and becoming viands." The rosebud mouth was the signature of an ethereal appetite; for women especially, whose low-set sleeves in the 1840s made eating a trial of grace, the stomach was meant to be publicly implausible. Byron's dictum was exaggerated by "a Native of the United States" writing in 1827: "I must own I cannot bear to see a pretty woman, not merely eat, but eat at all; and only wish that the act, like many others, could be performed without being observed."[43]

"Among the high classes," wrote a contributor to *Graham's Lady's and Gentleman's Magazine* in 1844, "the *mode* is rather shadowy, the form being more cared for than substance. . . . Among the *lower* class substance is a more material matter." But the shadowy mode had slipped into the dresses of schoolteachers and Lowell mill girls as well as society belles. In the parlors of urban tradespeople, cheap lithographs of ballerina Fanny Elssler (far thinner than life) danced above the vertical lines and restrained curves of Greek Revival bureaus and Gothic steeple clocks. The American Art Union in 1850 sent all 18,960 of its subscribers an engraving of long-necked, thin-ankled, tight-waisted Anne Page being courted by Abraham Slender in the *Merry Wives of Windsor* (Act III, Scene 4). It would have taken not a sharp eye but a good memory for any subscriber to realize that Slender was meant to be a numbskull and Anne Page an active country girl, for both stood in handsome nimbi of light, almost gracious, while the comic hero of the play, Sir John Falstaff— "in the waist two yards about"—was nowhere to be seen.[44]

The *Newark Daily Advertiser* in 1838 was most blatant about the shadowy mode: "We are decided admirers of leanness. Our greatest characters are usually little, attenuated men; stomachless, meagre, lean, and lath-like beings, who have spiritualized themselves by keeping matter in due subordination to mind. . . . Obesity is a deadly foe to genius; in carneous and unwieldy bodies the spirit is like a little gudgeon in a large frying-pan of fat, which is either totally absorbed, or tastes of nothing but the lard." No matter that neither Daniel Boone nor Davy Crockett nor Dolly Madison nor many another great American character was "stomachless, meagre, lean, and lath-like." Americans did see themselves this way. Their renewed concern with posture in the 1830s and 1840s drew on their self-image as thin and peculiarly unbraced: "The Yankee has not, like other nations, *one* distinctive posture. He sits—after a sort; —he stands—but never stands still; —he walks—'setting endeavor in continued motion;' —he runs, he ambles, he trots, he scuds, he wriggles, he hitches and he somnambulates." After 1820, use of the tape measure and manufacture of ready-made clothes would begin to regulate the posture of this man, just as a new genre of spinal contraptions would operate on the posture of American women. Neither standardized clothing patterns nor treatises on scoliosis would have been so persuasive without the common belief that Americans, being so lean, had need of firm measures for their shadowy forms.[45]

Europcan tourists in the antebellum era, like the novelist Thackeray, agreed that Americans were "lean as greyhounds." The men here seemed pale, thin, long, spindle-shanked, and the women very slight, gaunt, scrawny. Had those visitors mistaken for gauntness the fashionably pale complexions which sentimental young women arranged through alkaline diets of powdered chalk, burnt coffee or writing paper? Were they chauvinists comparing a narrow spectrum of bony city folk with the healthiest of European country specimens? Had Jacksonian fable or American fashion blinded them to the facts?[46]

Yes and no. The problem was one of scale. From the late 17th century on, American-born colonists and their American-born slaves were taller than their ancestors and their contemporaries in Europe and Africa. By the Revolution, native-born white soldiers had achieved an average height of 5 feet, 8 inches, an average that would stick through to World War II. White Americans were three or more inches taller than Britons in colonial times, perhaps two inches taller than most Europeans throughout the 19th century. Americans living in the South or in rural areas were generally half an inch taller yet.[47]

To Europeans, and to Americans accustomed to European models of fashion and beauty, the difference in height from one side of the Atlantic to the other was far more remarkable than any proportionate difference in weight or outline. And, at least during the first half of the 19th century, Americans seem not to have been gaining an extraordinary number of pounds. The evidence is scanty, since few thought to record their weights if once or twice they stepped up on farm or commercial platform scales. In 1850, Dr. Daniel Drake did weigh and measure 316 soldiers at Fort Mackinac, Fort Gratiot, and the Detroit Barracks. Their average height was 5 feet, 7 inches, average weight about 147 lbs. The native-born soldiers were slightly heavier than those of immediate English ancestry, lighter than those of German ancestry. (Drake expected them all to gain some weight as they reached full maturity around age forty; he did not consider the native-born to be underweight.) We have no decent earlier American data with which to compare those numbers, but contemporary European estimates of normal weight for height were entirely consistent with Drake's results. That is, white Americans were roughly the same weight-for-height as their European peers. Americans were just plain taller.[48]

Aided and abetted by the verticals in fashion, furniture, and Gothic Revival architecture, Americans appeared to themselves and to their guests as lean of frame. In the general absence of an aristocratic demeanor, they might also appear gawky or thin-legged, as in Felix Darley's 1856 drawings of La Longue Carabine, a.k.a. Natty Bumppo, Leather-Stocking, Hawkeye, the Pathfinder.

"No, no; deny your appetites, deny your appetites, and learn one virtue from a redskin, who will pass a week without eating even, to get a simple scalp," the Pathfinder cautions the old sea captain in the middle of the forest.[49] How could Americans see themselves as thin and gluttonous at the same time? Was gluttony mere metaphor, a convenient and customary target for moralists?

The Thin Glutton

Americans of all classes were taller precisely because they did eat more. They ate more meat and probably more fruit than their cousins in Europe or in Africa. They expected food more often. They had a more varied diet, at least on the coastal plains and during the summer. And when lean, abstinent Old Tippecanoe's partisans held a political rally on the banks of the Scioto in Ohio, four hundred women prepared 20,000 lbs of bread, 200 bushels of potatoes, 70 sheep, 80 slabs of bacon and 22 steers.[50]

"You are not much *asked*, not much *pressed*, to eat and drink; but such an abundance is spread before you, and so hearty and so cordial is your reception, that you instantly lose all restraint, and are tempted to feast whether you be hungry or not," the Englishman William Cobbett wrote of his year's residence in America in 1817–18. "And, though the *manner* and *style* are widely different in different houses, the *abundance* every where prevails." If Cobbett, accustomed to touring the poorest laboring districts of Great Britain, might be suspected of exaggeration, there was constant testimony from other less radical Europeans—so much so that as early as 1800 Americans had found "all foreigners who visit this country, Frenchmen, Germans, and even Englishmen, exclaiming against *our copious and everlasting* dinners." Etiquette assumed abundance; though Americans imitated European manners in other respects, they did not maintain that traditional reverence for the last scrap on the serving plate. By all means *take* the last piece: "It amounts almost to an insult toward your host, to do anything which shows that you fear that the vacancy cannot be supplied and that there is likely to be a scarcity."[51]

Recipe notebooks of American housewives and the recipes of specifically American cookbooks worked typically with large amounts. An 1810 plumcake required 3 lbs flour, 3 lbs currants, 1½ lbs lump sugar, ½ lb butter and 6 eggs. The Cook Not Mad, an 1830 advocate of moderation presenting "*republican* dishes and garnishing proper to fill an every day bill of fare, from the condition of the poorest to the richest," suggested an alamode of beef: a round of beef stuffed with ½ lb pork, ½ lb butter, the soft part of ½ loaf wheat bread, 4 hard-boiled eggs, and a gill of wine, highly seasoned with salt, pepper and cloves.[52]

It was the meat, the butter and the sugar that most overwhelmed observers. Per capita meat consumption for 1830–39 was 178 lbs a year, a level so far above any other country's that Americans themselves would not match it until the 1970s. From childhood on, Americans expected meat three or four times a day every day. When it did not come fresh, it would be hung beef or, more likely, salt or pickled pork. No wonder that Uncle Sam himself had begun in 1812 as Samuel Wilson, a Hudson River meatpacker.[53]

The meat was tough, fried or baked in butter or lard. The gravies were also butter or lard. "Mon Dieu! what a country!" exclaimed a French visitor; "fifty religions and only one sauce—

melted butter!" In the cities and among the wealthy, butter was spread thickly over potatoes and wheat breads; in the country and among the poor, butter sank into turnips and peas, buckwheat rolls, cornbread and unleavened Indian-meal biscuits.[54]

Meat, butter and cheap sugar came together in the American pie, "very white and indigestible at the top, very moist and indigestible at the bottom, and with untold horrors in the middle." American cookbooks from their start in 1796 devoted twice as many pages to sweet pies, pastries, sweet custards, cakes, cookies, sweet puddings and preserves than their nearest competitor and former model, the English cookbook. And if the French upper crust had the great pastry chef Antoine Carême with his towers of flour, starch, isinglass, sugar and yolks of eggs, all Americans had their pie. "We cry for pie when we are infants. Pie in countless varieties waits upon us through life. Pie kills us finally. . . . How can a person with a pound of green apples and fat dough in his stomach feel at ease?"[55]

"Paleness and pie": Americans were thin *because* they were gluttonous. Americans might eat a great deal, but they could not digest it. The English, on the other side of the table, digested well enough to elicit most of the major treatises on corpulence from 1750 to 1860. This contrast between the bloated imperial Englishman and the lean, go-it-alone American was lost neither on American cartoonists nor on the Scottish essayist Thomas Carlyle, who rhapsodized to Ralph Waldo Emerson in 1849, "How beautiful to think of lean tough Yankee settlers, tough as gutta percha with most *occult* unsubduable fire in their belly, steering over the Western Mountains to annihilate the jungle, and bring bacon and corn out of it for the Posterity of Adam!" Closer to home, however, that "most *occult* unsubduable fire in their belly" was indigestion.[56]

Americans ate too fast. A Russian compared them to sharks, a fellow Yankee (once again) to the anaconda: "The Americans are not epicures, but gluttons. They swallow, but don't eat; and, like the boa-constrictor, bolt every thing, whether it be a blanket or a rabbit. . . . It startles a foreigner to see with what voracity even our delicate women dispose of the infinite succession of dishes on the public tables." Meals took as little as 3¾ minutes, with some moments after for swallowing and spitting.[57]

Americans ate fast because, in taverns and boardinghouses especially, meals were served *table d'hôte*, all the dishes on the table at once, caught in the crossfire of appetites. They ate fast because they ate so much sugar and therefore had bad teeth, finding it painful, difficult or dangerous to chew. They ate fast because they ate without conversation, "serious, self-absorbed, and silent." They ate fast because they ate so often.[58]

In hotels on the American plan of bed-and-board, breakfast was at six, dinner at noon, tea at four, supper at six, with a light snack in the evening. In boardinghouses, breakfast was at eight: tea, coffee, bread and butter, potatoes, eggs, broiled fish, beefsteaks, hot cakes or fresh rolls. At eleven, soup and cold meat. At three, fish, flesh and fowl with vegetables and puddings, pies, fruit and cider. At seven, tea with toast, bread, butter and cakes. At bedtime, a little supper. The poor ate less regally and less regularly than the rich, but nearly everyone ate more often in the 19th century than people did a century earlier, when breakfast and dinner were supplemented at best by a meatless supper.[59]

Rules of graciousness and gastronomy were intended to divert Americans from so much food—or at least to slow them down. Put a fork with three or four prongs in the hand of frontiersman Harry Hurry and ask him to switch it conscientiously from right to left throughout the meal. Make it good manners to take small bites. Adopt the new mode of serving one dish at a time. When serving, do not overload the plate; when eating, leave something on the plate: "No genteel person eats more than half of anything."[60]

Etiquette worked no wonders with indigestion. Nor, it seems, did the new cast-iron stoves, which allowed for the preparation of food in smaller amounts and for better control of the temperatures for frying and boiling.[61] Americans ate quickly, ate much, and grew taller, but they grew lean. What they ate did not fill them out since it was never properly digested.[62]

If Americans could thus explain how they were thin *and* gluttonous, how can we explain their genuine hostility to Sylvester Graham, whose war against gluttony meant many a skirmish with indigestion? What was it that made Graham's system at once so much part of his era and so unnatural? Why not follow up the oxymoron of the thin glutton with the Grahamite paradox of a thin diet that fills one out?

Appetite and Abundance

When the chief American revivalist, Charles Grandison Finney, migrated to Ohio in 1836 to establish Oberlin College on pious, re-

forming and temperate principles, including Grahamism, he almost
instantly became one of "starvation's monarchs,"

> Who've proved that *drink* was never meant to *drink*,
>   Nor *food* itself intended to be *eaten*,
> That Heaven provided for our use, instead,
>   The *sand* and *sawdust* which compose our bread.

Even a man with such a mantle of celestial authority as Finney was
here ground down to sand and sawdust. Graham himself was called
Dr. Sawdust, and his disciples were known as members of "Tee-total
Fast Day Forever Associations," their mouths sewn up like corpses'.
Graham's insistence on coarsely milled flour, on unleavened breads,
on pure water as opposed to fermented drinks, on hard beds and less
sex made him seem a partisan of the grave. However much he might
talk Christianity, it seemed as if he expected nothing to rise. However much he might protest that he was restoring holy appetite, it
seemed that he was preaching a living death, thin ghosts in slow
time, stripped of the fat of the earth. This was the shadowy mode
taken to its extreme, like that Society for the Suppression of Eating
which had been facetiously registered as logical complement to the
Society for the Suppression of Intemperance. "Disease," the satirist
wrote, "lurks behind the fat sirloin, and there is Death in the tureen
of turtle-soup. Whenever I go to a dinner party, it seems to me that I
see in my mind's eye, the incarnate forms of Gout, Apoplexy, and
Fever, bringing in the dishes and coaxing their victims, 'just to take
one slice more.' "[63]

Out of the cold earth the Grahamite corpses came with a "preternatural buoyancy," far more puritanical than colonial Puritans,
who had eaten largely at funerals and again at Thanksgiving, lacing
their food with pepper from Salem, a major pivot in the Atlantic
spice trade. For Grahamites, "Mustard is murder; pepper is perdi-
tion"—and all feasting suspect. William A. Alcott, Graham's al-
terego and elder statesman of abstinence, published attacks on Sunday dinners, Independence Day binges and Thanksgiving gluttony.
Glum ghosts, these Grahamites and health reformers who could not
take pleasure in the celebration of abundance. Did not Americans
have a right to the fruits of their labors? It was not natural, in the
midst of a world of so much frontier and so little leisure, to consider
a loaf of stale bread and three tumblers of water sufficient merri-
ment.[64]

Oberlin College had to abandon the Graham diet in 1841 after rumors of mass starvation at the college aroused the townspeople. Students and faculty were scarcely starving on cold water, milk, wheat, rice, tapioca, sago, apples, a few vegetables and occasional slivers of fish or mutton, but this seemed a diet without backbone: no beef, no cider, no salt pork, nothing a man could sink his teeth into and survive. It was a peculiarly childlike diet of gruel and puddings, fruit, mush and dry bread.[65]

And this was most unnatural. Graham seemed to be turning away from maturity, fertility and the larger society of men and women toward the childlike, the asexual and the solipsistic. It was no mistake that many of his adherents were young men and women in boardinghouses who had come to the city only to find themselves betwixt and between. That "moral fury and mental exaltation resulting from abstinence" gave vent to ghosts in the pantry, lonely and transparent in their denial of hunger.[66]

Graham's contemporaries found his system unnatural precisely because he made Nature out to be ungenerous. Graham feared the possibility of unlimited goods, substituting for that the equally millennial possibility of unlimited Good. He wanted human nature to take up the slack by reverting to an image of happiness that did not demand so much from a tired earth. Perhaps he was right. While he was most active, flour prices had risen and the poor in the cities were less well-fed. Forced to a lower standard of living by the higher cost of housing and of household fuel, they were buying cheaper food and bakery bread made from less substantial flour. The average heights of common laborers were falling as their wages fell in relation to others between 1820 and 1860.[67]

But this was the New World, and those laborers were still of greater stature than the industrial poor in any other country. Depletion, exhaustion and age were unwelcome ideas, Jacksonian political epithets. Democrats called Tippecanoe at sixty-seven "granny," and the Whigs called Old Van at fifty-eight "a used-up man." Even Graham in 1836 invested in expansion: he had stock in the Delaware and Hudson Canal, the ideal portfolio for a man preoccupied with pure water and the alimentary passage.[68]

Jacksonians might embrace thinness as a style, but not as a way of life. If their body politics argued for a lean vigor, their devotion to abundance argued for a consuming appetite. Americans were not yet so fearful of abundance that they had to resort en masse to an abstinent, unsavory regime, or weigh out their food meal by meal, or watch their weight day by day. The reducing diets, the calorie counting, the bathroom scales lay in the future, where gluttony and thinness would seem to be the strangest of tablemates, where Melba toast, bran breads and Graham crackers would be fixtures on every diet chart.

At the end, Sylvester Graham was a failed, bilious romantic. His system had lain almost entirely with the romantic mode, demanding an immediacy of conviction, promising through diet and an act of will a sudden metamorphosis of the human being. A few had been transformed, but onward had been the course of that empire which some called the United States and others called Dyspepsia.

CHAPTER THREE

The Buoyant Body
in Victorian America

Long before Americans sought consistently to be thin, they desired a sensation of lightness, of buoyancy. The American Disease of dyspepsia was of such concern in the antebellum era because it was marked by chronic sensations of heaviness and sinking, sensations focused on the stomach and associated with gluttony. The most popular cures for dyspeptics—and for women whose "female problems" were often confused with dyspepsia—were meant to restore a sense of buoyancy. After the Civil War, in company with a shift toward a more active sense of the body in which energy was most at issue, the symptoms of dyspepsia were transferred to a new American Disease, neurasthenia or nervous exhaustion. In the process, the set of connections between indigestion, thinness and gluttony was gradually dissolved. Gluttony was free at last to be unequivocally associated with fatness, and fatness with heaviness.

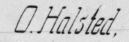

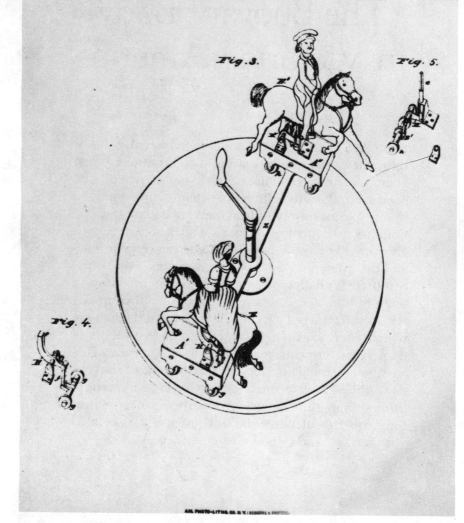

O. Halsted,

Exercising Machine,

Nº 3,480,

Patented Mar. 13, 1844.

Fig. 3.

Fig. 5.

Fig. 4.

Oliver Halsted's Exercising Machine, 1844, for relieving indigestion or dyspepsia

Bellies, Buoyancy and Women's Bodies

SOME SIX MONTHS before the world was to end, Oliver Halsted of New York City patented a machine for the treatment of dyspepsia. While Millerites awaited the return of Jesus in October 1844, Halsted foresaw the return of health. William Miller had located humanity within the last furious wheels of sacred chronology; Halsted sat man and woman upon mechanical horses moving on wheels in a tight circle, a sorry version of Ezekiel's chariot. As Millerites searched the skies for signs of the Second Coming, Halsted's operator would turn the crank at the center of the wooden platform, and man and woman would rise and fall on their canted and cantering horses.[1]

I juxtapose the millennial and the mundane in much the same manner as did Prof. Edward Hitchcock in his lectures to Amherst students in 1830. Hitchcock too was worried about dyspepsia, whose nausea, dry mouth, furred tongue, flushed skin, heartburn, nightmare and images of death would shorten by decades the lives of at least half the American people. Freed from the decay and confusions of dyspepsia, what might not his students do in this needful world? The apostles proclaiming the gospel had been eupeptics,

49

men of fine digestion; so the millennium itself could be brought on
only by eupeptics. "Oh, the light and influence, which they might
thus send out into the world, and down to posterity, would not, like
other emanations proceeding from a centre, spread and increase in
the slow ratio of the square of the distance and the time; but in a ratio so high, that the quadratics of the millennium could alone express and resolve it." A teacher of natural history, Hitchcock had extended the laws of physical illumination to flights of the spirit,
measuring apostasy by the darkness, heaviness and torpor of the dyspeptic. Overeating and the consequent indigestion brought on that
awful sense of weight which dragged down the soul. Dyspepsia dispelled would mean the soul unbound.[2]

Oliver Halsted meant his carousel as no Armageddon joust, but
he too hoped to restore a sense of buoyancy to the ailing body. Relieved of chronic dyspepsia by the joltings of a stagecoach, Halsted
had turned those unexpectedly therapeutic motions into a system of
massage from which he gained notoriety in New York while Prof.
Hitchcock was lecturing in Amherst. Halsted's system, as one critic
put it, involved tickling, pickling, ironing and throwing up the
bowels. He would tap at the solar plexus, bundle the stomach in
flannel cloths dipped in hot vinegar, pass a flat iron over the cloth,
then place his right hand on the lower part of his patient's abdomen
and push up. Using "tact," not force, he administered a series of
"gentle shocks" which seemed—the lower down the abdomen he
was obliged to go—more shocking than genteel. He therefore taught
his patients self-manipulation and, in 1844, invented his surrogate,
which transferred the most irregular if uplifting of human contacts
to a regular if wooden horse. Still, there was something suggestive to
such mechanical massage, since the woman had to rise astride, not
sidesaddle, for full effect.[3]

This were comedy if the same conflation of stomach and sex had
not also plagued other health reformers whose enemies made consistent innuendo of women's bellies. Such innuendo came in part
from an American prudery that fully abstracted the stomach, granting it nominal dominion over a much larger area from the thighs to
the neck.[4] It came in part from territorial claims which indigestion
made upon the uterus and the associated symptoms of hysteria, and
then upon the ovaries and the symptoms we now associate with Pre-
Menstrual Syndrome. It came, finally, from a widespread ignorance
of human anatomy, in particular of female anatomy. And it was
complicated after midcentury by more acute concerns with abortion, sterility and exhaustion.

A woman's stomach bore constant reference (as a man's stomach did not) to sexual functions. Many patent medicines directed against dyspepsia became specifics against "female weakness," the euphemism for menstrual problems. Any diet women undertook had at once a digestive and a reproductive meaning. We shall see throughout this book how often diet techniques and drugs are cousin to contraceptives and abortifacients. That horseback riding recommended since Dr. Cheyne as ideal exercise for the corpulent was thought also to promote miscarriage. Peter Puckerbrodt's 1832 recipe for an Improved Dyspepsia Bread depended for its "prophylactic qualities" upon white cotton rags, sawdust, a little chloride of lime, and plaster of Paris; it was rather a pessary than a droll alternative to Graham's bran bread.[5]

A woman's stomach, then, was completely freighted. "Dyspepsia Regina" had concentrated the sensations of personal weight in the pit of the stomach. Folklore and popular medicine made a single heavy bundle of tissue and fluid out of a woman's innards. Fashion slung layer upon layer of cloth from a woman's hips. Nature brought to bear the gravid weight of the fetus.

As the cures for dyspepsia aimed for the restoration of buoyancy (of the body, of the spirits), so in fashion and physiology, the kinaesthetic ideal was focused on the sensations of lightness and buoyancy. We are not yet arrived at any obsession with slimming, but we must follow the woman on Halsted's mildly bucking bronco to appreciate how the teaching of physiology to women, the crusade for dress reform, and the establishment of the water cure became means toward the release, if not the loss, of weight.

New Models of the Body: Volume Without Weight

"My mother told me often that I was a fright; that my skin was yellow as a squash, my nose large enough for two, and that my eyes were not mates." Set up to be a freak, Mary Sargeant Neal would set out to make the world whole. A short, thinnish, dark-haired bride of twenty-one in 1831, Mary Neal, now Gove, gave birth to one daughter, then had four miscarried or stillborn children. By 1837 she had embraced health reform and instituted a Grahamite boarding school for girls at Lynn, Massachusetts. The next year, struggling out of a cruel marriage, she became the first woman in the United States to give public lectures on female anatomy. She addressed large crowds of women, speaking against gluttony, tight-lacing, and self-pollution, that solitary vice whose prevalence she attributed to a repressive society which forbade women the full exercise of their powers. Like Sylvester Graham, she knew that only strict temperance could "roll back the polluting tide that is overwhelming our world with moral and physical desolation." Unlike Graham, she was courageous enough to illustrate her lectures with three-dimensional models of the sorely tried female body.[6]

Hers were not the first such models to be displayed by a woman.[7] Nor were hers the first models to appear in this country. Rachel Wells had modeled Siamese twins in wax in 1767; Abraham Chovet had lectured on anatomy in Philadelphia in the 1770s, using male and female wax figures with glass arteries and veins. And there had been for years small wax or wooden dolls modeled to the exact dimensions of fashionable women, who sent them to dressmakers in Europe.[8]

Even so, models in wax or papier-mâché were dramatic elements in the progress of women's physiological reform societies and in the establishment of a kinaesthetic of buoyancy and lightness. As increasingly articulated figures became available from European workshops, a woman's body could be seen to take on volume and depth without taking on appreciable weight, akin to those other buoyant, lightly framed structures which Americans were testing by midcentury—the balloon-frame house, the tiered riverboat, the precisely arched bridge, the crinoline. The marvel of the body was not its solidity or substance (Mary Gove hated to see fat people) but its architectural lift: how—like strut, truss or thin wire—muscle, bone and nerve held surface to center. By 1855 the Ladies Physiological Institute of Boston and Vicinity had acquired two embryos, a lobe of the brain, a skeleton, and a female manikin with nerves, viscera, and five hundred muscles open to view, showing the "nice dependencies and close relations of one to the other—All speaking to us, in loudest terms of a 'first Great Cause.'" A woman's "divine form" now had a deeper meaning; it was not all surface or seeming.[9]

This may explain the phrenological bust which the Institute also acquired. The science of head-reading depended upon a theory linking center to surface, giving psychological depth to the opaque contours of the human skull. Like the new American cartographers who were plotting far more revealing topographical maps in the 1840s,[10] phrenologists with their calipers were charting the cranium for a more revealing topography of human character. Each sentiment, propensity and intellectual faculty had its own latitude and longitude on the bumpy globe of the skull. Alimentiveness or Alimentativeness, the desire for food, lay just in front of the ear and below Acquisitiveness; the capacity to distinguish Weight lay just above the far corner of the eye, in tight company with the faculties for Size, Locality and Color. Those positions did not change from man to woman, since phrenology was ostensibly impartial in its anatomy of the sexes. A phrenologist's reading was based on the relative size and elevation of each of the 34, 35, 37 or 43 cranial territories. For women in particular, phrenology provided a set of authoritative measurements that were neither linear nor two-dimensional. In place of the superficial and petty calculations of neck, bust, waist and hips, they could have the deeper, more elevated calculations of Amativeness, Self-Esteem, Hopefulness, Wonder, Ideality and Wit, on a scale from one to seven. A woman might advertise herself in a matrimonial column by the size of her head and "nervous, 4; domestic propensities large, 6; selfish propensities full, 5; . . . reflective or reasoning intellect large to very large, 6 to 7."[11]

The world's foremost publicist of phrenology from the 1830s on would be Orson Squire Fowler, a student of Prof. Hitchcock, whom we have just heard on the subject of eupepsia and the millennium. If Orson Fowler skipped out on his ministerial studies to preach "the religion of bumps," he never broke step with the crusade for moral reform. His *American Phrenological Journal*, enjoying one of the largest periodical circulations in the country, reached as many as fifty thousand people East and West with Temperance homilies, dress reform advice, Grahamite propaganda and the old news that "gluttony is as bad as drunkenness, and *far* more prevalent."[12]

The distance between waxwork model and phrenological bust was not great. Sectioned and labeled, both were physiological emblems that truth will out, that the body after all cannot lie. Patted, pressed, measured and manipulated, both model and skull promised the active possibility of reform. A phrenological reading could change from year to year as one exercised one's best propensities or fought, as Hugh H. Hite did in 1853, against one's own "quite large alimentativeness." Similarly, the Ladies Physiological Society had gathered skeletons and waxworks in hopes that "the structure of the human form, shall come forth, in its loveliness not as now, marked and marred by deformity, disease and suffering, but shall appear in its completeness, harmonious in its proportions, perfect in its developments, fitted and trained for usefulness."[13]

This vision of beauty *had* appeared, twice in thirty years, only to lose her arms and then to be put in chains. A new Venus, evidently whole, was discovered on the island of Melos in Greece in 1820.

Like the earlier Venus de' Medici, broken during its Renaissance trip from Rome to Florence, the Venus de Milo suffered at the hands of men. In a seaside scuffle between French collectors and the Greek Orthodox priest who had bought the statue from a peasant, the Venus was said to have lost both her arms. Nonetheless, she became the archetype of feminine beauty until Hiram Powers's "Greek Slave" conquered America on a tour in 1847. Powers, who had begun as a waxworker for a Cincinnati museum, sculpted a classical nude with long waist and round breasts, her head turned away from the shame of the thin chains which hung loosely from one wrist at her lower abdomen, down across crotch and thigh, to her other wrist and the short column of an auction block. As a reminder of the recent Greek independence from Turkey, as a figure of bondage with a sad and distant expression, the Greek Slave became an exemplary and therefore tasteful nude.[14]

She was also remarkably weightless. The delicate chains could not drag her down, her hand on the column rested almost as afterthought, her one gracefully bent leg put no strain on the other. Aside from the hair pulled back tightly in a bun, she was strangely free from compulsion. Her beauty—and the gentility of her beauty— was due in great measure to her weightlessness, which made her at once graceful and chaste.

From phrenological bust to waxwork torso to Greek Slave, the most palpable projections of the human body insisted on a physical presence which despite its volume remained peculiarly light. That lightness, that buoyancy, was a sign of the harmony between the center of the body and its surface, a harmony presumed by phrenologists and preached by Mary Neal Gove. While dyspeptics slumped under the weight of their bodies, their bellies in pain and their skin dreadfully sensitive, the Greek Slave stood almost oblivious to her chains, rounded and calm, nearly floating.

Buoyant Bodies and Dress Reform

In photographs of the 1840s, when a sitting demanded a minute or more of absolute stillness, people seemed to set their features by patterns they had seen in drawing manuals or in books on how to read the face. Their heads often clamped to the back of the chair, they must have felt compelled by the camera's slow eye to concentrate on surface and to resist any motion from their depths which might contract a muscle or agitate a lip. Though framed by country arbor or classical columns, most subjects had to cope with a bustling urban world of superficial acquaintances, winking salesmen, smiling swindlers. They had learned as best they could how not to betray themselves with a grin or be cozened by an artful complexion. Photographers colluded here, posing people so that the timid appeared stern and the large-mouthed appeared only in profile.[15]

Photographic portraits aggravated a growing cultural suspicion of the countenance. By 1859 a health reformer would allege the thorough deceitfulness of the face. The burden of truthtelling lay rather with the body as a whole: "Not one man or woman in ten who lives as the People at large, will weigh as much as their faces promise. . . . Undressed [meat-eaters] look monstrous, with fleshy faces and gaunt bodies," while vegetarians had thin faces but nicely rounded bodies. The full body, not the flattering face, must be the locus of health and the index to character.[16]

For the People at large, as well as for health reformers, that full body was ideally a buoyant body. In theaters across the country, European ballerinas Maria Taglioni and Fanny Elssler toured to enormous acclaim, amazing audiences with the near-weightlessness of that new technique, dancing on point. Outside, women with small mouths and narrow waists floated above the waves on the prows of the light Baltimore clippers, and celebrated aeronauts like Eugène Robertson ascended to unimaginable heights in hot-air balloons while as many as four thousand watched from below. During the 1840 play "1940! or, Crumbles in Search of Novelty," men flew routinely in balloons. In lecture halls, masters of animal magnetism raised recumbent men breast-high with the tips of their forefingers.[17]

If dress reformers also desired an extraordinary buoyancy, they hoped still to restore a natural gravity to the female body. Buoyancy had to come less from the tailored artifice of hooks and metal eyes than from an active demonstration of the powers of a healthy body. The harmony of the center and the surface of the body must be achieved through a unanimity of parts rather than a painful compression or a supernal denial of the flesh, its volume and weight.

Amelia Jenks Bloomer, Deputy Postmistress of Seneca Falls, New York, must have been accustomed to the fine discrimination of weight and volume. Since the passage of the first low-postage act in 1845, postal letter rates had been based on weight, and new postal scales were being patented for the precise measurement of ounces.

Not that Amelia Bloomer or her friend Elizabeth Cady Stanton or
Stanton's cousin Libby Miller in 1851 were the first to protest
against the fuss, bulk and weight of women's clothing. Fashion history has had one long trailing hem of sumptuary laws, jeremiads
against excess (or immodesty), and caricatures of impractical elegance. Corsets and tight-lacing, designed visually to counteract the
pull of 8 or 10 lbs of dress material, had come under special fire by
the 19th century. No longer an exterior busk but a far more intimate
companion, the corset appeared politically as the aristocratic enemy
of free circulation, sexually as an incendiary stoking the flames of
Amativeness, scientifically as a boa constrictor deforming the spine,
and medically as the accomplice of dyspepsia, which produced "a
sense of constriction, as if a girdle was drawn tightly around the
body."[18]

On a tour of Europe, Elizabeth Smith Miller had been wearing
an ungirdled, unconstricting costume modeled after that worn by
women at water cure sanatoriums, a costume in turn modeled after
those Turkish trousers the Greek Slave would have worn after she
was sold. The long trousers with overskirt which Elizabeth Stanton
then designed for American women, and which she and Amelia
Bloomer wore in public, were not unlike the pantaloons and skirts
which young American girls had been wearing since the 1820s. A
woman critical of the Bloomer costume made just this association—
"think of the dress of a slim young lady of ten years old, on a grown-
up woman, particularly if she is rather fallen into flesh, and you'll
see how I saw a stout Bloomer look—certainly, that was not bloom-
ing." The criticism was well-taken, as the plump Elizabeth Stanton
would admit a few years later: "We knew the Bloomer Costume
never could be generally becoming, as it required a perfection of
form, limbs, and feet, such as few possess, and we who wore it also
knew that it was not artistic." But the costume, so far as it was neu-
tered and juvenile, did deny the heavy freight of a woman's torso. If
it was uncomplimentary to the fully mature woman, it did release
the center of her body from its cultural burden.[19]

The Bloomer was exemplary of the desires of many reformers to
put forward a woman who was at once buoyant and earthbound.
"We say to you, at your fireside, ladies, unhook your dresses, and let
everything hang loosely about you. Now, take a long breath, swell
out as far as you can, and at that point fasten your clothes." This release did not entail a new heaviness; the loose hanging in the first
sentence became a lift and suspension in the second. The Bloomer,

which revealed an adult with feet clearly connected to her center, meant ease of motion, more certain footing, *and* the buoyant steps recommended to young women by the great beauty Lola Montez. When the crinoline appeared in 1856, Amelia Bloomer would find little objection to abandoning her ostentatious trousers for "light and pleasant" wire hoops, which did away with layers of heavy petticoats.[20]

More successful than the Bloomer as a projection of volume without weight, the early crinoline also dispensed with much tightlacing, since in comparison to the width of the hoop most women's waists would appear infinitesimal. Fat or thin, a woman in crinoline extended an imperium about herself that implied a greater sphere and perhaps a greater freedom of action. Given the crinoline and its "wilderness of flounces," wrote an observer in 1856, "You will hardly be able to distinguish the embonpoint of one of your lady friends from the meagerness of the other." A tall, thin woman stands behind a short, wide woman in a large hoop skirt, both staring across to a dressing table mirror. "These Dresses are very well in their way," says one of the women in this 1857 *Harper's Weekly* cartoon, "but they make us all appear the same size. Why, a Girl might be as thin as a Whipping-post, and yet be taken for a Decent Figure."[21]

The crinoline was fashion's cure for dyspepsia and its whippingpost women. It lifted them up and billowed them out. "A beautiful Canadian or American girl comes nearer the popular idea of an angel than any being I ever beheld out of dream-land," wrote the Reverend David Macrae, visiting from Scotland just before the Civil War. "Pale features of exquisite symmetry, a delicately pure complexion, eyes radiant with intelligence, a light, graceful, often fragile form." But all was not hunky-dory in heaven: "American girls, however, are too generally pale and thin, and, what is worse, are generally *too* pale and thin. Every second or third face suggests delicacy and dyspepsia; and one does not like to think of angels as dyspeptic." Many had complained about the thinness of American women, who longed to be both rounded and "light, graceful, fragile." Macrae noticed their predicament: "The American girls themselves, I think, are nervous about their thinness, for they are constantly having themselves weighed, and every ounce of increase is hailed with delight. . . . Every girl knows her own weight to within an ounce or two, and is ready to mention it at a moment's notice. It seems to be a subject of universal interest."[22]

The crinoline, far better than the Bloomer, protected the illusion of roundedness and lightness, of volume without weight, even as 32,180 people weighed themselves at the Mechanics Fair in Boston just before the Civil War. Accustomed as we are now to making a primary equation between pounds and heaviness, I cannot too strongly emphasize that then the primary equation was between pounds and volume. Despite this first evidence for a popular interest in personal weight, we must resist any temptation to think that number of pounds carried any immediate or important association with fat or fatness. No one in antebellum society had befriended a height-weight chart, and the few physicians studying corpulence refused to underwrite any weight standards. The only common markers of weight were for infants (and these were mistaken) and for freaks, such as Daniel Lambert, the English giant who died in 1809 at 739 lbs, or Susan Barton, P. T. Barnum's Mammoth Lady, alive in 1849 at 576 lbs. Here too, in text, poster, waxwork and woodcut, the fascination was with bulk: the four or six men who could fit inside Lambert's suit, the sixty-two cubic feet of his coffin, the sixteen yards of cambric in the shroud of Miles Darden (dead at half a ton in 1857), the 6 feet, 2 inches around the hips of Rosina Delight Richardson (478 lbs in 1852). Nor did great bulk instantly imply a depressing heaviness: fat people were known for their buoyancy, their susceptibility to the raptures of laughing gas, and sometimes for their amazing grace on the dance floor. Great bulk might be as light as a thief in the night, if we can trust the story of a young woman in St. Louis who awoke near midnight to find a corpulent form struggling to climb in through her window, caught by the rear of his unmentionables. Her screams alarmed the neighborhood, but the fat man when apprehended was identified as her hoop skirt hanging on a hook near the window and inflated by the evening breeze.[23]

This story was retailed in 1856 by *The Sibyl*, a journal published by the National Dress Reform League. It was a curious story, for the crinoline became a nightmare only by virtue of the hook on which it was held. On such a slender hook hung the difference between dress reformers and women who were "slaves" to fashion. Both desired a healthy, buoyant roundness and an equivalent social domain. Both admired grace and volume without weight. Both wanted dress to be an effective expression of personality. Fashionable women in the 1850s, however, welcomed disguise and theatrics as means to an individual flair, while dress reformers sought a pious gravity and an honest movement from the center of the body to the surface.[24]

Buoyant Bodies at the Water Cure

At 5 feet, 4 inches and 100 lbs, Amelia Bloomer was slighter than the average woman on the Howe platform scales in Boston (124 lbs, 6 oz) or at the Maine State Fair (126 lbs, 5 oz). She would have been a good match for that male Reformer who wanted a mate whose "waist must be natural, her education solid, and her piety undoubted," if only she had not been so light. In the 1850s, as men also began to weigh themselves (averaging 146 to 152 lbs), they began to specify the weights of their prospective brides. Though they might be anti-slavery, anti-corset, anti-meat and in sympathy "with oppressed and suffering humanity everywhere," they all seemed to want, like HLW near Springfield, Massachusetts, "a form medium sized, well developed, erect, and plump (not gross, but full and round—I do not admire skeletons)." That is, their radicalism did not extend to a radically thin vision of female beauty. Avoiding the "tall, lean or lank-looking," they advertised for women of "good size" who were close to the average on the scale at the Maine State Fair. This meant, in the case of one man of 5 feet, 11 inches and 160 lbs, a partner of five-four and 120 to 140 lbs, and for another man of 5 feet, 10 inches and 160 lbs, a woman of shorter stature and 130 to 160 lbs. Turn and turn about, women of "progressive mind" held up as their model no other than the fashion-plate male escort of the 1850s, slim and long-bodied. Fida, a plain simple-hearted maiden, about medium height, full form, blue eyes, brown hair and a cheerful glow of health upon her cheeks, sought a dark-eyed, dark-haired socialist-spiritualist-vegetarian of medium height with slender form. Sophy Die-Away, a gay seventeen-year-old Southerner who could be ruled only by love, pined for a man 6 feet tall with a fine figure "but not at all fleshy."[25]

These personals are drawn from the *Water-Cure Journal* (published by the phrenological Fowler family). Hydropathic spas were strongholds of dress reform, Grahamism, Temperance, and the women's movement. The first National Dress Reform Association meeting was held at the Glenhaven Water-Cure. Mary Gove herself had taken the instrumental steps from physiology and dress reform to operating a hydropathic institute and training women as water cure physicians. Victoria, age thirty, 5 feet, 2 inches, 150 lbs, able to spin, weave, teach school and work in the meadow, was among other things a Temperance woman, an abolitionist, an advocate of dress reform and women's rights, and a firm believer in both phre-

nology and hydropathy.[26] Water cure, as we shall see, was perhaps
the most powerful method and certainly the perfect metaphor for
the pursuit of specific but unencumbered gravity. Of buoyancy.

Colonial Americans had never been partial to water. They had
imported their European fears of foul wells and miasmatic vapors to
the New but somehow Used World. As a drink for adults, water
ranked below beer, liquor, chocolate, coffee, cider and tea; for children it ranked below cider, milk, thin pap and small beer. As an internal medicine it was recommended for a clyster (enema) and as an
emetic for ridding the stomach of surfeit. Until about 1760, few
took the native medicinal mineral waters so much in vogue in gouty
England, nor did they use them afterward with the same modish
regularity as at Bath or Bristol.[27]

Water over the skin was no more popular than water down the
throat. Despite Puritan sermons on the healing pool at Bethesda
(John 5:2), bathing attracted no multitudes. Americans may not
have been unconcernedly or consistently unwashed, but adults
rarely experienced total immersion. Mrs. Drinker wrote in her diary
in 1799 after her first shower bath: "I bore it better than I expected,
not having been wet all over at once, for 28 years past." Aside from
some Baptists, sailors and fishermen, the adult experience of personal buoyancy (in water) was unusual until at least the late 18th
century, when a few public baths were opened and Nanking China
bathtubs appeared on the Eastern seaboard. Those first bathtubs,
however, were shallow affairs 6 or 7 inches deep, and 19th-century
cartoons preserved the image of a bath as a cold, cramped, quick ex-
cursion. When a larger, deeper tub was designed, filling that tub
(especially with warm water) was costly and time-consuming until
more effective municipal water systems were in place. By 1823, all
of Philadelphia (the Baptist center of the country) had four hundred
private baths. During the 1830s, hotels in Boston and New York first
installed baths or showers in their basements. Abigail Fillmore
would finally acquire a bathtub for the White House in 1851, and
the New York poor would get their first public municipal bath in
1852.[28]

Swimming was a rare accomplishment. More poets lamented a
drowning than swam the Hellespont. Even Joseph Rodman Drake's
winged elfin sprite breathes a prayer before diving into the waters
blue, where

> He spreads his arms like the swallow's wing,
> And throws his feet with a frog-like fling

—and is stung by a prawn, rubbed raw by a starfish, struck by the giant claw of a crab, and suckered by a leech. In 1846, James Arlington Bennet was still discoursing on swimming as if it were as arcane as Archimedes. It required "but little well directed action to keep the human body afloat," he wrote, citing Ben Franklin, who had encouraged people to place confidence in the power of water to support them, for "it is not so easy a thing to sink as you imagined." Especially for fat people, added Bennet, who must be "both extremely cowardly as well as clumsy, to get drowned at all."[29]

Mary Gove in 1843 was a drowning woman. She was coughing blood in 1839, and four years later she had been reduced to "infantile weakness." She learned of the water cure from the English reformer Henry Gardiner Wright, who had been a patient at the original water cure spa in Gräfenburg (Austrian Silesia), where the peasant Vincent Priessnitz had fashioned a *summa theologica* of the virtues of water. By varying the pressure, density, temperature and direction of water, and by careful designation of the posture and orifices of the ailing patient, Priessnitz substituted water for every orthodox drug and medical technique. The full daily treatment of a dyspeptic, for example, might include wet sheets for sweating, a two-minute plunge bath, twenty to twenty-four glasses of water, two enemas, two sitz baths, and wet bandages around the neck, chest and abdomen. Herself healed by a comparable regime, Mary Gove in 1846 was down to one bath each day and a wet bandage around her abdomen.[30]

We are back, as we should be, to bellies. In the translation of the water cure from Europe to the United States, the (generalized) stomach became the center of operations. European water cures at midcentury were directed by men and patronized in the main by men whose chief complaints were syphilis, gout, catarrh and joint diseases. Patients ate large amounts of food and drank liberally of local mineral waters. The social orders mixed somewhat freely, but their tone was socially conservative, with an understanding that no acquaintance struck up at a spa could be used to advantage on the outside.[31]

In the United States, much was different. Water cures were occupied preponderantly by women complaining of dyspepsia, uterine disorders, "infantile weakness" or nervous debility, and consumption, in that order. Diet was controlled: usually small vegetarian meals with pure, fresh water. The social mix was quite as wide as in Europe, but friendships made at spas became for women in particular an enduring source of emotional, social and political support. And the tone was hardly conservative. Amarintha, thirty-three, advertised in the *Water-Cure Journal* for a "plain, honest, sensitive, anti-all-sorts-of-slavery man; also anti-war, inclined to Hydropathy and Vegetarianism, who is or tries to be practically a Christian, not a bigot or sectarian."[32]

The American water cure was in fact a refuge from an oppressively patriarchal environment. Although two male physicians, Russell T. Trall and Joel Shew, had introduced the water cure in 1843 in New York, American establishments were often managed by women. Twenty percent of water cure physicians and many more on the water cure staffs were women. Dress reformer Harriet K. Austin, trained by Mary Gove, ran the largest of the establishments, the Dansville Water Cure, with her adoptive father, James C. Jackson.[33]

The water cure was equally an escape from an exhausting, heroic medical regime. One Mr. Goss had tried change of diet, change of scenery, mineral waters, tonics, silver nitrate, asafoetida, iron, quinine, soda, ipecac, brandy, friction with a flesh brush, nitric and muriatic acid baths, blue (cathartic) pills, prussic acid and Sands's sarsaparilla before he reached the water cure and an end to his dyspepsia. Of the 3,379 patients treated by 1858 at the Glen Haven (New York) Water Cure, 3,006 (89%) had previously used opium, 2,923 (86%) calomel, a mercury derivative, and 600 of the women had submitted to caustic burning. Given the customarily massive doses and widespread use of constipating sedatives, compensating laxatives and mercurial purgatives, we need hardly refer to hurried meals, fried foods, spoiled meats or corseted stomachs to explain the prevalence of dyspepsia in American society, and we may appreciate how comforting must have been the relative calm of the water cure.[34]

The cure was a ritual of renewal. Crossing the threshold, you surrendered yourself to a different and slower time. You did not hurry; you dressed more freely and spoke more openly. You had no cause to suspect the abuse of confidences. In this world you knew that all bounties were honest. Completely at rest, you could put yourself completely at risk. The success of the cure depended upon the extent of your Crisis, that painful effusion of waste and age from your body. Water, the universal solvent, could work within you like "the fountains of the great deep." The wetpacks, the plunge baths, the hip baths, the head baths, the sitz baths, the showers, the injections into vagina and rectum, the steaming and the sweating, all of this water could free you of morbid matter if you gave yourself up to it. The Crisis would proceed through uneasiness and insomnia to high fever, but at the end there would be visions of a new body. Before leaving, you would share these visions, make sense of them as a personal, social and spiritual healing. When you left you would feel lighter and younger. "If the water-cure had done nothing more than establish the fact that the glow and joyousness of early life are things which may be restored after having been once wasted," wrote novelist Harriet Beecher Stowe, "it would have done a good work."[35]

Glen Haven, New Lebanon Springs, the Eastern Hygeian Home—these were floating islands halfway between childhood and maturity, between domestic circle and bounding main. On these floating islands women dealt with floating bodies—a queasy stomach, a prolapsed uterus, an unwanted pregnancy. Abortions had become increasingly common since the late 1830s; by midcentury there was perhaps one aborted fetus for every five or six live births in the United States. Neither common law nor common medicine discriminated between pregnancy and the "obstructed flow" of menstrual problems until the fetus quickened in the fourth or fifth month. The same treatments used to restore menstrual flow could be used to procure abortions—including the hot sitz baths, water or vinegar douches, and vaginal injections common to all water cures. Respectable married women could feign dysmenorrhea and obtain emmenagogics from physicians. They could consult clinics explicitly devoted to female difficulties, such as those publicly advertised by Mme. Restell in New York City, Boston and Philadelphia from the 1840s to the 1870s. Or they could go off to a water cure, where the typical regimen, unaltered, might well terminate their pregnancies. Dr. Trall, who taught water cure at his Hygieo-Therapeutic College in New Jersey, himself perfected a self-injecting syringe for abortions, which he considered acceptable until shortly before labor. Water cures were not principally dedicated to abortion, but with their social climate and their ritual Crises they could relieve women of those burdens which they had no wish to carry to term.[36]

The water cure restored the natural gravity of women by releasing them from cultural double binds. The activist Catharine Beecher, who stayed at thirteen water cure spas, would return from them each time inspirited enough to do battle with an American culture that kept thrusting women forward as national moral symbols while thrusting them back toward kitchens and static parlor theatricals. There was a middle earth of politics and business, of law and the professions, in which women needed grounding and mobility. At the water cure, they could accomplish with their bodies what they had still to accomplish in society at large: they would gain weight *and* feel lighter. Santorio Santorio himself had declared this the ideal: "To feel the body heavy, when it is actually light on the balance, shows a worse state of health, than to feel it weighty when it is really so. On the other hand, to feel it light, when it is really heavy on the balance, shows an excellent state of health."[37]

This was a good definition of that buoyancy so much at issue in this chapter. Generations before Americans began to think of lightness in terms of pounds on a scale, they were in pursuit of a *sensation* of lightness. The water cure with its ritual immersions made buoyancy as thorough an experience as possible. Patients floated, like women at country pools in contemporary paintings, halfway between childlike purity and mature sensuality.[38] Their Crises resolved the contraries, made them whole and gave them a sense of community. And a sense of faith.

In faith (as in dieting), no disappointment, however great, is final. This chapter began with the world about to end in 1844. After 1844, many Adventists revised their calendars and reread the times. If the End had not come, 1844 did signal a last historical stage, a period of scrutiny and symbolic judgment of an equally disappointing America whose Protestantism and republicanism might have destined it to be the redeemer nation. But America had failed, sapped by Catholicism and slavery. Those who made the most of this explanation were Seventh-Day Adventists, who disabused themselves of the Catholic Sunday and returned to the original (and therefore millennial) Sabbath. While Mary Gove, now Nichols, became in the early 1850s a Fourierite, a Memnonian utopian and an advocate of free love, the Baptist preacher John Preston Kellogg and his wife Mary became Seventh-Day Adventists. They were and would remain Temperance workers, abolitionists, and subscribers to the *Water-Cure Journal*, but they moved down the road apiece to work with James and Ellen White at the Adventist press in Battle Creek, Michigan. In 1863, after spending three weeks at "Our Home On the Hillside," the Dansville Water Cure, Ellen G. White had a prophetic vision of "God's great medicine: water, pure soft water." Her vision would propel John Harvey Kellogg, son of John Preston and Mary, to the forefront of American hydrotherapy and another son, William, to the—but no, we are not ready for them quite yet. A war has come.[39]

The Civil War as Movement Cure

Northerners at the onset of the Civil War saw it as a healing crisis. The canker of slavery, like dyspepsia, was "dark, discouraging and cheerless in its progress. . . . It will neither kill the patient nor depart from him." The slavery agitation, said Lincoln in his famous "House Divided" speech in 1858, "*will* not cease, until a *crisis* shall have been reached, and passed." This was medical language. The apocalypse was fitted to a vision of a therapeutic millennium. Indeed, the war might literally cure dyspepsia. Ralph Waldo Emerson wrote in May, 1861, anticipating the conflict: "What a healthy tone exists! I suppose, when we come to fighting, and many of our people are killed, it will yet be found that the bills of mortality in the country will show a better result this year than the last, on account of the general health: no dyspepsia, no consumption, no fevers, when there is so much electricity, and conquering heart and mind."[40]

If anything, the war was to be a Movement Cure. National calisthenics. As the country had grown more urban and commercial, and as a cult of domesticity had closed in around middle-class women, exercise had become a category of activity distinct from both work and play. The more distinct, the more therapeutic. Ben Franklin in 1742 had recommended "now and then a little Exercise a quarter of an Hour before Meals, as to swing a Weight, or swing your Arms about with a small Weight in each Hand; to leap, or the like, for that stirs the Muscles of the Breast." Eighty years later, such gentlemanly exertions seemed rude and unsystematic. From Italy, Switzerland, Germany and Sweden had come systems of graduated calisthenics designed to straighten the spine, strengthen the muscles, expand the lungs and improve the circulation. Exercise was everywhere incorporated into the programs of health reformers, phrenologists and physicians. This meant less rocking and more creeping for the infant, vaulting and wrestling for boys, running and square dancing for girls, a three-mile morning walk for women, a full gymnastic series for men. Theodore D. Weld, abolitionist and Grahamite, rose at six, washed in cold water, then walked, ran, jumped and hopped for an hour before breakfast. Mary Gove Nichols taught girls to romp without fear and to welcome that lean tissue known as muscle. Catherine Beecher advised an hour of vigorous exercise each day so that women might shake off the chronic weaknesses brought on by sedentary habits and tight clothes. Women's rights, dress reform and exercise were so closely meshed that the modified Bloomer never disappeared from the women's gymnasium.[41]

Exercise maintained the centrifugal tendency of the healthy body. It flung the poisons out of the system. There were seven million pores to the surface of an average man. From these pores must issue 2 lbs of insensible perspiration each day, as Santorio Santorio had taught. A first sign of disease was slowed perspiration and the stagnant retention of "thin acrid impurities." The human body was meant to be in motion, rejuvenating itself inside and out. It was no inert structure; skin, blood, nails, hair, bone and muscle were daily transformed. Between the sweating surface and the digesting center stretched 450 muscles working to keep the body from turning in upon itself and becoming heavy with constipation. Surface and center had much the same need of muscle. As Catherine Beecher wrote, "the lining of the stomach and intestines is in fact only a continuation of the outer skin." A freely perspiring skin, well exercised in fresh air, was tantamount to a fluent gastrointestinal tract.[42]

Movement could therefore cure dyspepsia even as it maintained the harmony and buoyancy of the body. Phrenologist Andrew Combe, almost as widely read as his extremely popular phrenologist brother George, made explicit the connections between dress reform, exercise, digestion, buoyancy and health: "If the lively and bouncing girl, whose loose and unconstrained attire admits of the freest motion and fullest respiration, passes in a few months from the exuberant and playful indulgence of her feelings, intellect, and muscular system, to the quiet and composed inaction and confined dress of a sedate young lady, who never walks out, except at a measured pace to school or to church, is it really wonderful that her stomach and bowels should begin to act with less vigor?" Nor was it any wonder that while young men marched off to a critical, calisthenic and cathartic war, young women found a Movement Cure of their own.[43]

Their sergeant-at-arms was Dioclesian Lewis, a portly 6 footer whose 200-plus lbs biased him against small men and small women who indulged their own frailty. Like the Baptist Campbellites whom he and his mother joined in the 1830s, Dio Lewis believed that with a radical return to primitive principles, the millennium would make its appearance. His mother a seamstress, Dio worked in a scythe factory, taught school and then studied homeopathy after a year at Harvard Medical School. In Buffalo in 1849 he practiced medicine, published the *Homeopathist*, and married. In 1851 his wife contracted tuberculosis and was given up for lost. Her weight dropped from 116 to 80 lbs. A corsetless Episcopalian, she was persuaded by Dio to return to first principles: long walks, fresh air, flannel clothing. She survived to share with him a long robust life as he lectured on the Temperance circuit, toured clinics in Paris, and founded the Boston Normal Institute for Physical Education (1861). In 1864 he built a Female Seminary in Lexington, Massachusetts, installing Theodore D. Weld as headmaster. Out from Boston and Lexington during the next years would stream hundreds of teachers of physical education, expert with wooden rings, wooden dumbbells, beanbags, clubs, wands, and Dr. Schreber's Pangymnastikon, the matériel of the New Gymnastics.[44]

Unlike the regimented drill common to parade grounds and to many European systems of calisthenics, the New Gymnastics was centrifugal. Solo motion was outward from the center of the body to its periphery, as if the body were its own evangelist. Such motion called for lighter apparatus, which Lewis refined from German (*Turnverein*) equipment or which, like the beanbag, he invented. He claimed that his apparatus gave full play to every muscle and was suited to both sexes and all ages. The exercises were done to music in 8/16 time in physiological order, from thrusts to lunges to bends to turns. Everyone wore flannel and strong shoes and, he boasted, everyone moved freely.[45]

Unimpressed by the "muscle-mania" of men in gyms hefting 40-pound dumbbells, Lewis promoted instead a thoroughgoing vigor and elasticity. In well-received books and lectures, he encouraged moral as well as muscular tone. While he spoke against "such a compound, doubled and twisted, starched, comical, artificial, touch-me-not, wiggling curiosity" as Miss Seraphina Flamingo, he campaigned also against the despair of indigestion and the sin of overeating. "I used to know a good man," he wrote, "who tried hard to be a Christian, but failed because he ate too much dinner." There should be calisthenics for the jaw, too: it should take six minutes of mastication to eat a Graham cracker. Two meals a day instead of three would relieve the stomach of that iron wedge of gluttony. Less food (but more meat), less sleep and more exercise would reduce the fat, waddling, wheezing "anti-going-up-stairs sort of people" to ship-shape.[46]

Ship-shape did not mean a skittish sloop. Lewis was worried that American women were shrinking due to their lack of exercise, their corsets and indigestion. As long as she did not have what another re-

former called the "squaddy uneven roundness of an obese," a large
woman weighing 140 to 160 lbs was proof of women's innate equality with men. Lewis was equally upset with nervous, irritable little
men; were American men also on their way to Lilliput? During the
Revolutionary War, he noted, when fifteen of the most prominent
leaders weighed themselves at West Point, only one was below 200
lbs.[47]

Again, our modern calculus, weight = heaviness, does not apply.
And the modern dancer would be surprised at the inflexibility of the
New Gymnastics. Most exercises were done in place to a strict
rhythm, the chin tucked in toward the neck and the spine almost
rigid. Lewis liked the erect body, the book balanced atop the head,
hard thin pillows at night. At home, the ingenious Pangymnastikon
allowed for a hundred different exercises within a confined space.
The New Gymnastics had few twists or full extensions, none of the
spirals or contractions which another crusading Graham would in-
sert into the modern repertoire. When New Gymnasts did cross the
gymnasium, they moved to the outlines of feet stenciled on the floor
or to the geometry of the square dance. Shocked by the free rotary
whirl of the lewd waltz, Lewis ultimately preferred push-and-pull
to the unbounded play of muscles.[48]

In fact, the New Gymnastics was most remarkable not for its
freedoms but for its precise figural reproduction of the oppositions
of civil war. Among Lewis's proudest innovations was his series of
exercises in which partners pulled against each other with a wooden
ring between them. Across thirty pages of images of linked men in
his *New Gymnastics*, the walnut ring of union was tried and tested.
Such partnered oppositions were the culmination of his gymnastic
curriculum and the final steps toward an elastic body.[49]

Grounding the Body: The Rest Cure

The Civil War did not fulfill any promises of cure through crisis or
opposition. The war was conducted by dyspeptic, asthmatic or ma-
larial generals and fought by a rank-and-file which grumbled along
on coffee and hardtack, raw salt pork and soaked beans. When they
had no salt (a special problem for the Confederacy), they used gun-
powder on their hell-fired stew. They sliced off chunks of dried
("desecrated") vegetables and drank Gail Borden's new "conse-
crated" milk. The Union health manual told soldiers to put in their

mouths no solid food larger than half the last joint of their little finger, and to chew slowly and well. They were to wear flannels at all times and to have exceedingly regular bowel movements. Nonetheless, about as many soliders died from intestinal ailments (typhoid, diarrhea, dysentery) as from battle wounds.[50]

On the field after one battle, Oliver Wendell Holmes, that Autocrat of the Breakfast Table, "picked up a Rebel canteen, and one of our own—but there was something repulsive about the trodden and stained relics of the stale battlefield. It was like the table of some hideous orgy left uncleared, and one turned away disgusted from its broken fragments and muddy heeltaps." That war which in the beginning Holmes had seen as a harpoon driving through the "defence of blubber" to strike at Northern sensibilities had quickly become a glutton's undigested nightmare. The war did not seem to make things whole. Thirty years earlier, Prof. Hitchcock had envisioned the same battlefield: "May no one be compelled, after twenty or thirty years contest with dyspepsy, to look back, and see the lopped-off fragments of himself, strewed over the field of combat. O, such experience has all of death in it, but the last pang. Nay, it is death protracted, repeated, multiplied, concentrated." And that was what the poets saw, wherever they looked, North or South, during the Civil War: not a redeeming crisis but "the worn spirit," "ghastly trenches," "the stump of the arm, the amputated hand." Exhaustion, fragments and shadows.[51]

Americans needed a rest. Gradually, over the last third of the century, nervous exhaustion would displace dyspepsia as *the* American disease. Exhaustion had been seen before, most often at water cures, but after the Civil War it gained a notable currency and a new name.

"Neurasthenia," explained Dr. George Beard in 1869, and again in 1879, 1880 and 1881, was a want of force. Unlike anemia, it was due not to weak blood but to frayed nerves. Its causes were as numerous as its symptoms. Indeed, it would be unavailing to list the symptoms—Beard spent page after page doing just that, always to his own exasperation. In a sense he need not have bothered; the symptoms were the same as for dyspepsia. Beard himself was conscious enough of the historical transition from dyspepsia to neurasthenia to show how, by physical laws of inheritance, dyspepsia in a grandparent could turn up as neurasthenia in a grandchild.[52]

Those grandparents back in the 1830s had already noted that dyspepsia was the torment of every class of "brain-worn" persons.

The laboring poor seemed to have truer appetites and stronger digestions than students (especially female students), "literary men, officers of state, dealers in scrip, daring adventurers, and anxious and ambitious projectors of improvements." The American Art Union sent out reproductions of country scenes to improve the digestion of dyspeptic businessmen whose labor "wearies without strengthening the body, because it makes the inside instead of the outside of the head sweat." The more caught up were people in the sheerly mental aspects of modern urban life, the more their animal parts were unsettled.[53]

Their grandchildren after the Civil War suffered the same irritability, lack of concentration, insomnia and weakness, but by 1880 the prime diagnosis would be nervous exhaustion. In 1869, just as neurasthenia became a clinical entity, a woman was termed dyspeptic when she had "intense throbbing in her neck, difficult breathing, dull pains in her side, near her heart, throbbing and pain in small of back, dizziness when stooping, black and blue spots appearing on face, headache often, can walk but little." Soon she would be a certifiable neurasthenic. This was much less the discovery of a new disease than a refocusing of therapeutic concern from the stomach to the head, from what was ingested to what was communicated. At root, dyspepsia was a personal problem; neurasthenia was a social disease.[54]

The generational shift from one American disease to another had several sources. Shiploads of young immigrants from Ireland, Central Europe and China in the antebellum era, then from Southern and Eastern Europe after the war put into question the vitality of "native" American stock. The immigrants seemed impressively fertile, marrying early and raising large families. Was the "native" stock exhausted? Had the emotionally and mentally taxing life of prosperous Americans affected at last their sexual capacity or their social inclination to reproduce? Native-born white women complained more of chlorosis or the "green sickness" (anemia, amenorrhea) and resisted definition as breeders. Eleven percent of the women born in this country between 1860 and 1880 never married, the highest proportion in American history. When women did marry, they had fewer children. Contemporaries worried loudly about the exhaustion of the "race," all the more likely as frenetic industrial sewing machines and office typewriters drew young women away from the calm home.[55]

The brain itself was caving in. In 1856, the journalist Robert Tomes had observed that "dyspepsia, nervous disorders of all kinds, and insanity, are so much more abounding in the United States than in any other country, as almost to become national characteristics." There were six times as many people labeled insane in 1880 as in 1850. When Charles Guiteau pleaded insanity in his trial for the assassination of President Garfield in 1883, George Beard agreed (against the tide of outrage) that Guiteau *was* insane. Though there were somatic distinctions between exhaustion and insanity, the American climate—its dry air, its extreme temperatures, its implosive technology—conduced to both.[56]

Above all, it was the social climate that brought on exhaustion. Neurasthenics were troubled by noises and visual presences. Beard eagerly acknowledged the new phobias of his era—agoraphobia, claustrophobia, phobophobia (fear of fears)—while pinpointing a new disorder, neurasthenic asthenopia, or irritable eye, which no glasses could help. Although inflammation of the eyes had been a regular complaint at water cures before the Civil War, the subsequent surge of newspapers and news made the eyes the peculiar victim of modern society, with its telegraphs and rotary presses. The visual field was becoming as cluttered as a late Victorian parlor, busy as a Wild West circus, as illusive as stereoptic pictures. There would be 350,000,000 advertisements in American newspapers by 1807. One's powers of attention were almost certain to be exhausted by such a flood of color, news and puffery. The irritable eye could be but the metonym of a sensational fatigue. Neurasthenia became a defensive act of drastic, selective inattention.[57]

There was yet another, less obvious reason for the shift from dyspepsia to nervous exhaustion as the national disease. More older people were walking around. In 1840, less than a third of those born would survive to age sixty-five; by 1900, half would. The Civil War took the lives of 10 percent of all white males aged 18–45 and wounded another 5 percent. In its aftermath, one would be more likely to encounter "used up" people with the typical marks of age in a vitamin-poor society—palsy, bent backs, dim sight, arthritis, mental debility. Originally, "fogies" had been wounded military veterans; now the old themselves became "fogies," and laws required their retirement. Out of the factory and off the judicial bench, they were to live quietly, disengaged and, as it were, recuperating. Their food would be the food of childhood and sickbed, their lives secluded.[58]

The cure for neurasthenia was exactly this, as if nervous exhaustion and old age were equally chronic. While exercise, fresh air and low diet (less food) had been prescribed for dyspeptics, the neurasthenic was put to bed and fed. Since neurasthenia, like dyspepsia, was a protean malady that "does not affect any particular vital organ, but flies about among them all, giving a little twist and pull to each, seriatim," the cure had to be systemic. The systemic model for dyspepsia had been the waterway (canals, alimentary passage, pores); for neurasthenia it was the electrical path (telegraphs, networks of nerves, eyes). Therapy therefore did not aim at unclogging but at relaxing the current. Sylvester Graham had hoped to relieve overstimulation by purifying the system; George Beard used marijuana, bromides, opium, massage and electricity to steady the nerves (he meant this literally) and to strengthen them. Neurasthenics would be rejuvenated by returning them, through sedation and seclusion, to infancy.[59]

The most successful nerve doctor was not Beard but novelist and physician Silas Weir Mitchell, who had worked in a Union hospital for nervous diseases and had become an expert on nerve injuries, only to suffer a nervous breakdown himself. During the war he had seen sixty thousand injections of morphine given in a single year; ten years later he would become a Professor Morphia.[60]

Mitchell's treatment, the Rest Cure, was imitated on both sides of the Atlantic. He placed his patients in opaque wombs of darkness, sleep, milk, massage, gentle electrical currents and sternly enforced boredom. The body, the mind and time itself were suspended while the patient lay inches away from trance, a sleep-eater, gaining weight, trusting in a higher power.[61]

That higher power was Mitchell himself. Though almost as many men as women were diagnosed as having nervous exhaustion—it struck hard at working-class men and at the New England gentry—and though the diagnosis was convenient to both sexes and most ages,[62] Mitchell treated primarily respectable young women. His personal ability to dominate these women made his rest cure what it was. Unlike the water cure, which relied upon a personal crisis and a communal restoration, the rest cure was authoritarian. Taking advantage of the full compliance he demanded, Mitchell drew his patients back to infancy not to uncover primal anxieties (as would his European admirer Sigmund Freud) but to reshape their characters. He was the flesh-and-blood incarnation of his fictional "Character Doctor," whose business it was to "furnish characters to those who need them." Neurasthenia so paralyzed one's will and so weakened one's ability to express oneself that any cure entailed a wholesale reconstruction of character. Strong-minded women like

Charlotte Perkins in 1885 eventually resisted such self-surrender. Others used the experience to ground themselves.[63]

I seriously intend the pun. Neurasthenia was *nervous* exhaustion because its fatigue was not grounded. It was a suspended, almost incorporeal exhaustion. Neurasthenics could not bear the weight of their own hands or the touch of anything heavier "than the brush of a butterfly's wing."[64] Their bodies weighed *on them* because they could not transfer that weight to the earth. The rest cure anchored them to the world with grounded currents and forced feeding. To gain weight under such a regimen was to return to one's proper medium. This weight, unlike the weight gained at the water cure, was meant to be ponderable. The ideal body was not the buoyant body but the body electric, at once fixed and energetic.

The Release of Gluttony

As the physical, emotional, sexual and moral symptoms of indigestion were transferred to neurasthenia, gluttony was progressively disassociated from the problem of thinness. Neurasthenics were portrayed as thin and losing weight, or as picky and trifling nibblers. High feeding was a cure, not a cause, of nervous exhaustion. Gluttony could at last be unambiguously associated with fatness (fleshiness). And personal weight would mean at last what we have been waiting for it to mean: poundage, not volume.

If I have obstinately delayed a direct discussion of cures for obesity in the 19th century, it is because Americans also held back. Indeed, I have yet to trace the several steps by which fatness and heaviness became generally reprehensible. But our patience will be rewarded. When, finally, we come to the diets, galvanic belts, calisthenics and electrical rollers for reducing, they will be astonishingly familiar. In the historical shift from dyspepsia to neurasthania, as gluttony was sheared off from thinness, nearly every one of the cures for indigestion would be paraded anew as a cure for fat.

With Sylvester Graham the groundwork had been laid for the romantic mode of dieting, the instant transformation of the body from within by acts of abstinence and moral courage. With Mary Sargeant Neal Gove Nichols, who became a lifelong Catholic in 1857, the groundwork has been laid for the ritual mode, that slower, more painstaking metamorphosis of the body by outside powers: water, electricity, the strong hands of massage and authority. The nobleman Luigi Cornaro was the exemplar in the preceding chapter; Graham even edited his treatise. Here the exemplar has been the scientist Santorio Santorio, of whom S. Weir Mitchell was a most admiring student.[65]

Oliver Halsted's merry-go-round has taken us across an apocalypse to the news-racked and high-strung. It has taken us from dyspepsia to neurasthenia, from the buoyant body to the body electric. All we need to do now is fly.

CHAPTER FOUR

The Balanced Body at Century's Turn

With the advent of powered flight, modern dance, scientific management and home economics, a new kinaesthetic ideal appeared, insisting on a dynamically balanced, centrally controlled body. Rather than buoyancy, Americans sought to master the spiral and flow of things—in the body, the home, the factory, and the national economy itself, for which there was also a new model concerned rather with abundance than with scarcity. Neither the new kinaesthetic nor the new economic model was tolerant of excess; no longer did the political arena or the social world accept the fat person as a healthy, influential person. Slimming became an acceptable strategy for dealing with the problems posed by abundance, gluttony (or "overnutrition") and the "dead weight" of fat. Strategies for reducing were often those which had been used before against dyspepsia, now that gluttony was associated clearly with fatness and the "disease" of obesity.

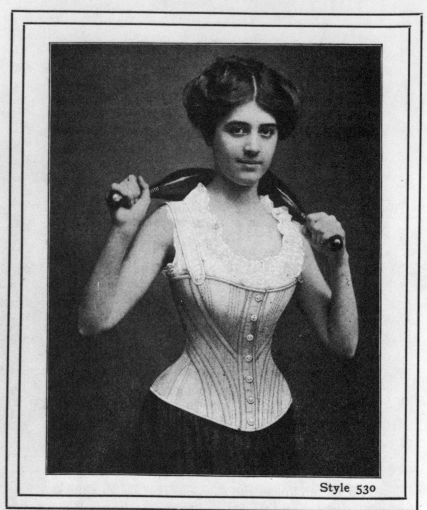

Style 530

Exercise

fails of its purpose when respiration is retarded by a stiff and rigid
corset. The benefits that accrue from healthful activity are enhanced
many fold by a Ferris Good Sense Corset Waist. For the woman who
plays golf, tennis, or rides a wheel, for the woman who loves good health
and takes pride in her personal appearance there is no garment equal to

Ferris Good Sense Waists

26

*The more elastic corset, for the more athletic, more balanced woman, from
a Ferris Brothers Co. catalog, c. 1900.* Courtesy of the Margaret Woodbury
Strong Museum, Rochester, NY.

From Buoyancy to Balance

"BETTER THAN A BICYCLE, a merry-go-round, and a shoot-the-chute all combined," said reporter Grace M. Gould after touching down on Maine soil, July 11, 1897. She had been up for perhaps ten minutes in a giant biplane kite, 26 feet of muslin and spruce from wingtip to wingtip. In September another reporter skimmed for nearly a minute over the Indiana dunes on a biplane glider, enjoying "about the same sensation felt by a man when taking his first ascension in an escalator. There is the queer feeling of being lifted from beneath."[1] Neither the woman nor the man compared the experience to rising in a balloon or floating on water. This was a new kind of lift, controlled and directional, a technology less of release than of command.

Flight—sustained heavier-than-air-flight—was a question not so much of buoyancy as of balance, and the bicycle was the key. Steadily improved since 1866, when foot-cranks were added to what had been a hobbyhorse on wheels, the bicycle by the 1880s had become more graceful and less precarious, "such that the rider propels it mostly by a part or the whole of his weight, instead of only by muscular thrust." In 1896, a New York editor foresaw that "the flying machine problem is liable to be solved by bicycle inventors," for "to learn to wheel one must learn to balance." While others from Berlin to San Diego were sweating to get maximum lift from minimum structure, the Wright brothers in their bicycle shop in Dayton were preoccupied with the inherent stability and responsiveness of the machine itself. That led them to a reconsideration of data on lift and drag, and to a possibly unique insistence on a mechanical on-board control system, so that the flyer like the bicyclist had instant, absolute mastery of the motions of the craft.[2]

The straight-line flights of the two brothers at Kitty Hawk in 1903 were therefore of less consequence than their 1904 flights at Huffman Prairie. As the historian Tom D. Crouch has shown, when Wilbur Wright banked slowly over the Ohio field and returned in a full circle to his point of departure, powered flight had come into its own. Beekeeper Amos Root, watching the thin biplane with its two propellers, compared it to "a locomotive that has left its track, and is climbing up in the air right toward you—a locomotive without any wheels . . . but with white wings instead."[3] Even as an observer, Root chose to talk not of floating or buoyancy but of power and command.

The command came from the sensitive center of the structure, where the pilot held a wing-warping lever linked to a movable rudder in one organic system of control.[4] Such controlled flight was the culmination, in the realm of heavier-than-air machines, of the same motion toward which pathbreaking American dancers were headed at exactly the same time in their heavier-than-air bodies.

Early gliders had been isolated gestures, single poses taken through space, much like the 1880s performances of young women practicing Delsartean gymnastics, a program of training by which each inner feeling must well out from the center of the body in its truest gestural form. Taught first to French actresses and opera singers, Delsartean movements were popularized in America as a genteel dance-theater and used also as a remedy for "abdominal obesity." A homeopathic physician recommended them for the great mass of harried Americans: "Delsarte says, 'be graceful; stop this tremendous hurrying; don't be so rigid and so firm; don't be so intense; relax; let down; don't go to sleep stiff on the pillow and lie in a cramped position, but see how heavy you can make your head, back and limbs; let go.'" Like the man hanging from the glider, the Delsartean woman had to learn to relax (she would take lessons in falling), to sense equilibrium, and to follow the natural momentum of her initial impulse. Like the glider flight, Delsartean motion was usually short and self-consciously dramatic.[5]

In the 1890s, glider flying became at once more daring and more technical, as did physical education in women's colleges and Chautauqua summer camps. While glider pilots measured wind speed and wing stress, young women were run through standardized tests of strength, endurance, muscular coordination and speed. Charles W. Emerson at his influential College of Oratory in Boston combined Delsartean motions with a new emphasis on free gymnastics as means of strengthening the center while freeing the periphery. "The ideal effort is to throw the arms with all the power of the person, and at the same time to maintain perfect repose of body." Poise would put the body "in exact relation with the law of gravitation." If only the glider pilots could have managed this. . . .[6]

As Wilbur Wright banked over Huffman Prairie, two American dancers had come to a similar appreciation of a strong, flexible torso controlled from an organic center. Both had been blessed with Delsartean training; both had experienced the athleticism of traditional American stage dancing, with its jigs, clogging and acrobatics. Neither of the women was thin or delicate, neither was trying like ballerinas "to create the delusion that the law of gravitation does not exist for them." Indeed, Ruth St. Denis and Isadora Duncan were intent on making as much as possible of the aerodynamics of the centered, balanced body. In 1904, enthralled by the portrait of the goddess Isis on a cigarette poster, Ruth St. Denis was beginning to plan out her dance "Radha," transferring from Egypt to India only the setting but not the origin of her movements, which grew rhythmically from the pulsing of her bare midriff. Meanwhile, Isadora Duncan, enamored of Greek statuary at the British Museum, was standing for hours, hands pressed to her solar plexus, waiting upon the source of all true motion. St. Denis and Duncan would use their bodies in dance as the Wrights used their aircraft in flight, not as supernaturally buoyant or balletic miracles, but as dynamically balanced structures. From them would issue the model of physical motion as a subtle spiral, a spiral equally crucial to the design of the Wright biplane, whose lateral balance was decided by a helical twist across its cambered wings.[7]

The controlled spiral bespoke aptness and economy of motion, efficiency of expression and an internal command of torque. Neither the "winged gospel" of the flyers[8] nor the Hollywood choreography of the modern dancers suddenly compelled Americans to reread their bodies, but the same desires for economy and efficiency, command and flow, which were so obviously changing the forms of motion in flight and in dance were at work changing the experience of movement and attitudes toward fat and weight in the larger society. During this kinaesthetic transition from buoyancy to balance, fatness became literally upsetting, unnecessary weight an intolerable burden. The best body would be an aerodynamic body, curved but slender, controlled but light.

The first flying machines derived from sketches of men settled on or under huge flapping wings. As they became more practical, airplanes lost their formal resemblances to living bodies and became instead models of certain kinds of motion. Similarly, Frederick W. Taylor's new discipline of scientific management required that the human body become unobstrusive, a series of abstracted motions rather than a particular mass. The scientific manager in the factory could subdivide and replot the physical tasks of every job so that every effort was part of a smooth series of motions, the human body a perfect consort of the machine. Workers were not to trust their lifetime of experience with their own bodies, since they had bad habits of movement which obtruded on the balance and timing of the entire plant. It was the plant that was the organic entity and for which Taylor devised time cards, centralized task-accounting methods, and a system of internal regulation for the immediate control of the flow of the work.[9]

In 1883, Taylor had begun using a stopwatch to analyze the work of laborers and machinists so as to eliminate "all false movements, slow movements, and useless movements." His stopwatch techniques segmented motion and time and then, by reducing the prescribed intervals between the segments, made motion apparently smoother. But the separate movements were still beads on a string, akin to Delsartean posing, to short glider flights, and to the serial frame photography by which Eadweard Muybridge was capturing humans running and jumping.[10]

As such serial photography became the motion picture, so Taylor's time studies led to the more fluid motion studies of Frank B. Gilbreth, who used the movie camera and the flow chart to analyze movement without arbitrary stops and starts. To Gilbreth, as to the flyer and the modern dancer, motion was trajectory, and "Perfect Movement," his 1912 wire sculpture, was a controlled spiral. Gilbreth's dedication to the *line* of motion was most starkly expressed in his cyclographs of moving parts of the body. By attaching an electric light bulb to the pivot of motion, framed against a dark background, he could obliterate the extraneous flesh and leave only bright white paths through space. The body when sighted in its essence was now an articulated spine and a line of travel. We have moved from the Victorian kinaesthetic ideal of volume without weight to the 20th-century kinaesthetic ideal of energy without volume.[11]

This coincidence of kinaesthetic values in high technology, industry and the arts of the body was critical to the appearance of the American culture of slimming. Together, flyers, dancers and efficiency experts were preparing the way for a society intolerant of fat. The flyers, of course, had the greatest visibility, rural and urban, and the greatest draw of rich and poor, man and boy, woman and girl. The efficiency experts had the greatest power, manipulating work environments and industrial pace. The modern dancers in the long run had probably the greatest effect, as their principles of movement became part of the cinematic code and established the standards for the motor education of most young children.[12]

Between 1880 and 1920, gluttony (freed from its association with thinness) would be bound to fatness, fatness to inefficiency, inefficiency to lack of energy and loss of balance, and imbalance to overweight. This knot of relationships would hold as well for housewives as for dancers, in the home as in the heavens.

Domestic Economies

As a custom of frugality, as a habit of forethought, domestic economy was nothing new. But as a system of household science, as a means for precise internal regulation, domestic economy instilled a truly new fear of abundance which extended from the larder to the human body itself. While housewives had long been accustomed to the world as a rich, messy space of spontaneous eruptions, plentiful attachments and supervening bodies, home economists urged a clean, lean, purposeful flow. Their world was no less full, but in their world, energy overcame volume. It was the difference between the random violent thwongs of the old carpet-beater and the directed vibrations of the new electric vacuum cleaner. It was the difference between Sylvester Graham's idealized homely hearth and Lillian Gilbreth's "time-saving" circular kitchen at the Brooklyn Borough Gas Company Exposition.[13]

"The true economy of housekeeping is simply the art of gathering up all the fragments, so that nothing be lost," Elizabeth Fries Ellet wrote in her early text, *The Practical Housekeeper* (1857). "I
mean fragments of *time*, as well as materials." It was this fear of losing track, of surrendering to "the dominance of things," that lay behind every step toward scientific method the home economists took.
In 1882 Mrs. Hopkinson of the Mothers Club of Cambridge read a
paper on Accuracy, by which she meant personal honesty and fidel-
ity: exactness applied to the world of things must redound upon the
self. "Here is the source of discontent," wrote novelist and cookbook
author Mary Terhune the same year. "Our daughters fit loosely into
their places in our homes."[14]

She was on the money. The number of women with jobs outside
the home tripled during the last third of the 19th century. Not only
were black (freed) women and unmarried immigrant women enlarging the public work force; young native-born white middle-class
women were leaving home to become teachers, nurses, stenogra-
phers, department store clerks, telephone operators and typists,
whose keyboards would be redesigned for greater efficiency by
Frank and Lillian Gilbreth. Formal laboratory training in household skills was intended to certify housework as an estimable profession and so secure a new fit between modern woman and modern
home. Nationwide there were thirty college departments of domestic science by 1900. And while the number of women in the food
processing industries rose from less than a thousand in 1850 to sixty-
four thousand in 1900, Juliet Corson, Maria Parloa and Sarah Tyson
Rorer were directing cooking schools in New York, Boston and Philadelphia.[15]

The muscle of domestic science was flexed in the kitchen. Here
one fought off the fear of abundance and the golem of waste. Elsewhere in the house, furniture might assume an economy of forms—
a piano that became a sofa, a sofa that turned into a bathtub, a
bathtub that collapsed to a traveling bag, a lunchbasket that expanded into a table, a table that unfolded into a lounge chair, a
lounge chair that extended into a bed, a bed that turned into a piano.[16] That elasticity of form reappeared in "hygienic" garments—
the chemiloon (chemise and pantaloons), the Emancipation or Union Suit, the Delsarte Bicycle Corset, the Nuform Corset, the W. B.
Reduso Corset for large women, the self-adjusting or Health Preserving Corset ("Sing a song of Corsets / With such elastic springs, /
Just a dozen patterns, / Pretty healthful things").[17] But it was in the

kitchen that the most complex transformations would take place and where, therefore, the world of things would be most triumphantly mastered.

Almost on its own, the kitchen had been changing. Since Sylvester Graham's time it had shrunk by half, lost its fireplace, gained a cast-iron stove fueled by wood and then by coal. Its white plastered ceiling was lower, its windows curtained, its walls cupboarded, and its paint a lighter shade. In tenements and small prairie homes, the kitchen remained the living center for the family and the entry point for friends, but in larger houses and apartments it lay behind vestibules, parlors, drawing rooms and dining rooms. Food came to dining tables through magical partitions not unlike the spirit cabinets of mediums. On the distaff side of the partitions the magic was increasingly mechanical. Most of the heavy, specialized tools for cooking over flames had vanished; from their hooks hung can-openers, portable meatgrinders, double boilers and rotary eggbeaters, all patented since midcentury.[18]

Home economists wanted to put this lighter, smaller kitchen at the hub of a symmetrical floor plan. The kitchen would be command central, out of which would flow the heat, the hot water, the food and the energy of the home. The housewife would calculate, measure, combine and oxidize across a level, continuous working surface while a clock ticked meaningfully on the scrubbed wall. This was kitchen as brisk machine shop or, in so many photographs of cooking schools, as spartan laboratory. In *Six Little Cooks: or Aunt Jane's Cooking Class*, Elizabeth S. Kirkland's little helpers learned exactly what was a half-pint, how to weigh out the ingredients for a creamy sauce, and when a tablespoon was meant to be heaping. Kitchen lore became domestic science as Aunt Jane made precise those operations which for so long had been ruled by pinches and smidgeons. Girls learned their intermediate arithmetic by studying the photograph of a woman standing at a mechanical bread cutter which cut off a slice at every turn of the wheel. If a retail 5 cent loaf of bread is 11¼ inches long and the slices are 5/16 inches thick, how many inches of a loaf will be cut off by 18 turns of the wheel?[19]

Scientific cookery, orderly and industrious as the first cafeterias (1893) and automats (1902), could transform poverty into riches. In 1867, before the onset of real domestic science, a woman would write of *A Wife's Effort at Low Living Under High Prices*. In 1879, with real domestic science in view, Juliet Corson would teach cook-

ing to the wives of workingmen and distribute fifty thousand copies
of her *15¢ Dinners for Families of Six*. New England women in the
1880s organized People's Kitchens for good cheap food, on the
model of European soup kitchens. By 1890 it had become possible to
conceive of *Liberal Living Upon Narrow Means*. At the Rumford
Kitchen of Chicago's Columbian Exposition of 1893–94, scientific
cooks served 20-oz luncheons for 30 cents. In 1896, well-off but exi-
gently charitable women conducted poverty suppers, donating their
normal expenses to the needy while testing how far a single dollar
could go toward feeding a party of twelve. They had a dollar meal
of tea, bread, apple sauce, butter, potato chips, tongue, cake, cookies, sherbet, milk and nuts—and thought the repast wholesome if a
bit spare.[20]

In 1899 Melvil Dewey, founder of the first schools of Library
Economy, said he would catalog Home Economics at 339, a number
previously reserved for pauperism; since pauperism resulted from a
disregard for home economics, there would be no cataloguing problems. Dewey was delivering the opening address to the first conference of the National Household Economics Association. The conference had been organized by the sanitary chemist and civil engineer
Ellen Swallow Richards, who treated the stomach "as if it were a
thing apart . . . an inanimate machine, and a very simple one at
that," and by Melvil Dewey's wife Annie Godfrey Dewey, who kept
detailed weekly time budgets and punctilious domestic records of
buttons, canned fruit, household guests and the number of meals
each had eaten.[21]

Such ritual economy would be the force lifting the poor "from
beneath," like the escalator (invented 1892) or the ferris wheel
(1893). Economy was a redemptive force, since crime was born of
an empty stomach and drunkenness "from the constant gnawing of
an unsatisfied stomach caused by not having the proper foods properly cooked."[22] If the poor understood nutrition and followed the
lead of science, they would discover that they too had the resources
to transform their lives. Like other Progressives urging the scientific
management of waterways and forests,[23] home economists were advocates of dynamic equilibrium and an internal regulation: balanced diet, domestic expertise. Annie Godfrey Dewey's perpetual
accounting was a means of keeping tabs on the welcome-but-
unwelcome swell of things, while her husband's decimal system literally put tabs on the explosion of printed materials after the Civil
War. The huddled masses in the United States were poor not because
there was too little but because there was too much.

From Scarcity to Abundance: "Over-nutrition"

The historical shift in models of movement from buoyancy to balance was geared to a shift in economic models from scarcity to abundance. Like the home, which was now a center less of production than of consumption (as Ellen Swallow Richards was well aware), so the problem at large was one less of supply than of demand. Mary Baker Eddy's Christian Science and Madame Blavatsky's Theosophy posited a deity of infinite generosity, a God of Supply. Physical culturists, starting with Dio Lewis, argued against the old idea that exercise exhausts: "Writers speak of our stock of vitality as of a vault of gold, upon which you cannot draw without lessening the quantity; whereas it is rather like the mind and heart, enlarging by action, gaining by expenditure." Images of the human body and the body politic as closed systems would never entirely vanish—they were most imprinted on the physiology of sex and the politics of tariffs—but they were slowly obscured by images of plenty.[24]

The national economy had been growing at an accelerated pace since 1840, leveling off only in the last decades of the century. In 1866, during a mild depression, the Oberlin economist Amasa Walker was already concerned about the kinds of consumption ("mistaken, luxurious, public, reproductive"), though more concerned with acts of self-denial that could turn wealth back to industry as capital. All classes had "some need of non-necessaries," but this must be an "harmonious, temperate, and well-proportioned luxury." Ten years later, in the midst of a more severe depression, the laissez-faire economist David A. Wells saw that the country was hurting "not because we have not, but because we have; not from scarcity, but from abundance." The main economic issue in the 1880s was the surplus in the Treasury and what to do with it; national elections hinged on debates over lowering the tariffs or spreading the wealth by changing monetary bases from gold to silver. The problem was overproduction and underconsumption. "In the midst of plenty," wrote William Hope Harvey in one of the most widely read pamphlets of the 1890s, "we are in want." While women dispensed hearty economical meals at the Rumford Kitchen of the Columbian Exposition, the worst financial panic in American history was shutting down 172 state banks. Just after the Exposition closed, "hungered and half-starved men" were banding into armies to march on Washington. Even so, by 1897 Simon Patten, co-

founder of the American Economic Association and the American
Academy of Political Science, was basing his economic analysis on
the fact of abundance.[25]

Social critic Thorstein Veblen saw this abundance and fretted
over luxury and conspicuous consumption in his *Theory of the Leisure Class* (1899). Muckrakers and settlement workers knew this
abundance personally but were furious that it had not made its way
to tenements or slums. Railroad agent Behrman died of this abundance as novelist Frank Norris drowned the fat man in a downpour
of wheat in *Octopus* (1901). Simon Patten, confronting this abundance, wrote against "over-nutrition."

Overnutrition was the true menace. While undernutrition was a
social problem of distribution and equity, overnutrition was an out-
moded personal habit. With so much of everything in view, why
hoard? Overnutrition was an atavistic response to abundance. It
created surplus nervous energy, which worked itself out through
selfish vices. The well-fed had to learn to channel all excess into the
"pleasure of right actions" and social work. Balance, command and
flow were critical to the survival of democracy under such a deluge
of goods. Ellen Swallow Richards took this theory at full value: "I
believe, with Professor S. H. Patten, that the well-to-do classes are
being eliminated by their diet, to the detriment of social progress,
and *they* and *not* the poor are the most in need of missionary
work."[26]

What was overnutrition or taking-without-needing among the
well-to-do[27] was seen as profligacy among the poor. Thus Wilbur
Olin Atwater's twenty-year campaign against "the conceit, let us
call it, that there is some mysterious virtue in those kinds of foods
that have the most delicate appearances and flavor and the highest
price." Atwater (whom Simon Patten read closely) was writing as a
chemist about the "pecuniary economy of food." Given that "the
cheapest food is that which supplies the most nutrient for the least
money," he deplored not the poverty of the poor but their mismanagement of resources, their poor habits of cooking and shopping.
Poor men ate unnecessarily expensive cuts of meat, while their wives
threw away all the trimmings. Americans, Atwater contended, were
sloppy with their food because of its native abundance. They let
themselves be deceived by that abundance and the gross weight of
their portions.[28]

Inspired by the work of German physiologists, Atwater during
the 1880s began his own nutrition research. Like Frederick W. Tay-

lor estimating the number of foot-pounds of work an ideal man could do in a day, Atwater sought mathematically to proportion fuel to work. Men doing moderate physical labor required 3,000 to 3,600 calories and 120 to 130 grams of protein daily. Unfortunately, Americans wasted a fifth of their protein and fat, and then they overate, mistaking bulk for energy. To stem that foolishness, Atwater drew up tables converting foods into fuel or nutrient units, then figured the ratio of nutritive value to retail cost. A pound of milk was more economical than a pound of beef; round steak was as good as tenderloin, mackerel as good as salmon.[29]

Sylvester Graham had intimated that good bread and pure water were sooner spiritual than physical substances, but Atwater it was who thoroughly stripped food of its body. In the style of the Gilbreth cyclograph, Atwater's charts reduced the smell, taste, texture and weight of food to an essential nutritional line against a dark backdrop of labor. Were we today less accustomed to tables of proteins and calories, we might find it implausible that the son of a Temperance minister could entirely reconstrue the meanings of foods without reference to taste, ethnic tradition, or social context. Yet that is what Atwater did—not because it is what capitalists or scientists always do, reducing the world of things to inventories, classes and laws, but because the ranks of numbers made munificence appear manageable. The numbers may have seemed attractive because capitalists and scientists had been laboring to make the world commensurable, but Atwood befriended them because "things cannot always go on thus." The soil would become exhausted, the population dense. Abundance played on our confidence, lulling us into a false sense of security. The more there seemed to be, the more deadly the illusion of an inexpendable wealth. Atwater's tables of quiddities—essential nutrients, calories per serving—were to restore a sense of proportion by exposing the naked spine of our food. With the help of the Department of Agriculture, the millionaire Andrew Carnegie and a generation of "scientific" cooks, Atwater was so successful at this balancing act that he reset the nutritional standards for the nation.[30]

No matter that he was wrong about the wastefulness of the poor.[31] No matter that he exaggerated the protein needs of the working person, downplaying fresh (expensive) fruits and vegetables and playing up a diet deficient in what would soon be called vitamins.[32] No matter that home economists using his tables welcomed the new steel-milled de-germed flours, which required baking powders and more sugar but seemed purer, or the extracted, condensed foods, which promised but rarely delivered the essences of things.[33] No matter that neither he nor most home economists saw the problem of waste as a problem of social scale; while some feminists like Charlotte Perkins Gilman made plans for cooperative kitchens, domestic science was dedicated primarily to the individual household, isolated and conjugal.[34] No matter that long-term planning and bulk-buying were unrealistic for the growing number of single working women in "efficiency" apartments with tiny kitchenettes, or for working-class families whose breadwinners could rarely anticipate a full year of constant wages.[35] No matter that such economy presumed a logistical flow and a "respect for inexorable law" alien to those whose lives were most open to the interruptions of illness, industrial accidents, strikes, seasonal layoffs and winter cold.[36]

Whatever the *post hoc* critique, the American crusade against fatness had begun. Fatness was awkward, imbalanced, inefficient, uneconomical. Fatness meant overnutrition, the center of the body out of control. The crusade against fatness arose not from a specific concern with fashions in clothing but from a far more general concern with fashions in consumption.

The Social Decline of Fat People

Despite the reputation for gluttony enjoyed by Diamond Jim Brady and his banqueting partner Lillian Russell, the tables of the Gilded Age were turning against fat. The famous Fat Men's Club of Connecticut, founded in 1866, foundered in 1903, by which time Russell herself, epitome of middle-aged voluptuousness, had been bicycling to recapture the lithe figure of her early stage career as "airy, fairy Lillian." Captain Bush of Hoboken, dining moderately at the annual gathering of the Fat Men's Association in 1879, had been on a diet for fourteen months and had lost 140 lbs.[37]

Fat men and women were increasingly self-conscious, and society was more embarrassed for them. Cartoons showed them to be at odds with the scale of modern life: a fat man dwarfs a hotel bed or a Pullman sleeper, a fat woman plugs up the aisle of a streetcar or the compartment of an elevator, a fat couple peers up a narrow staircase or hesitates in front of a turnstile. Boies Penrose, the Pennsylvania political boss and grand eater, could not fit into a theater seat. President Taft got stuck in his White House bathtub. *City Life*, an 1889 board game, gave Number 13 The Capitalist a large middle, a round face and the power to Take 3 From Pool, while Number 6 Fat Man was sadly inert. "Surplus fat," Mary Norton Henderson wrote in *The Aristocracy of Health* (1906), "is to be avoided as an embarrassment to all the internal economy." By 1910 a fat man was thought to have committed suicide owing to his shame at his bulging girth. Even in death, the "areolar tissue or fat is often the cause of much embarrassment to the embalmer, as decomposition may set in here, causing gases to accumulate under the skin."[38]

This embarrassment blushed from language itself, as euphemisms for obesity ran thin. "Stout," once a fine word for all ages, had become ambiguous if not uncomplimentary. "Fat" had become an "ugly word," wrote a middle-aged woman from her Morris chair in 1907, but was there "no substitute? no gently suggestive, delicately insinuating euphemism? Plump, now? From my youth up I was that. Stout? Obnoxious adjective, barely tolerable as a noun." "Chubbiness" pertained to healthy children, "chunkiness" to runaway slaves and then to street toughs. Around midcentury, "dumpy," "pudgy" and "tubby" had emerged, none of them quite as pejorative as "porky" (1860s), "sod-packer" (1880s), "jumbo" (1880s, from the Gullah for elephant), or "butterball" (1890s). A man might have a potbelly or, after 1879, a bay window, but Thomas B. Reed, portly Speaker of the House, proclaimed: "No gentleman ever weighs more than 200 pounds." Fatty Arbuckle as Sheriff "Slim" Hoover summed up the situation just before the final curtain of *The Round-Up* in 1907: "Nobody loves a fat man."[39]

Certainly not the life insurance companies. Since the 1830s, life insurance agents had extracted larger premiums from people of great width. When medical examinations became mandatory, examiners filling in standardized forms became stricter with overweight applicants. One physician in 1873 cut short his examination of a "stout, healthy-looking man of 62" solely on account of the applicant's overweight (5 feet, 3 inches, 182 lbs). The *Medical Record* editorialized on the doctor's behalf, noting that the overweight man later admitted to having had two apoplectic attacks in the previous four years. As the proportion of elderly in American society rose, examiners were more inclined to look askance at the traditional weight gain with age, and in the 1880s the principal medical authorities on life insurance agreed that those rated up for corpulence were generally "a very bad class of lives."[40]

Judge William Howard Taft applied for life insurance around 1900. At 6 feet, 2 inches and 275 lbs, he had—as his application indicated—"some tendency to obesity." His insurance agent (self-interested, surely) deposed: "The Judge is not a fat man but a big man . . . his flesh is hard and solid." Taft's medical examiner in Cincinnati wrote, "This risk, not withstanding the large over-weight, is rated a 'first class.'" The insurance agent was making the older equation between Big Man and big body, a social equation tested by Taft on his trip to Japan in 1900, where an entire village turned out to push him uphill in his rickshaw "and gathered in crowds about me, smiling and enjoying the prospect of so much flesh and size." But the medical examiner was in the vanguard, granting Taft a good bill of health *despite* his weight, and Taft was fully aware of his weight as a problem. He had warned his prospec-tive wife, "I shall worry you so much with my appetite that you must gain strength to meet the trial." By 1905, often sleepy, embar-rassed to be seen riding a horse, he was promising Helen that "I will make a conscientious effort to lose flesh. I am convinced that this undue drowsiness is due to the accumulation of flesh." In a year he was down from 320¾ to 250, but in 1909 as President he was back up to 355 lbs, "a big blond man who had been molded between two six-foot parentheses, bulging . . . in the middle, his trousers wrin-kled . . . his coat bumpy."41

Fat no longer seemed so protective and reassuring, even in the biggest of Big Men. It was as messy and loose-ended as Taft's admin-istration, or as childish as "The Fat Baby," a 1908 Pathé Frères fea-ture in which Ed. Dunkhorst, "the Human Freight Car," played a great overgrown kid. While Teddy Roosevelt had his "tennis cabi-net" and was doing daily calisthenics, the stolid Taft was lampooned in 1906 as a fat peacemaker setting foot in Cuba and upending the island, in 1909 as a Kewpie Doll and as Billy Possum playing golf: "It's a Great Game for us Fat People, Isn't It." Fat did not establish authority or define an inviolate personal ambit; it invited conde-scension and familiarity, as when Chauncey Depew, Senator from New York, patted Taft's stomach and asked, "What are you going to name it when it comes, Mr. President?" Fat implied not the asser-tion of power but its false promise or its miscarriage.42

Political disrespect for fat had been mounting since the 1880s. There had been lost opportunities: Zachary Taylor, Millard Fill-more, Ulysses S. Grant, and Chester A. Arthur all had paunches as Presidents. But the politician then seemed meant to carry some weight; the Jacksonian thin man was in abeyance. In 1882 Grover Cleveland's supporters, faithful to the old Big Man image, were un-afraid of advertising their candidate's large frame and inclination to corpulence. Cleveland's opponents, however, for the first time since the Jacksonian era, considered his 250 lbs a vulnerable weakness. Cleveland in 1885 was "The Apotheosis of Phlegm," insensitive as any pachyderm; in 1896, during his second term, he was "The Fat Knight,"

> . . . rare reformer fat, gelid, glum, grave,
> Steatopygous, shallow, sham, solemn, stolid,
> Firm "sot in his ways," self-satisfied, solid;
> His triumphal trait, chiefest characteristic.

"Not from such," wrote the characterologist Joseph Simms in 1889, "but among the slim and active, must we look for regeneration of the world."[43]

Mrs. Grover Cleveland, meanwhile, was lending her figure to the promotion of Sulphur Bitters, a digestive medicine. It would be folly to pretend that the depreciation of fat suddenly changed the eating habits of Americans, poor or rich. Large meals, for those who could afford them, did not disappear overnight. The 75-cent special at Fred Harvey restaurants in the late 1870s included tomato purée, stuffed whitefish with potatoes, a choice of mutton or beef or pork or turkey, chicken turnovers, shrimp salad, rice pudding and apple pie, cheese with crackers, and coffee. The imposing Secretary of the Treasury William Windom dropped dead immediately after eating and speaking at Delmonico's annual banquet of the New York Board of Trade and Transportation in 1891; he had just delighted his audience with the news that the floating tonnage of the United States was far in excess of any other nation. When life insurance medical directors sat down to their banquet in 1895, they had clams, cream soup, kingfish with new potatoes, filet mignon with string beans, sweetbreads and green peas, squabs and asparagus, petits fours, cheese with coffee, and liqueurs to follow. Historians and novelists have featured such meals as comic or conclusive proofs of the hypocrisy of the Gilded Age, whose orators discussed economy or moral reform while consuming enormous plates of food. To the contrary, as posh affairs went, those seven- and eight-course dinners were obedient to a newly economical etiquette: they were two or more courses and thirty to sixty minutes shorter than formal diners of the previous era, and their portions were smaller. From the 1880s on, as the social elite honored a growing proportion of diners in their fifties and sixties, and as middle-aged men and menopausal women were urged not to eat as they had when young, the menus of banquets gradually diminished in length and breadth. Diamond Jim Brady was notorious for his gargantuan meals not because he was the champion of an esteemed sport but because he was one of a dying breed.[44]

And his dining companion, Lillian Russell, why had she begun working out with barbells and punching bags even as she was starring in "The American Beauty" in 1896? Why was the fat comedian George K. Fortescue on stage at the Fifth Avenue Theater in 1884 as Well-Fed Dora, burlesquing Russell's well-rounded rival, Fanny Davenport? Why was Davenport herself taking "amazingly long walks" and dieting at just this time? Were they not, in all their flesh, splendid nymphs like those in Adolph William Bouguereau's "The Nymphs and Satyr" (1873), a famous French painting carried across the United States on the boxtops of Hoffman House Perfecto Cigars?[45]

The truth is, they were caught betwixt and between. By the 1880s, Bouguereau, monarch of French academic artists, was painting adolescent bathing girls and slim prepubertal cupids. The perfect figure for a teenager, according to Mrs. Susan C. Power's *Ugly-Girl Papers* (1875) was "all curves, but slender, promising a fuller figure." Girls passing from the "plumpness of childhood into the ugly age of development" should not end up as "overripe pears." "On the whole," wrote Dr. Emma E. Walker thirty years later in her "Pretty Girl Papers" for the *Ladies Home Journal*, "it is better to be too thin than too plump, for an excess of fat may cause serious mischief. It makes one heavy and awkward, and finally the 'fat walk'—the waddling gait you know so well—develops, and I beg you to avoid this!" "The precise medium between corpulence and leanness is hard to attain and harder to keep," wrote the feminist physicians Daniel G. Brinton and George H. Napheys; "so that if this matter attracts a good deal of attention, it is nothing more than right, aesthetically speaking, that it should." By the turn of the century, Madame Qui Vive (Helen F. Stevans Jameson), writing for the *Chicago Times Herald*, would admit that "I once heard of a woman to whom the idea of gaining or reducing flesh had never occurred, but she died before I got a chance to look at her."[46]

The problem was that "women are now young longer than they are beautiful," wrote Drs. Brinton and Napheys. Demographers might agree. As longevity increased, Americans tended to understate their ages, like Prudence Jones,

As thirty as ever a woman owns—
As thin as a spectre could be with her bones

and also a prude who "held for a sin all plumptitude." The English satyrical raconteur Frank Harris, who spent much of his youth on the make in America, found that 'as my youthful virility decreased, my love of opulent feminine charms diminished and grew more and more to love slender, youthful outlines with the signs of sex rather indicated than pronounced." Traditional pornographic poses of older, stockier men with younger, thinner paramours were redrawn with greater gentility by Charles Dana Gibson in the 1890s, while bicycles-built-for-two paired more athletic men with hardier women. There was something to this lubricious gerontology. Older men would recall the steel-engraved ladies of the antebellum era, while younger men would remember the sturdy nurses of the Civil War. Late-century concerns with father–daughter incest and social agitation for laws raising the age of consent were further evidence for a close relationship between patterns of aging in America and the double image of beauty. The older (and far-sighted) looked toward a tender, floating youth, while the younger (and near-sighted) appreciated a more balanced maturity.[47]

But the slender, innocent girl and the full-blown, confident woman were soon shadowed by a third figure, "pale, impure, wicked, voracious, consumed with pride, full of revenge, greedy for power and gold" and taut of line. This *femme fatale* was also redrawn, subdued and pinioned, by Gibson, by Harrison Fisher, and by Howard Chandler Christy, most of whose "girls" were taller, prouder, more commanding than the men around them. If they were not dying Camilles or Mimis, that is because the tubercular aesthetic was itself dying out, and it had never been as much a part of the American scene as of the European. If they were not deadly Salomes or Judiths, that is because they were restrained at their center by a belt, a tucked shirtwaist and a steam-molded corset which gave passion little leeway. The serpentine abandon of the European *femme fatale* became in America the controlled spiral of the Gibson girl turning on or just out of the reach of her admirers.[48]

From the end of the Civil War (and, soon, the end of the crinoline) to the end of the century, American beauties hovered between adolescence and maturity, between the seductively naive and the ambitiously seductive. The two images (and, later, their shadow) coexisted on the stage and under the big top, in stereographs and lithographs, across museum walls and exhibition billboards, on posters and postcards, in advertisements for soaps and corsets. At the Columbian Exposition in 1893, the title page of the brochure on *Art and Handicraft in the Woman's Building* presented exactly this double model of beauty. On the one side stood a painter, a Gibson Girl with slightly disheveled hair, her left foot poised on top of open tomes, her body towering over a spinning wheel; across from her, a third her size, a Greek woman in antique gown stood sculpted on a wooden pedestal.[49]

These images coexisted within the ranks of the genteel and within the working class. (The rule of thumb that the poor love full bodies is drawn from the wrongheaded but handy belief that the poor are profligate.) And they coexisted in fashionable costume, which demanded a tightly laced juvenile waist in the midst of the padded busts, large bustles and long trains of the 1870s and 1880s. As the crinoline had been fashion's remedy for dyspepsia, so the bustle was its remedy for neurasthenia. The bustle drew the ungrounded body down, filling it out and forcing it into a stern diagonal from bosom to rump, the swag of its drapery and flounces insisting on a weighted forward motion. Yet this was a composite motion, a matronly sweep and a maidenly lunge, accommodated by newly elasticized corsets. The 1890s hourglass figure in shirtwaist, belt and skirt completed fashion's shift from buoyancy to balance and torque, but it did not settle matters in favor of one or the other image of beauty. Rather, it hinted at the prospect of yet another, a woman whose body could handle with grace the improvisations of bicycling and shooting-the-chute, whose movements could seem natural before the instantly disarming snapshots from Kodak Brownie cameras, whose perfumes had to be stronger because she was never in the same place for very long. This woman, neither adolescent nor matronly, was a-borning with the modern dancer and the first aviators, and we shall meet her soon in the person of Susanna Cocroft. Meanwhile we may catch a glimpse of her at New York's Globe Theater in 1911 as "The Slim Princess." In the Kingdom of Boriveenia, a woman must be fat to be married, but Princess Kalora is so thin that she makes French fashion models look obese. Her tutor, Herr von Schloppenhauer (= Mr. Slop-about), sings "I like 'em plump" with a fat-girl chorus in Act I, but he has failed to fatten poor Kalora on two years of health-resort food in Albania. Her terrible plight is eventually resolved when an American captain of industry, Pike from Bessemer (home, of course, of industrial efficiency), at length proposes to Kalora and takes her back to the New World, where slim, resilient women stand guard over toothpowder, straight-front union suits and breakfast food.[50]

The Bouguereau nymph and the Big Man were being squeezed from many directions within American society—industrial, architectural, linguistic, annuarial, political, gastronomical and aesthetic. The squeeze was not perfectly coordinated, but it was steady. There was much denying it, little escaping it. Fat would not long withstand this cultural pincer movement—on the left, a new kinaesthetic ideal promulgated by flyers, dancers, efficiency experts and home economists; on the right, a new economic model preoccupied with abundance, consumption and overnutrition; at the center, moving up slowly, a new definition of food in terms of units of energy. Now, at last, it makes sense to write about the culture of slimming itself.

Slimming

When one Dr. George N. Niles of Atlanta celebrated fat in 1910, the *New York Times* saluted him with a sideswipe: "At Last a Physician Rises Up and Seriously Defends Surplus Flesh; Which Should Comfort Thousands." Declared Dr. Niles: "Fat is like a housewife who, though not apparently earning anything, by her care and industry conserves the fruits of her husband's labor, enabling him not only to support the domestic establishment, but also to lay aside a surplus."[51] This obnoxious comparison was not at all what home economists had in mind. Everywhere, home economists wrote and spoke against fat. They skimmed fat off soup, trimmed it off meats and scooped it from the frying pan. "All food . . . should be as light, porous, and free from fat as possible," commanded Maria Parloa of the Boston Cooking School. "Dainty cooking, not such as tempt men to gluttony, is what our housewives should study," dictated Sarah Tyson Rorer.[52]

It was to Mrs. Rorer above all that women looked in the 1890s for advice about reducing. Herself not slim, Mrs. Rorer matched *Human Nature*'s 1898 profile of the domestic woman: clean-featured but rounded, receptive and touched with lace. She was truly a transitional figure, midway between the double-chinned, plump-fingered "old-fashioned New England housewife" cooking at an ancient brick oven and the new "home manager" in the Apple-

croft Efficiency Kitchen, her body as spare and carefully ruled as
her account books. If Mrs. Rorer was a Spiritualist and a housemis-
tress, if she wore full silk dresses at her cooking demonstrations, she
was equally the pharmacist and engineer, pushing cookery toward
science so that "weights, measures, temperatures and exact time
could always be given, and not so much left to the *judgment* of the
cook." She was also the acknowledged authority on food—more eminent than her younger contemporary Fannie Farmer. She wrote
fifty-four cookbooks; her *Philadelphia Cook Book* sold 152,000 copies by 1914. She wrote the kitchen column for the *Ladies Home
Journal* and trained more than five thousand girls at her Philadelphia Cooking School. She created bargain dinner plans for the poor
and endorsed pure food investigations, time-saving foods, standardized measures. And she detested fat.[53]

"An excess of flesh," she wrote, "is to be looked upon as one of
the most objectionable forms of disease, and must be treated as
such." Transformed from a simple physical presence to a malevolent
entity, fat took on the features of the bacterium, bred on waste, infiltrating the body to feed on it: a deadly parasite. "The disease of
obesity—for it certainly is a disease—creeps on so slowly that the individual becomes thoroughly wedded to the form of life producing it
before he realizes his true condition." Men would tend to eat too
much meat, women too much starch, sugar and butter. Then "the
whole machinery will be overtaxed, joints will swell, feet will begin
to shuffle, and the mind will become inactive. . . . The end comes
quickly."[54]

The answer to fat was, as in the rest of domestic economy, a willful suppression of abundance: avoid alcohol, malt liquors, potatoes,
rice, bread, butter, sweets and most fatty foods; get up from the table hungry; cut out a meal a day; do not nibble; stick to 40 oz food
and 55 oz water daily. Saccharin (available since the 1880s) might
be used as a sugar substitute, but you were better off learning to
do without the taste entirely. From Highmore, South Dakota, Mrs.
W. R. N. wrote that all her family was inclined to flesh and wished
to reduce. She wanted to know "the kind of food that is satisfying."
That was the rub, Mrs. Rorer wrote back: this question of *satisfying*, when fleshy people ate so much more than *necessary*. The scale
of desire was at issue here; fat people carried with them "a living
death" because they were never satisfied. Dieting must be an act of
internal regulation, the balance and control of desire.[55]

There was little new here in terms of reducing techniques. Nor should we expect great novelty from such a transitional figure as Mrs. Rorer. Like many others, she was in the midst of transposing to the "disease" of fatness the traditional host of cures for dyspepsia.[56]

Cures for dyspepsia, as we have seen, were as various as its symptoms. Soon, however, the variety of treatments for fatness would exceed that for dyspepsia, in part because fat seemed so easy of solution and therefore vulnerable to any number of therapies, in part because fat was actually so obdurate that any approach had to be tried, and in part because theories about the formation of body fat were at a loss to explain why what seemed so easy to forestall was so hard to dislodge. In each therapeutic frame—the medicinal, the dietary, the calisthenic, the psychological—treatments for obesity built upon older ideas about indigestion while advancing newer ideas about physical economy.

MEDICINES

Medicines, prescription or patent, took up the familiar digestives, cathartics, emetics, diuretics and laxatives to dissolve and then expel the unloved fat. Digestives became Berledets (boric acid, corn starch, milk sugar) or Human Ease (sodium bicarbonate and lard); sassafras tea became Densmore's Corpulency Cure; mineral waters became Lucile Kimball's powder (soap, Epsom salt, washing soda). Arsenic, previously administered to stimulate the flow of digestive juices, became an adjunct against fat because it sped up the system; it was used by 1910 in an obesity tablet compounded with strychnine, caffeine and phytolacca. Phytolacca was pokeberry, a well-known emetic and purgative which Dr. W. W. Baxter observed to be a reducing agent for plump migratory birds. From his rural acuity came Phytoline for sedentary human beings, dissolving fat, stimulating "vital cellular physiological action," upgrading fatty tissue to muscle and sweeping away all waste.[57]

Phytoline was a hustling, bustling kind of medicine, as most anti-fat medicines were meant to be. It worked energetically and purposefully, "with a special selective action on fat cells," akin to the ideal domestic servant cooking or cleaning with dispatch and loyalty. But such servants, so much desired, were hard to come by. Middle-class housewives, increasingly their own workers, responded avidly to the appeal of medicines that promised to work inside their bodies as they themselves had to work inside their houses. In 1906, the Star Book Company of Chicago was wholesaling 11,300 confidential letters seeking help for obesity from Dr. O. W. F. Snyder and 6,055 letters sent in response to obesity ads run by the Howard Company. Hattie Beal & Co. opened 238 pieces of mail each day in response to ads for its weight-reducing program and Slenderine medicine with which "you at once become master of your own body. You CONTROL your weight ever after." F. J. Kellogg's Safe Fat Reducer had drawn 112,697 responses by 1914. The names of anti-fat medicines appeared on "the dead walls of old abandoned barns all over the country in letters three feet long, on the face of rocks visible from the passing railway train in characters still larger." Testimonials came from traveling men as well as housebound women. Now that the fat man had no defenders, was denounced by physicians, resented by tailors, scorned by novelists, lampooned by cartoonists and cruelly ribbed by bus conductors—or so wrote a contributor to the *Living Age* in 1914—now fat men too admired the virtues of Richard Hudnut's Obesity Pills, whose box carried the logo of a little man as round as the world.[58]

DIETARIES

Once they had made the rounds of ipecac, camphor (as an appetite suppressant), potassium acetate (a diuretic), digitalis (a stimulant), Chichester's Corpus Lean and Dr. Gordon's Elegant Pills,[59] fat women and men would turn grudgingly to diet, which demanded of them more will power. A young man, "disgustingly corpulent," had moved into a Graham boardinghouse in 1838, hoping thereby to find relief from "shortness of breath and uncomfortable dullness," but he left alarmed at the changes in himself or in his fare. Nonetheless, Graham's spare diet, directed against gluttony and indigestion, was steadily redirected against obesity, appearing either as Graham crackers and apples, or as brown bread and tea, or as gluten crackers and soda water, or as whole wheat bread and fruit, or as the perennial dry toast.[60]

In 1745 one physician had figured that the human body was composed of 60% gluten; by the 1890s physiologists figured 60% water and 5 to 6% fat by weight (the normal woman with a slightly larger proportion of water and of fat than the normal man). The proper scientific diet, then, would seem to need to deal as much with liquids as with solids. But confusion reigned here. Obesity had only recently been separated out from gout and dropsy, both of which had customarily been treated with mineral waters, and yet everyone knew that boxers, jockeys, and long-distance walkers severely limited their liquid intake in order to "fine down." Should one treat fat as bloat and insist on a dry diet, or should one use liquids to wash out the system and dissolve the fat? Water stimulated hunger but also swept food through the system faster and prevented constipation, so should one drink at meals or not? "Can water be called fattening?" one woman asked Mrs. Rorer in 1894. No, wrote Mrs. Rorer, but her answer was perplexing: Water keeps the figure rounded and plump; water drinkers as a rule are plump; we are 75% water and should stay that way, for the sake of our kidneys.[61]

If water was perplexing, milk was a riddle. While S. Weir Mitchell was fattening neurasthenic women with whole milk at sanatoriums, Philippe Karell, physician to the Emperor of Russia, was using whole milk to cure hypochondria, migraine headaches, edema and obesity. He confessed that he could not explain milk's effect, but effective it was, and widely promoted against obesity. Milk was something of a domestic miracle, comforting yet energetic, the very model of home economics. The use of the milk diet to put on fat and take it off was characteristic of this transitional stage between dyspepsia and obesity, where many treatments became peculiarly amphibious.[62]

There was less immediate confusion but eventually more heated controversy over solid foods. Justus von Liebig, the most influential of German organic chemists, claimed at midcentury that nitrogenous (albuminous, protein) foods were dedicated exclusively to the repair of muscular tissue. Under no condition could the body transform protein into fat. Since the body was always reconstituting itself, protein was always necessary and never stockpiled. Starches and sugars (carbohydrates) and fats were fuel foods. Like other fuels, they could be stored as surplus. Once stockpiled as fat, they sincerely resisted any return to a useful life. Meats were proteid and easily digestible; grains were carbonaceous and less digestible; butter and oils were fatty and least digestible; and vegetables—some were indigestible and passed right through as pure bulk, others could be turned into fat. Which ones? "As a rule," wrote Alice Worthington Winthrop for *Harper's Bazaar*, "all vegetables which grow underground are fat-forming,"—as if fat grew in darkness and flourished out of sight.[63]

Proteins were light, modern, active, responsive, alert and ra-

tional. Fats and starches were heavy, historical, passive, slugabed
and sentimental. Proteins had jobs to do and they did them; fats and
starches gravitated toward the soft life, the sinecure and nostalgia.
This nutritional allegory was played out across most of the popular
reducing diets of the late 19th century. The allegory led dieters away
from the calming starches of the dyspeptic's dinner toward the lean
beef of the athlete's training table. The allegory relieved them of
that ancient anxiety over the spare diet as a debilitating diet. Now it
would seem that the diet and the dieter could be both light and
strong.

   Mr. William Banting, a fashionable London undertaker who
had made the Duke of Wellington's coffin, lived several doors down
from Berry Brothers & Rudd, whose large vintners' scales served to
weigh the likes of Lord Byron, Beau Brummel, and the fundaments
of the English aristocracy. From his earliest years, Banting had "an
inexpressible dread" of growing fat, but in his thirties fat crept upon
him nonetheless. He tried to row away from it, but rowing whipped
up his appetite. The same for sea air, bathing, horseback riding and
Harrogate waters. Purgatives and diuretics did not work at all;
ninety Turkish baths drained off a grand total of 6 lbs. Fat clung to
him like barnacles, those most oblivious of parasites. By the age of
sixty-five he weighed 14 stone 6 (202 lbs), could not tie his shoes, had
to climb down stairs backward, and was growing deaf. He consulted the aural surgeon William Harvey, who recalled a lecture by
the French physiologist Claude Bernard on excess sugar (glucose) in
the liver of diabetics. Since many diabetics were fat, and since Banting's deafness was due not to any disease of the ear but to adipose
matter in the throat pressing upon the eustachian tubes, Harvey prescribed a diet free from farinaceous (starchy) and saccharine (sug-
ary) foods. Banting took so well to lean meat, dry toast, soft-boiled
eggs, and green vegetables that he lost 35 lbs between August 1862
and May 1863. Few men, Banting wrote, had "led a more active
life—bodily or mentally—from a constitutional anxiety for regularity, precision, and order," and he had finally found them all in 21–
27 oz solid food and 30 oz liquid daily, with a special (alcoholic) cordial in the morning and grog for a nightcap. On September 12,
1863, he stood 5 feet, 5 inches, weighed 156 lbs and could walk
proudly face forward downstairs. Six months later he had reached
150 lbs and clear hearing. Exultant, Banting wrote out and printed
up his good news, giving away the first 2,500 copies of his *Letter on
Corpulence* and issuing by public demand a fifth edition within a

year. At his death in 1878, more than 58,000 copies of his diet book had been sold, and Banting had become "banting," the new participle for reducing.[64]

"Banting" was as much American as English. By the 1880s, American physicians found Banting's banting the most common method of dieting to lose weight. The laity had adopted it by word of mouth, and it had entered into the lore of cooking schools. Its popularity was a neat prologue to the proteid passions of Atwater's pecuniary economy. Stripped of its antiquated cordials and grogs, Banting's diet fitted not only the nutritional allegory of Protein versus Fat but also the American economy's slow swing away from pork and lard toward beef and its by-product, oleomargarine.[65]

Trimmed further, Banting's lean meat became the legendary American Salisbury steak. Dr. James M. Salisbury (1823–1904) had begun to put the art of therapeutics into order in 1854 with a study of baked beans. He was trying to locate the nutritive principles behind health and disease by living on one food at a time. After three days on beans alone, as he wrote, "light began to break." Using a microscope, he proved that bean food did not digest well; rather, it fermented and filled the digestive organs with yeast, carbon dioxide, alcohol and acetic acid. He hired six hale and hearty men to feast for days solely on baked beans, with the same poor results. Stomachs could not take to beans, as they could not take to thirty days of oatmeal porridge. He continued his experiments, feeding two thousand hogs to death on various diets and studying cholesterin (cholesterol). During the Civil War, as a nutritional consultant, he prescribed broiled beefsteak and coffee to ward off camp diarrhea. The Union Army asked him to devise an army ration, but the manufacture of a Salisbury dessicated food was cut short by Union victory.[66]

After the war, Salisbury published his *Microscopic Examination of the Blood* (1868), inspected skin diseases and fungus, treated nervous diseases and consumption, and arrived at a therapeutic system that purified the blood, improved digestion and, almost inadvertently, reduced weight. Beans, with the double-walled sacs and gases of the typical legume, had been the clue all along. Their gases paralyzed the stomach wall; their skins clogged the alimentary canal. Paralytic diseases, tuberculosis and dyspepsia, claimed Salisbury, were caused by gluey, fibrous deposits in the body which thickened the mucus and blocked the intestinal canals. Beans, peas and many other foods left long, tacky streamers of themselves in the body. Even meat could be dangerous. Not just its fatty veins but its connective or "glue tissue" and cartilage could clasp internal organs in the fatal embrace of embolism or tumor.[67]

The remedy was hot water and "the muscle pulp of lean beef made into cakes and broiled." Salisbury explained: "hot water washes out the slimy stomach, gets it clean enough from bile and yeasty matter to digest lean meats, which give maximum of nourishment with minimum of digestive effort." Well-done lean beef, the only single food on which a human could live for long without harm, was good for the three years it would take to bring a patient back from the last stages of tuberculosis. And "Never mind the shrinkage in weight. It is natural and absolutely necessary, for the reason that those foods which upholster, or make fat, are the very ones which produce the disease."[68]

Salisbury had personally worked through the eras of indigestion and neurasthenia to come at last to obesity. Outside and inside, the fat body was a sick body. So viscid an agent of death was fat that lean beef had to be minced and scraped from the sides of the American Chopper before one could be sure that it was safe. While a physician was wondering whether "the coming American is to digest his food himself at all, or whether it will not be digested for him outside his body, and administered ready for absorption and assimilation," Salisbury was transforming banting into an industrial process. The large-scale processing of cattle in the stockyards of Chicago (laid out for better flow by engineer Octave Chanute, patron of the Wright brothers) had its counterpart in the new meatgrinding equipment of Salisbury's Cleveland kitchen. A diet of broiled beef pulp and hot water was far more than a cosmetic act of reducing; it bespoke a scientific reform of the body, a kind of physiological trust-busting. The spirit and the flavor of the new diet made eating tantamount to precision tooling and domestic economy.[69]

Popular and enduring as the Salisbury steak was and is, his reducing plan required "a repulsive and ostentatious observance of details, a nauseating and monotonous diet, and a disregard of the claims of the palate which cannot fail to disgust." This, however, was an English and old-fashioned critique. Skeptical modern Americans thought Salisbury's 3 lbs of lean beef and six pints of hot water daily just plain too much food, especially for women, who required 20 percent less food than men, according to Atwater. For women there was another very popular diet, which explicitly promised domestic economy.[70]

The "No-Breakfast Plan," wrote Dr. Edward Hooker Dewey from Meadville, Pennsylvania, in 1896, would *"emancipate your lives from one-half of the slavery of your kitchens."* Morning hunger was "morbid want," breakfast a pleasureless, habitual eating which led to indigestion and illness. What was morning sickness but a woman's "protest against putting food into a morning stomach"? Even the most restless sleepers and active dreamers had little need of breakfast. Only true labor could summon true appetite, and true appetite asked but one light meal and one regular meal each day. Not three meals, then, but one and one-half. Freed from the drudgery of breakfast and the groaning board of two other full meals, Mrs. P., a farmer's wife of 220 lbs, lost 45 lbs of "absolutely dead weight."[71]

Dead weight: a strange notion to apply to a living body, unless one were under the spell of allegory and that dead weight were fat. Dead and yet dangerous, fat was becoming ghoulish. It crept up on the sly, then settled in like a thick, malevolent fog. We have come some distance from the ghostly *thin* disciples of Sylvester Graham. Now it was fat that drew the hearse.

MUSCLE WORK

As a ghastly presence, "chronic, gradual, progressive, persistent" fat would seem less easily disposed of by will power, minced beef and true appetite.[72] Protein might ward off future fat, saintly abstinence might spread its temporary charms across the present, but what could either do with the pasty ghosts of Thanksgivings past? Diets were holding actions, and Prince Otto von Bismarck, the German Iron Chancellor, had never much liked holding actions. Grown to an unwieldy 244 lbs in the summer of 1883, Bismarck became for Americans as well as Europeans the prime example of the Big Man who had to learn that political force and personal weight were not coextensive. Suffering from neuralgia, insomnia, edema and depression at the age of sixty-eight, Bismarck yielded to the authoritarian regime of his 101st physician and lost 60 lbs in less than a year. Reinvigorated, Bismarck in 1884 set Germany on its colonial march through Africa while maintaining his own exercises under the constant supervision of Dr. Ernst Schweninger, whom Bismarck gratefully elevated to a German professorship.[73]

The Schweninger cure was actually the Oertel cure, which relied as much on graduated exercises as on a low-carbohydrate and restricted-fluid diet. Indeed, Dr. Max Joseph Oertel called it his "terrain-kur." At his Munich sanatorium he had laid out a series of paths in colors coded for the angle of incline, with level paths in red and the steepest in yellow. A fat patient's recovery was a pilgrim's progress from the bloody slough to the golden summit.[74]

So the Schweninger cure, which was the Oertel cure, which was the terrain-cure, was actually the training cure. It had been described in most detail and with most celebrity in English by Sir John Sinclair in *The Code of Health and Longevity* (1807), again by Walter Thom in his 1813 account of the exploits of the great pedestrian Capt. Robert Barclay Allardice, and again by Archibald MacLaren, fencing master at Oxford in the 1870s. By MacLaren's time, trainers offered their runners, rowers, gymnasts and boxers more fresh water and vegetables, but the dieting table was still set with stale bread, lean beef or mutton, and little salt. The differences were that dieters ate much less of the same things and geared their exercise to a civilian life.[75]

It was this laboring at labor which would shake the "dead weight" of past fat, very much as pilgrims shook sin from their shoulders—and with the same puritanism, for however much classical physicians had acclaimed the strenuous tussle and heave of sex, modern dieters were dissuaded from such license. What then was good exercise? Dr. J. L. H. Down put a fat patient to turning the handle of a mincing machine. (Was this after all the secret to the success of the Salisbury diet?) Others pedaled bicycles. Mountain-climbing was superb, but city-dwellers might take an elevator to the twentieth floor of a skyscraper and jump down the stairs one at a time. The Kaiser chopped wood at Sans Souci to lose weight, while American women in small apartments were rolling on the floor in loose clothing twenty times before their no-breakfast and twenty times after their evening lemon juice. At home on rainy days, there was the 30-foot dash across the room or the Sargent Health Jolting Chair to exercise the arms, legs and internal organs. Oppidan economy extended to a host of exercising machines; some were later used in penny arcades, others were sideshows in themselves (the Gifford portable health-exercising and gymnastic apparatus became a rowing machine, chest bars, horizontal bars, a bed, a crib with lateral motion, an adjustable table and a chair).[76]

Most often there were calisthenics to "regain muscular control of the abdomen," that pivot upon which the modern dancers placed such trust. These calisthenics were rarely inventive, but they came

now with messages about efficiency and regularity rather than pleasure and eupepsia. If allegorical fat lingered between the living and
the dead, then exercises had to be daily and perpetual. "Corpulency
should not be met by a so-called short cure. . . . The cure should last
as long as life and should merely consist in putting the muscles to
their natural use."[77]

For many, muscling in on fat was still a dubious proposition.
Banting had given it up when it made him hungrier; Americans had
used calisthenics to improve digestion and *increase* the weight. "It
does seem illogical, doesn't it?" agreed Dr. Emma E. Walker in her
"Pretty Girl Papers" in 1905. How could exercise both put on and
take off weight? The answer had been given in the *Ladies Home
Journal* four years earlier: "That which tears down fatty tissue
when given vigorously will build up tissue when given lightly." Such
an answer was as unsatisfying as Philippe Karell on the milk cure or
Mrs. Rorer on whether water was fattening. It was all the more unsatisfying when musclemen like Eugene Sandow and physical culturists like Bernarr Macfadden and Jørgen Peter Müller were promoting vigorous exercise to *build up* a healthy body.[78]

Those who made the most of the ambidexterity of exercise were
masseurs and masseuses, whose techniques at once built the body up
and broke it down. Called friction or shampooing and borrowed in
the 1830s from Hindu and Arabic sources, now it was known as
massage or movement cure and imported from Northern Europe
and the Sandwich Islands. Employed in the 1830s to cure dyspeptics
and in the 1870s to calm neurasthenics, by the 1890s it was primarily for the thin and the obese. By pounding out the fat from between
the tissues while provoking interior respiration (oxidation) and se-
cretion, the masseuse forced the body to burn fat that was "dead
weight" and put in its place "a fresh class of fat altogether," healthy
and responsive. Kneading and squeezing a great roll of fat "as
though it were dough," the masseuse became the body's home economist and efficiency expert. Massage transmuted potential energy
into kinetic, explained Thomas S. Dowse in 1890; massage effected
"dynamical exchanges." In plain language the masseuse was the
body's civil engineer.[79]

I write "masseuse," not "masseur," because of a swift change in
the gender of the skill. In 1885, one masseur advertised in the Chicago business directory. In 1886, three masseurs. In 1905, with 105
listings under massage, three-quarters were for masseuses. Across
twenty years, the massage business had shifted from a man's to a

woman's profession and from the athletic to the therapeutic. Chicago did not offer the 260 different schools of Japanese massage, but like the Japanese, American masseuses turned much of their handicraft to the abdomen and the small of the back. Those regions demanded a softer touch and a redirection of energies: less Scandinavian hacking, more clockwise spiral flowing strokes from the center outward.[80]

The steady pressure of the good masseuse was soon Taylored to the machine. In 1914 Peter J. Peel opened his first reducing salon in Chicago, featuring Gardner Reducing Machines which enveloped his male clients in two sets of adjustable rollers and did an especially smooth job on the abdomen. Gardener machines reached women at W. F. Taylor's Corset Shop in San Diego and at the Bush Sanatorium in Louisville. Coach Amos Alonzo Stagg at the University of Chicago employed a similar machine to treat the charleyhorses of his athletes. In 1916 *Modern Hospital* was impressed with an electrical ring roller reducing machine with helical springs of tempered steel and rollers mounted on ball bearings, which could scud up and down the body eighty times per minute.[81]

Something quite peculiar was going on here. Efficiency was getting in its own way. If the reducing of fat called for physical exercise, efficiency called for least effort. From calisthenics to massage to electrical apparatus, the fat person was being led down the same primrose path as the housewife with new electrical appliances. Could one reduce weight by *eliminating* work, or reduce work by adding more machines?[82]

The penultimate example of this confusion of the effortless with the effective was electrotherapy. In its elementary form, it was yet another holdover from such cures for dyspepsia as Dr. Christie's galvanic belt advertised in 1849. George Burwell's 1892 Boston boncontour obesity belt had 100 to 150 electrically charged magnetic-ore discs laid between denim, Shaker medicated flannel and satin. The electricity would dissipate fat more safely than medicines, more permanently than diets, and more cheaply than a French massage.[83]

In its complex form, electrotherapy *was* a French massage. Since 1900, Dr. Jean Alban Bergonié had been perfecting "passive ergotherapy," a controlled means for producing "muscular work artificially by electrical excitation." Fixing electrodes to the seat and back of a reclining chair, Bergonié ensconced the fat patient in the chair and settled other electrodes on wet towels over the thigh, under the calf, across the abdomen and on the arms, all held in place with rubber bracelets or bags of sand. A current of 50 milliamperes run through this electric chair would contract the patient's muscles one hundred times a minute, strong enough to raise the body even under 40 kilos (88 lbs) of sand. Properly managed, the one-hour sitting could be the equivalent of a ten-mile run in a heavy sweater. "All this without the intervention of the will, and almost without sensation, the patient being occupied during the treatment with his own thoughts or with the book he is reading."[84]

This was a fairy tale cure: safe, "aesthetic" exercise without fatigue, suitable for those with weak hearts, wrenched backs, puffy joints or anemic constitutions. Men and women could gain strength without fortitude, lose weight without will power. George Beard and S. Weir Mitchell had applied electricity to steady the nerves; Bergonié and his many American imitators thought of electricity as a dynamic force and applied it to the muscles. The stern authoritarian manner of Mitchell and the equally authoritarian manipulations of the masseuse had become the impersonal authority of the dynamo. The more "modern" the cure for obesity, it seemed, the less the patient had to do.

MIND WORK

Electricity short-circuited any resistance on the part of the fat person. Cooperation had been the sticking point for medical therapy, dieting and calisthenics. Dr. Salisbury had noticed that his patients did not know how to use their nerve force economically; they consumed it as they consumed food. He could not trust their will power: "Will-power, or voluntary mental effort, affords neither a balance-wheel nor a safety-valve to check this waste." His patients were rather to learn to relax and make themselves into "passive, interested machines." Settle down in an easy chair, he instructed them, with the palm of the right hand on the forehead and the palm of the left over the back of the neck, your eyes fixed on a small object, your breath easy and slow, to a count of forty-nine. Then move the right hand to the pit of the stomach and the left to the small of the back. The right palm was a positive pole, the left negative, and "by thus placing the palms of the hands over the various nervous centres or plexuses, a vital current is directed back into the body." Here, between the palms of the hands, massage turned into mesmerism and mesmerism into psychology.[85]

The Lambert-Snyder Health Vibrator in 1906 promised 15,000 vibrations to the minute to reduce constipation, indigestion and obesity. It had no electrical parts, no wheels, no cogs, no springs. It worked—if it worked—because the body was a battery drawing on the energies of the universe. But, as Salisbury had suggested and as partisans of Mind Cure and New Thought made clear in the 1890s and early 1900s, energy could flow only through a body that was relaxed. Mind Cure's deific All-Supply and New Thought's laws of corresponding vibrations seemed to confound self-help and self-abandon, making a virtue of receptivity. With practice, however, the unconscious could be tapped like an oil well; after the first gusher, one learned to control it. Call this method of control meditation, self-hypnosis or mind therapy, it could be as practical as it was transcendental. Sip some water, advised Dr. Alice M. Long in 1908, and say to yourself, "As the organs of assimilation and elimination are now properly performing their respective duties, the blood is circulating normally, all waste is being carried away and my weight is decreasing. I am growing lighter and lighter each day. Each week I shall lose two pounds. My food is assimilating properly, all waste is being carried off and I am growing better in every way."[86]

We have arrived at the ultimate economy: thinking fat away. This should not be confused with wishing fat away. Dr. Long's sentences were framed in the language of science and ritual; weight would disappear gradually and with (unromantic) composure. The patient invocation of All-Supply depended upon a disciplined relaxation. If this were paradox, it was the paradox toward which efficiency experts always tended when confronted with a heavy, stubborn body: more control but less strain. We should be little surprised, then, if the paradox were solved by conjuring up the flow of the unconscious. This flow within the mind might be channeled like the flow of work in a factory or the flow of electricity through an induction coil into a fat body on a reclining chair. Indeed, the electrical currents passing through that body in ergotherapy were so weak that Bergonié's method was far closer to mental persuasion than it was to physical exercise. The psychological treatment for obesity took electricity's fairy tale as far as it would go: all flow, no fat.[87]

In every case, as medicines, diets, calisthenics, and electrical/ psychological tactics were transposed from indigestion to obesity, the old-but-new cures were etched with the social and kinaesthetic programs of industrial efficiency and domestic economy. Abundance had always to be restrained and directed from a powerful and yet relaxed center. "In every case," Annie Payson Call wrote in her influential Mind Cure book, *Power through Repose* (1892), "it is equilibrium we are working for." Not the denial of gravity—not floating or gliding—but the use of gravity: "The more the weight is *thought* to the feet, the freer the muscles are for action," and thus "the motive power of the body will seem to be gradually drawn to an imaginary center in the lower part of the trunk." From this center, as dear to Isadora Duncan as later to Martha Graham, would come "the true economy of force."[88]

Age-Old Remedies and Impermanent Cures

I have dealt *seriatim* with the medicinal, the dietary, the calisthenic, and the psychological, but this is not to imply that people proceeded from one sort of treatment to the next in proper single file. The truth was a mess. People set out to lose weight anyway they could, regardless of compulsive historians, and they mixed everything up. They dieted one way, exercised another, dosed themselves with this and that, gave themselves pep talks or learned to relax. They did not always know about the most up-to-date drug or accept the diet most compatible with their cultural *weltanschauung*. They jumbled eras as well as genres.

We can see all this in the continued popularity of the age-old remedies against fat: acids, soap, lotions, tobacco, tea, salts. Most of these dated back to the Romans. The tobacco cure (as a sialogogue or spit-inducer) was attributed to the 17th-century scientist Giovanni Borelli, the Castile soap cure to the 18th-century physician Malcolm Flemyng, but such attributions simply gave a pedigree to the anonymous. The most popular remedies—vinegar, lemon juice, soap pills—lingered at the backs of household recipe books or in the colored powders, tablets and lozenges of patent medicines. Russell's Anti-Corpulent Preparation in 1889 was mainly citric acid; Jean Downs's Get Slim in 1914 was a New Yorker's form of pink lemonade; Every Woman's Flesh Reducer was a Chicagoan's bath powder with citric acid, Epsom salts, camphor, alum and soda. A woman in 1694 would rub her skin with vinegar and then apply a reducing ointment of fullers' earth, white lead, henbane juice and myrtle oil; in 1907 she would apply Absorbit Reducing Paste with oxbile, beeswax, lard, oil and perfume, or Fatoff, 90% water and 10% soap.[89]

Then, with no sympathies whatsoever for the orderly historian, these folk remedies would be tumbled in among the most modern cures. The Dr. Turner Triplex System of Flesh Reducing (promoted by the same company that sold the Neal Reducing Belt and the To-Kalon Keapshape Reducing Corset) was at least quadriplex: a low-carbohydrate diet with saccharin tablets, phenolphthalein (laxative) salts, brisk walking with deep breathing, and evaporated condensed milk with traces of ginger. Marjorie Hamilton's Quadruple Combination System of Fat Reduction was actually sextuple. If calendar girl Hamilton modeled a reducing program without "Drugs, Medicine, Sweating, Turkish Baths, Massage or Sweat Belts, or Appliances, or Nerve-Racking Exercises, or Starvation Diet," her cure did entail enemas, the juice of half a lemon twice daily, Indian club exercises, Kissingen mineral waters, a modified Banting diet, and Healthtone Obesity Powder (sodium carbonate, Epsom salts, Glauber salts and saltpeter).[90]

Orthodox physicians were hardly less indiscriminate. While they unanimously denounced the use of vinegar and the overuse of laxatives and purgatives, they were not loath to work with all genres at once or to prescribe medicines that differed only in name from the herbs and mineral waters of lay healers. Dr. E. S. McKee of Cincinnati made these Olympian but common recommendations in 1891: "Treatment requires, of course, rigid diet. Hydrocarbons [carbohydrates] must be eliminated to give place to albuminoids [proteins]. Alcohol must be interdicted. Exercise, household duties, gymnastics, or massage cannot be neglected. Electricity, both in the form of general faradization and the intrauterine use of faradic current, is of value." He also advised laxatives, sea baths, mineral waters and hydropathy.[91]

Such all-encompassing therapy stemmed in some measure from the confusions incumbent upon the shifting of cures for indigestion over to obesity, but it stemmed in greater measure from the impermanence of any single cure for overweight. "Everything you ever tried, I tried," Lucile Kimball confided in 1914. "I went through exercises, rolled on the floor, cut down my food, gave up sweets, fats and starches, wore elastic clothing, tried electricity, massage, osteopathy, vibration, hot and vapor baths, swallowed pellets, capsules and teas—*gained as rapidly as I lost*." She herself was hawking red pepper, menthol, bitters, aloes (a cathartic), soap, Epsom salt and washing soda. These came through the mails in pink and brown tablets and a bath powder, but a disguise was not a cure.[92]

The more vehement the campaign against fat, the more resistant fat seemed to be. If efficiency demanded the shedding of "dead weight," fat began to encroach upon "the heart, the liver, the spleen, the kidneys, and even the *Brain* itself," turning a person into "a revolting, waddling, quivering caricature and monstrosity." If economy of force demanded a dynamic equilibrium, fat began to move in vicious circles: you could reduce it by calisthenics, but exercise aroused appetite, and satisfying the appetite restored fat; you could use stripping agents like acids and hard soaps, but these made you thirsty, and drinking increased your bloat. Here was a merry-go-round indeed.[93]

"The fat is there, and will show itself," wrote diet doctor N. E. Yorke-Davies. He was referring to the uselessness of corsetry and tight-lacing, but he might just as well have been summing up the prospects of all the different slimming techniques. Brought over from London to treat William Howard Taft in 1905, Yorke-Davies was successful . . . for a while. Then Taft gained the weight back.[94]

Before World War I, before the advent of flappers, bobbed hair and short skirts, powerful new models of the human body in motion and of the industrial process in action had promoted ideals of physical movement and consumption that had no place for fat. Fat had then become ghostly, a slow menacing poltergeist, obnoxious, sometimes deadly. Were there no new methods to deal with fat in the body as there were new methods to deal with waste in the factory and the home?

Yes there were.

CHAPTER FIVE

The Regulated Body

Between 1880 and 1920 appeared four slimming techniques that were not inherited from older remedies for dyspepsia. These techniques—fasting, Fletcherism, calorie-counting and thyroid medication—were nicely compatible with the new kinaesthetic ideal of a dynamically balanced body. Each dealt with gluttony and fatness as if they were problems of flow. Each had a different means of economy by which to command that flow. Fasting, an assertion of spiritual economy, was an act of immediate regulation: the refusal of food. Fletcherism, or slow chewing, was an act of mediate regulation at the portal of the body. Calorie-counting depended upon a more internal regulation of flow by balancing intake against the energy consumed within the body. Thyroid pills directly regulated the internal metabolism itself. All four techniques dealt with abundance as if it were a threat to the system, a moral as well as a physical danger.

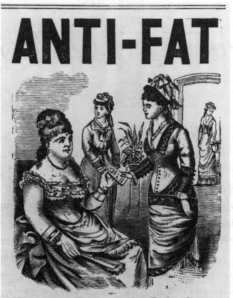

ANTI-FAT

The Great Remedy for Corpulence

ALLAN'S ANTI-FAT

is composed of purely vegetable ingredients, and is perfectly harmless. It acts upon the food in the stomach, preventing its being converted into fat. Taken in accordance with directions, **it will reduce a fat person from two to five pounds per week.**

"Corpulence is not only a disease itself, but the harbinger of others." So wrote Hippocrates two thousand years ago, and what was true then is none the less so to-day.

Before using the Anti-Fat, make a careful note of your weight, and after one week's treatment note the improvement, not only in diminution of weight, but in the improved appearance and vigorous and healthy feeling it imparts to the patient. It is an unsurpassed blood-purifier and has been found especially efficacious in curing Rheumatism.

Advertisement from Harper's Weekly *(1878). Allan's Anti-Fat was the first popular obesity drug compounded with* fucus vesiculosus *or bladder-wrack, whose iodine content might remedy what would soon be called thyroid insufficiency or a slow metabolism.* Courtesy of the National Library of Medicine

Fasting

MOLLIE FANCHER could read books with their covers shut. She could decipher torn bits of an old mining report through a scaled envelope. She could live without eating.[1]

In 1864, "brilliant, pretty, petite, cultivated" and about to graduate from high school, she had fallen from a horse and broken some ribs. Scarcely recovered, she caught her dress on the steps of the Fulton Street horse trolley and was dragged ten or fifteen yards down the road. She went into spasm and paralysis, lost her sight and her ability to swallow. Tended by a wealthy aunt, she lay in bed shaping wax flowers and embroidering watchpockets, one hand stuck rigidly behind her head. In nine years her sight returned and her muscles began to relax, but still she did not eat.

Her psychic powers seemed the consequence of her fasting, which had ennobled her as common invalidism would not have. Even after fourteen years without so much food "as an ordinary healthy girl would eat in forty-eight hours," she had "faultless features neither wrinkled nor drawn nor wasted." Her ashen complexion only complemented her trances and her second sight.

The Reverend Joseph T. Duryea, a Presbyterian minister, came

115

often to her house at the corner of Myrtle and Downing streets in Brooklyn. He scrutinized her soul and found it impeccable. Four physicians, examining the rest of her, were satisfied of the prodigy. Astronomer Henry F. Parkhurst kept a complete record of her astonishing condition. James B. Smith, builder of the Equitable Life Assurance Building and the American Museum of Natural History, stood by her for years. In 1878 Dr. J. R. Buchanan, soon to marry a clairvoyant, lectured before the Brooklyn Conference of Spiritualists on Mollie Fancher's powers of apprehending objects at a distance. In 1879 Dr. William A. Hammond published his *Fasting Girls*: like the others, Mollie Fancher was an hysterical fraud.

Since at least the 4th-century Desert Fathers, Christendom had entertained saints, holy women and fasting virgins whose moral authority was drawn from the dry cache of asceticism. With the model before them of Jesus in the wilderness, adolescent girls in particular had taken to forty-day fasts, which drifted into months and then years. In the Catholic world, fasters became visionaries and devotees of the Blessed Virgin, living on the fragrance of flowers or thin communion wafers. Protestant fasters were rather the monitors of national piety, like Jane Hodge in England, who stopped speaking and eating in 1669, saying that she was fasting for the sins of the people and was the savior of the nations. The most recent of these monitors had been Sarah Jacob, the Welsh fasting girl, daughter of farmers in Carmarthenshire. At the age of ten, after a bout with scarlet fever, she felt a pain in the pit of her stomach and ceased taking food. She drew the notice of the neighborhood, the county and then the country, as men and women made pilgrimage to her, guided by placards at the nearest railway station: "Fasting Girl" and "Shortest Way to Llethernayadd-ucha." She lay abed dressed as a bride, a wreath of flowers around her brow, rows of gifts displayed on shelves in front of her. But the longer she fasted, the rosier and plumper she looked. Skeptical doctors mounted a "serious watch" on December 9, 1869. One week later she was pale and ill, but her parents insisted that she go on. She died of starvation the next day.[2]

There was collusion in this girlslaughter. The English fasting woman Ann Moore in 1813 had also been closely watched, but she had relented after nine days and confessed to being fed through wet towels and her daughter's kisses.[3] Now, however, Sarah Jacob, her parents, the attending physicians and the pilgrims had too much at stake not to see the ordeal through to its end. It was less a question of losing face than of losing faith. The body had become the guarantor of the spirit, and it must not lie.

When Dr. Hammond indicted Mollie Fancher on the grounds of hysteria, he was saying that the body could very well lie, whether put up to it consciously or unconsciously. Yet we must look further than that ever-so-convenient diagnosis of hysteria to understand how Mollie Fancher had come to be invested with such powers as a truth-teller.

American Puritans had fasted in moments of great undertaking (sailing to the New World, declaring independence) and in moments of great peril (earthquakes, epidemics, wars). Between 1620 and 1750, 691 fast-and-humiliation days were called in New England to ask God's blessing or to beg God's mercy. Fast-day sermons became a principal vehicle for the elaboration of the Puritan theology of the covenant by which God and people were bonded together in a holy mission. During calamitous times, the sermons pointed to a covenant forsaken; during prosperous times, to the dangers of selfishness ("The Fatter the Soil, the Ranker the Weeds") and of pride ("*Vessels* excessively and most richly laden, do often sink with over-much *Weight*"). In the 19th century, fast-day sermons pointed especially to that intemperance or slavery which threatened to disrupt all covenants. But there were few references to gluttony in any of those sermons, and the actual fasts were less physiological than spiritual gestures to "rent, unnaile, and unglue thine affections from the world." Fast days demanded neither a gloomy countenance nor, usually, total abstinence; rather, one was to put off eating until noon and then to eat without relish. By 1846, fasting itself had been so neglected that the Protestant Episcopal Church thought to publish explicit rules, citing as epigraphs Matthew 4:2 (Jesus in the wilderness) and I Corinthians 9:27 ("But I keep under my body, and bring it into subjection"). According to the New York diocesans who wrote the guidelines, many had never learned how to fast and so had never begun, or had begun but failed. They had failed because they had demanded too much of themselves. In general, fasting must be incremental, a series of small self-denials in the company of much prayer. No single act of discipline must become the focus of concern, especially not food, which should be handled with restraint at all times. At the fast table, one might skip breakfast or skimp on the main meal or simply hold oneself to plain foods. Fasting did not mean starving.[4]

Total abstinence, indeed, was not admirable. American "walk-ing skeletons" like P. T. Barnum's Calvin Edson had no mantles of piety thrown about them by the public. Vegetarians and Graham-ites had assumed those mantles only to find themselves wearing the gastronomer's new clothes. "That is a poor mystery of gastronomy," wrote one critic in 1837, "which feeds the eyes and leaves the stom-ach famished." Vegetarians themselves had disapproved of Jervis Robinson's starvation diet for dyspepsia; a gill of water and three 1-oz Graham crackers daily were just too little for life.[5]

Even the marvelous fasting girls were not expected to feed on air. Popularly, fasting referred to abstention from solid foods, that is, from meat, bread, cereals and starchy vegetables. Fasters could and did take fruits, greens, juices, teas, whey, mineral water, tobacco and opium without being reckoned cheats. The Fasting Girl of Lan-cashire, Ellen Sudworth, had been surviving since 1871 on a diet of soups and puddings. Mollie Fancher herself managed to swallow fruit pulp and juice. It was likely that this sweet, soft diet brought on the tooth decay that compelled doctors to yank all her teeth; had she wanted to, she could no longer break her fast.[6]

Mollie Fancher was not fasting to remind Christians of their sins or to stave off an imminent disaster. Rather, her fasting was an asser-tion of power, a force in and of itself. She was by virtue of her fast both virgin and dynamo. Unlike the neurasthenic woman under the rest cure, confined to the bed and diet of an infant, Mollie Fancher was mistress of her world in the same way that a somnambulist has mastered the night. Mollie was not the first fasting girl, but she was one of the first in the United States to draw from fasting itself a spiri-tual authority. Fasting had begun its slow transformation from the negative to the positive. Now that physicians were more often feed-ing up their convalescents than putting them on low diets, fasting could be detached from invalidism. It was about to come into its own in nice counterpart to the campaign against fat.

The controversy over Mollie Fancher was a new turn of events. Dr. Hammond issued two challenges to her: the first, that if she could read the words on a $1000 check placed inside an envelope, she could have the check; the second, that if she allowed herself to be watched round the clock for a month by physicians of the New York Neurological Society, and if she fasted "perfectly," he would give her another thousand dollars.[7] This fasting "perfectly"—i.e., without any food or water—was a novel demand. Once fasting had become an intrinsically empowering act, Hammond had the right (nay, the duty) to require that it be pure and thorough. His two challenges were actually inseparable: to question Mollie Fancher's psychic powers was to impugn the purity of her fast, and to suggest that her fast might be fraudulent (because imperfect) was to dismiss her claims as a teller of hidden truths.

Henry S. Tanner understood. When Mollie Fancher refused "for decency's sake" to submit to the surveillance of a male medical establishment, Dr. Tanner offered himself as a chivalrous substitute, "to show the power of the human will, and to prove to materialists that there is something beside oxygen, hydrogen, and carbon in the brain." He believed that "mental action is not a mere function of the brain" and that by force of will during a long fast he could absorb atmospheric oxygen and electricity.[8]

Born in Tunbridge Wells, an English middle-class spa town, Tanner emigrated to the United States in 1848 at the age of seventeen. He became a carriage maker and was married in 1853. His wife helped him manage a fruit store while they both studied at the Eclectic Medical Institute in Cincinnati. (One of the teachers there at the time was J. R. Buchanan.) After their graduations, they practiced as physicians and ran electrothermal baths in Ohio. Henry Tanner became convinced that people ate too much and that the solution to stomach problems and inflammatory diseases was fasting. He took up the habit of week-long fasts, but his independent wife declined to join him in his abstinences. She was, however, subject to his experiments with food. He was sure that character was modified by what one ate: carrots made one fidgety and sly, turnips amiable, French beans irritable. He fed his wife 3 lbs of French beans daily; sure enough, she became so irritable that she threw a jug at him. When he tried turnips, she sued for divorce and left for Duluth and three square meals a day. He followed her. She left for Wisconsin. By 1877 Henry Tanner spoke of himself as a bachelor. In Minneapolis, Tanner became a Temperance lecturer and proprietor of a Turkish bath. Under the watchful eyes of two doctors, he also undertook a successful fast of forty-two days, during which he had Pauline visions.[9]

Now he was in New York, unable to agree with Hammond on the terms for the supervision of this new fast in honor of Mollie Fancher. The problem was that Tanner, a homeopath, and Hammond, a regular or "allopathic" doctor, owed their loyalties to different medical camps, and fasting was one subject calculated to raise the hackles of the regular medical establishment. First off, it reeked of lay healing.

Next it seemed an unpleasantly familiar throwback to a previous generation of regular doctors who had believed in starving a fever and who called most illnesses fevers. Further, Tanner's fasting appeared to be a Midwestern populist attack on Eastern prejudice; Tanner could exploit the popular beliefs that just three days or eight days without food would ordinarily be fatal and that common people in extraordinary situations—trapped in mines, caves, avalanches—could survive by faith alone. If Tanner succeeded in his proposed forty-day fast, he would give the skeptical, imperious East its comeuppance while defending the virtue of a small, crippled clairvoyant woman in Brooklyn who had refused to truckle to prurient urban bigwigs. Finally, fasting for forty days and nights would roil the already muddy waters of medical theory. Tanner himself had learned at school that ten days without food was the limit of human endurance. Dr. Alonzo Clark, President of the College of Physicians and Surgeons in New York, would say at the end of Tanner's fast: "Any man who has reached middle age, and is in sound health can fast for forty days, provided that he takes water." But most regular physicians were not so blasé, and some "seemed to feel that Dr. Tanner was a dangerous and revolutionary person, whose success in going without food ten or twelve days would overturn something or other—no one knew just what or just how."[10]

So Henry Tanner, a short, stout man, fifty years old and 157½ lbs, began his fast at noon on June 28, 1880, in Clarendon Hall on East 13th Street in New York City under the constant supervision of "irregular" physicians, who would take his pulse and his temperature with great regularity. Hearing that Dr. Hammond regarded water as a food, Tanner changed his plans for the fast after thirty-six hours and began to abstain from all drink as well. On the sixth day, Hammond warned that Tanner was liable "to become insane at any time, and I'm not sure that his mind is not a little unbalanced now. He might possibly live thirty days without food, but he can't live ten days without water." On the ninth day, Tanner was weighed at a corner saloon and found to have lost 14 lbs. By the eleventh day, regular physicians were also observing, as were hundreds of visitors who now had to pay 25¢ admission to see the haggard Tanner. Tanner was allowed to gargle with water, but the amount he gargled was measured before and after; he bathed and applied wet towels to his head, but he did not drink. On the thirteenth day, Tanner said he no longer desired to eat or drink, but he did want to hear Moody

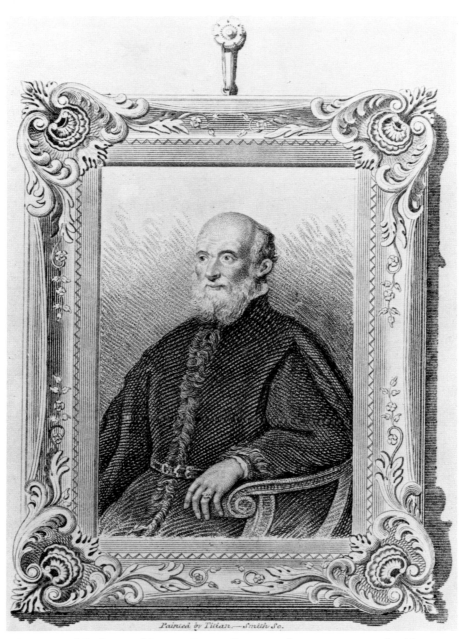

Portrait of Italian nobleman Luigi Cornaro, from a painting by Titian, reproduced in *Sure Methods of Attaining a Long and Healthful Life* (London, 1826). Cornaro's 16th-century treatises on rejuvenation through an abstemious diet established the modern prototype for the romantic mode of dieting. Cornaro died at the age of ninety-one in 1566.
Courtesy of the National Library of Medicine

Portrait of health reformer Sylvester Graham, from J.H. Trumbull's *Memorial History of Hartford County* (1886). Graham's dietary regimen was stark enough for his followers to become the first American group of weight-watchers—in order to prove that a simple diet led not to a wasted body but a robust life. No full-length portrait of Graham exists: was Graham, like modern dieters, wary of exposing his body to an historical scrutiny? *Courtesy of the U.S. History, Local History and Genealogy Division of the New York Public Library, Astor, Lenox and Tilden Foundations*

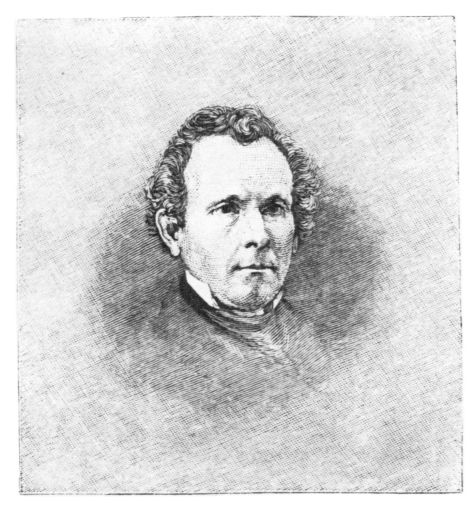

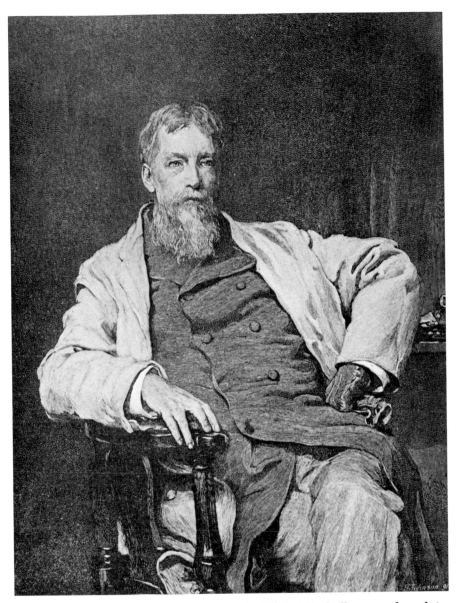

Painting of 19th-century physician S. Weir Mitchell, reproduced in *Century* (1891/92). The doctor's authoritative, uncompromising demeanor here is exactly as it must have been with the neurasthenic patients enduring his Rest Cure. Weir Mitchell intimidated his patients into immobility and fatness; the Rest Cure was but the most dramatic example of the mid-19th-century shift in therapy from the "low" (scant) feeding of the sick to "feeding them up." In the process, gluttony was gradually freed from its common associations with indigestion and thinness.

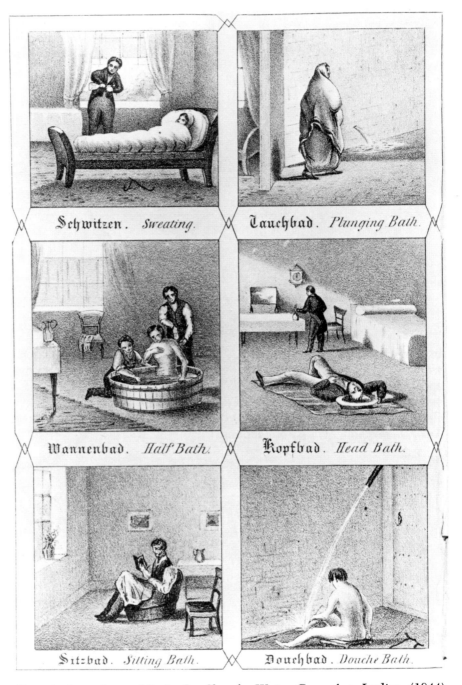

Schwitzen. *Sweating.* — **Tauchbad.** *Plunging Bath.*

Wannenbad. *Half Bath.* — **Kopfbad.** *Head Bath.*

Sitzbad. *Sitting Bath.* — **Douchbad.** *Douche Bath.*

Frontispiece from Marie L. Shew's *Water-Cure for Ladies* (1844), obviously borrowed from German sources and often reproduced. Note the variety of postures in which the water cure was worked. To restore a person's sense of buoyancy, one had to reorient that person within the world, from all angles and from all perspectives. *Courtesy of the National Library of Medicine*

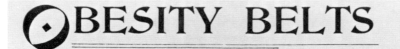
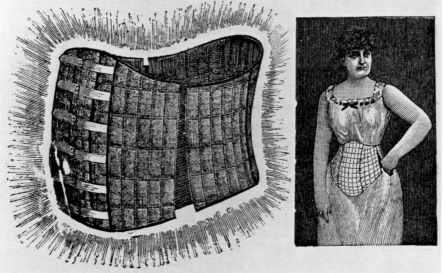
From Burwell's *Obesity and the Cure* (1892). The belts had 100-150 electrically-charged magnetic-ore discs laid between two layers of denim, covered on the inside with medicated flannel, on the outside with satin. The electrical charge dispelled intestinal gases, dispersed tumors and disintegrated fat. As it has been since the late 18th century, electricity was both a universal solvent and an energizer—just what the fat, sluggish person needed. *Courtesy of the National Library of Medicine*

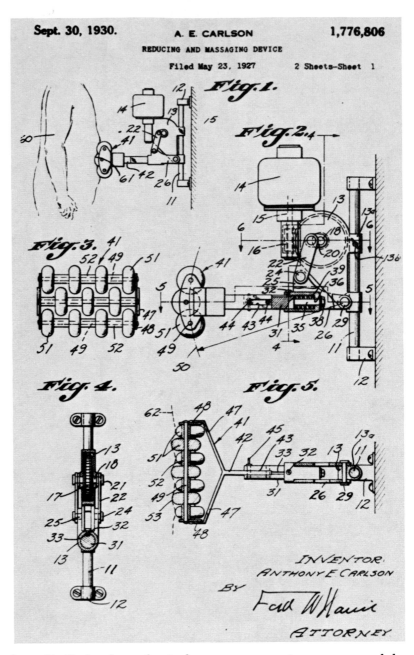

Sept. 30, 1930. A. E. CARLSON 1,776,806

REDUCING AND MASSAGING DEVICE

Filed May 23, 1927 2 Sheets—Sheet 1

Fig. 1.

Fig. 2.

Fig. 3.

Fig. 4.

Fig. 5.

INVENTOR.
ANTHONY E CARLSON
BY
ATTORNEY

Anthony E. Carlson's mechanical masseur swung in an arc up and down the abdomen, alternately compressing and releasing the fat. All the action here was inside the machinery itself; the fat was inert. Like electricity, massage was meant to dissolve fat and energize the body; massage, however, was neither as subtle nor as penetrating as electricity, so the masseur could never claim the same powers over fat as the electrotherapist.

and Sankey hymns sung by Sabbath School children. On the fifteenth day—his fourteenth ostensibly without water—he had to relent and resume liquids. By the seventeenth day, friends were advising him to desist since he had already proved himself, and D.A.P. near Peekskill, New York, was writing that "the eyes of this Whole Village is on your great Undertaken."[11]

Tanner had drawn wider attention than that. From across the country came gifts of Indian clubs, patent mattresses, flowers, slippers, roast beef, bottles and cans of milk and baby food. From Canada came a tiny bon-bon box with tinier vials of gin and claret, two Lilliputian crackers, morsels of smoked beef and a miniature silver spoon. He received, screened for contraband, three or four hundred pieces of mail a day: news of a fasting kitten, the story of a man in 1835 who had gone three weeks without water, a proposal of marriage from a Philadelphia woman if he should live, an offer from a Maine museum to stuff him if he should die, and from Mollie Fancher a letter whose contents he would not reveal. This "Starvation Comedy," as the *New York Daily Tribune* called it, this "wrestling match with the invisible fiend of hunger," was taking in $30 to $50 a day in admissions by the fourth week. Women were serenading Tanner at the piano, and newspapers in London were printing special daily dispatches on his condition. Dr. Marion Sims, the famous American ovariotomist, wrote from Paris to wish Tanner success. Down to 126½ lbs at the end of July, Tanner drew even larger crowds and soon had a communication from Hammond granting the integrity of the fast and asking Tanner to stop at once. Tanner went on.[12]

During the final week, at least six thousand people paid to stare at the tired, touchy body of Dr. Tanner. On August 7, the fortieth day, he weighed 121½ lbs. His red corpuscles had scalloped edges, his white cells looked squeezed together, but outwardly he was in better shape than most had expected. When he broke his fast at noon in the crowded hall, he ate a quarter of a peach, drank a glass of rice milk, then devoured a Georgia watermelon. "He eats like a pig," commented one spectator, and some immediately suspected a ruse. There had been much debate on what to feed him this day. Zwieback, beef tea, milk, watermelon were possibilities, but no one had been prepared for the half pound of broiled beefsteak and the half pound of sirloin he had consumed by suppertime. Tanner gained 19½ lbs in the next three days. Within a month he was back on the lecture platform trying to persuade audiences "that they should rely upon the recuperative power of the self and nature; not upon burnt toads, mercury and arsenic."[13]

Tanner was the first American hunger artist. He would gradually be forgotten—so forgotten that *Appleton's Cyclopaedia* would put him in his grave in 1896 while he had yet another twenty-two years to live.[14] But we must grant him his place, with Mollie Fancher, in the culture of slimming. From 1880 to World War I, hunger artists took to a theatrical extreme that willful economy which was so much and so paradoxical a part of the Gilded Age. Americans followed the fasts of the famous European hunger artists Giovanni Succi and Stefano Merlatti. Large crowds flocked to see Succi during his twenty-eight-day fast in New York in 1888 and his forty-five-day fast in 1890, his longest ever. Meanwhile, New Yorkers were mocking the "Two Tons of Fat on Exhibition" at Bunnell's Museum, poking and shaking the fat men's fat "just to see it shiver."[15]

Ambivalent about surplus and its waste, its heaviness, its sprawl, Americans were finding more drama in starvation than in gluttony. The new techniques of flash photography in the 1890s would turn a stark light on the thin bodies in tenements and opium dens, while A & P Tea Company ads made fun of men walking little dogs and losing sight of them under their massive bellies.[16] Fat bodies out of control no longer appeared powerful or competent. Hunger artists battling appetite, fighting off desire, waxed noble in the very midst of their waning.

Long fasts could be the means of regaining control of the body, a therapy at once moral and physical. The same day that Tanner began his fast, Agnes Dehart out on Staten Island began a thirty-one-day fast to rid herself of stomach ulcers. C. C. H. Cowan of Illinois fasted forty-two days in 1899 to shake a chronic catarrh. Spiritualist Milton Rathbun of Mount Vernon, New York, told his friends in 1900 that he was too fat and would fast for forty days. In 1902, Mrs. Emma Wacker starved out a dropsy after forty days' fasting in Ohio. By 1903 the *New York Daily Tribune* was asking, "Is prolonged fasting becoming a fad?" as Edward De Forest in Pennsylvania was on the thirty-ninth day of his fast against stomach disorders. In that same year Dr. William S. Wilkinson of Augusta fasted fifty-seven days to cure his dyspepsia, and Bernarr Macfadden hired Madison Square Garden to prove that eight athletes after fasting seven days could break world records. The Garden was packed as

Gilman Low became so strong through fasting that he could lift 1,000 lbs more than one thousand times in 35 minutes, 34 seconds.[17]

For young women, fasting led rather to attempts to lift familial weights and social oppression. Like John Zachar of Racine, Wisconsin, whose fifty-three-day fast in 1888 was meant to establish equity between himself and his father after a dispute over property, women could use the fast as the fiercest form of domestic economy.[18] Anorectics, first recognized at the turn of the century as a distinct class of patient, worked their passive aggression within the family, eventually losing out to themselves—as did Jennie Hill of Akron, fifteen, who died in 1885 after fasting twenty-five days on small bits of oranges and water, to the puzzlement of her parents and physicians. Kate Smulsey in 1884 and Marie Davenport in 1904 fasted to show that females could go the New Testament distance, like Dr. Tanner. In 1910, Clare De Serval was known as the "Apostle of Hunger," fasting in a glass box hermetically sealed except for air windows covered by fine metal gauze. But the true apostles of hunger were the women suffragists with their hunger strikes.[19]

There had been earlier hunger strikes by women prisoners in Russia who wanted their babies back, but Marion Wallace Dunlop, an English artist, was evidently the first to use fasting for explicitly political purposes. Jailed in the summer of 1909 for her suffrage protests, she refused to eat until granted status as a political prisoner. Her jailers, surprised, tempted her with fried fish, bananas, and hot milk, but at last felt constrained to release her after eight days of stubborn starvation. During the autumn, faced with more suffragists on hunger strikes, British authorities resorted to forced feeding using tubes, jaw clamps and stomach pumps. The moral victory each time belonged to the women, but the pattern of abstinence and brutality would be repeated in the next four years in England and again in 1917 in the United States, where women had been picketing the White House for the right to vote since mid-January. By June they were being arrested for obstructing traffic. In September, as longer sentences were meted out to persistent pickets, Alice Paul and Rose Winslow led the imprisoned suffragists in a hunger strike, in ironic counterpoint to a 1910 suffrage slogan, "An ounce of persuasion precedes a pound of coercion." As with the English, the American hunger strikers were first cajoled and then force-fed.[20]

At a critical point in the struggle for women's rights in the public world, fasting had become identified with virtue, feeding with violence. Forced feeding in 1917 was as close to rape as any medical procedure could be. Lucy Burns was stretched out on a bed, naked, and held rigid by five warders as a doctor pushed a tube up her left nostril and then down her throat. The food pumped into her felt like a ball of lead in her stomach. Dragged to the psychopathic ward, Alice Paul was force-fed like this three times a day for three weeks. Rose Winslow vomited and screamed during the feedings, lay gasping long after. "Don't let them tell you we take this well," she wrote, her nose bloody, her throat raw. "We think of the coming feeding all day. It is horrible."[21]

From Mollie Fancher to Rose Winslow, the long fast had become high theater. While fatness and gluttony seemed in the most flattering of lights no more than sociable, leanness and abstinence had taken on a new, sometimes heroic seriousness. And if the spotlight fell on the extraordinary discipline of the hunger artist or the indomitable spirit of the hunger striker, then the shorter fast, the more everyday abstinence, the "No-Breakfast Plan" or the smaller meal would begin to seem possible for the rest of us—and reasonable, virtuous, even empowering. When Upton Sinclair wrote on "Starving for Health's Sake" in May 1910, *Cosmopolitan* got more positive letters in response than to any previous article in the magazine's history. Half a year later Sinclair was still receiving letters agreeing with him that fasting was "the key to eternal youth, the secret of peace and permanent health" by which the body would come to its ideal weight. When he was a boy, Sinclair recalled, his family had been very skeptical of Dr. Tanner's fast. Now even the ordinary person, like the three women on Long Island or the hotelier in North Dakota, had begun to fast. From Norwich, Connecticut, C. C. Haskell conducted a correspondence school in fasting, across the state from the original site of the now defunct Fat Men's Club.[22]

Fletcherism

Horace Fletcher was a well-rounded man. After a youth spent on whaling ships and in the Orient, he had made his fortune in San Francisco as a manufacturer of printing ink and an importer of Japanese art. He was a marksman, an athlete, a painter, and for a while the manager of the New Orleans Opera Company. He was fat.

Or rather, as an insurance company told him around 1895, he was too heavy for his height. He was 5 feet, 7 inches, but his weight fluctuated between 198 and 217 lbs. His application for life insurance was denied. For the next three years, Fletcher tried and failed to reduce his weight. As a last resort, forty-nine years old and still fat, he considered going to medical school to learn the secret of reducing, but his friend Edward Hooker Dewey advised him to experiment first and study later. Fletcher did, experimenting with an epicurean regime recommended to him by the owner of a snipe estate and truffle preserve. In June 1898 he weighed 205 lbs. Four months later he was down to 163 lbs, and thereabouts he would remain until his death in 1919.[23]

As a marksman, Fletcher had invented a technique of snapshooting without waste of effort or ammunition. He applied this to eating: the ammunition was food, the effort was digestion, the teeth pulled the trigger. Chewing was like taking aim.[24]

The analogy was not all that good, since Fletcher's new method of eating was neither rapid nor effortless. The "Great Masticator" practiced an "industrious munching" or one hundred chews to the minute. Most low-fiber foods could be dispatched in less than thirty seconds of chewing per mouthful, but shallots, for example, could take seven minutes. At dinner, Fletcher might slack off to 2,500 chews over thirty minutes, but generally a meal could be dispensed with after fifteen or twenty minutes and twelve to fifteen mouthfuls. Chewing, or fletcherizing, would convert "a pitiable glutton into an intelligent Epicurean."[25]

Fletcher was a hunger artist who counted movements of the jaw instead of days on a calendar. His was the slow fast of "a stomach trained down so fine that it was like a pair of apothecary's balances, sensitive to the least inharmony." Even milk and soups had to be chewed before being swallowed. One undigested morsel of food could rumble through the stomach and intestines like a bull in a china shop. This was Fletcher's image, but it came out of the long corrida of dyspepsia.[26]

Labored chewing had been directed against indigestion for many years. The English physician William Kitchiner in 1822 had specified thirty to forty munches for each mouthful of meat. Across the Atlantic, Sylvester Graham believed that natural foods would oblige people to exercise their teeth and prepare each morsel properly for the stomach, but he did not wax arithmetical. Dio Lewis proposed six minutes for the eating of a Graham cracker. In 1885 another whole wheat cracker was put on the market with the specific appeal of being impossible to swallow without great jaw service. It was called, honestly, the Educator Cracker. The two men who proposed an Eat-Your-Food-Slowly Society in 1888 must have welcomed that hard, square cracker.[27]

Horace Fletcher did, though his brother later wanted to manufacture a competing line of biscuits to be known as "Fletcherets."[28] Fletcherets, however, would have been targeted against gluttony rather than dyspepsia. After his 1898 weight loss, Fletcher spoke, wrote and rode bicycles in a health campaign that merged the social dharma of economy with the private drama of the fast. He made the eating of less food into the formidable pretense of eating more, just as scientific cooks arranged a similar magic in the efficient kitchen. Chewing foods until liquefied demanded a commitment to an almost mechanical molar precision, but Fletcher, like Atwater and other nutritionists, was intent on the essences of things. If hunger artists literally consumed themselves, Fletcherites consumed only the best of what was not themselves, and in so doing they made the best of themselves.

By 1910, Fletcherism had spread from the middle-class patients of "No-Breakfast" Dewey to the posh tables of New York high society and to the cells of Sing Sing Prison. Bank employees were organizing a Fletcher Club for efficiency at lunch and on the job. John D. Rockefeller wrote out a "Confession of Faith in Dietetic Righteousness": "Don't gobble your food. Fletcherize or chew very slowly while you eat." A satirist noted that "Half one's friends suddenly began boasting that they were living on twenty cents a day and never felt better. They breakfasted off a cup of diet food, lunched on a nut, and dined on a concoction of vegetable juices with a banana as a pièce de résistance." Mrs. Rorer advised her nervous readers to chew each mouthful fifty times. There were "munching parties" in England run by the stopwatch to ensure that guests spent five minutes on each morsel, and from London the American novelist Henry James was writing to novelist Edith Wharton about "the divine Fletcher," who had renewed the sources of his life. "Am I a convert? you ask. A *fanatic*," he replied when his friend Mrs. Humphrey Ward asked about the Fletcher system. "Grapple it to your soul with hoops of steel." Theosophists and orientalizers reading the sutra on eating discovered that Fletcherism was no less than the liberation of *prana* (energy) from food. In Buffalo there was a daily Fletcherite "communion service" in Miss Palmer's kindergarten, each child devoting twenty minutes to a single cracker.[29]

Fletcher himself was on the executive boards of the National Council of Boy Scouts and the Health and Efficiency League of America, which he had cofounded with the economist Irving Fisher, Dr. John Harvey Kellogg, and S. S. McClure, editor of *McClure's Magazine*. He wrote for the *Ladies Home Journal*, *Good Health Magazine*, and the U.S. Army Medical Department on the method "of attaining economic assimilation of nutriment and immunity from disease."[30]

Immunity from disease? Yes, that too. Like fasting, Fletcherism promised a ritual purification of the body. Perfect chewing, like perfect fasting, made the body clean as it made it light. The throat was ordained a filter, not a gullet; anything unable to be swallowed by physiological reflex at the back of the throat was never meant to be swallowed at all. Given the work of the teeth and the saliva, "If we swallow only the food which excites the sense of taste, and swallow it only after the taste has been extracted from it, removing from the mouth the tasteless residue, complete and easy digestion will be assured and perfect health maintained." The more predigested the food flowing into the stomach, the less chance of strained intestines, constipation and a disrupted internal economy. We must all be "Competent Chauffeurs of our own Corpoautomobiles," and our exhausts must be inoffensive.[31]

Fletcher verged on coprophilia. He weighed his feces (2 oz) and described them in dull detail. Healthy excreta were small and ashy, with "no more odor than a hot biscuit." Since perfect chewing did away with most bulk—Fletcherites were forever pulling fibrous residues from their mouths—"there will be no invitation to discharge waste oftener than once in four or five days, when the response will be immediate, easy and final." Fletcherite "mouth thoroughness" was also an industrial education of the bowels. "By George!" Fletcher exclaimed when criticized for his phrase "Dietetic Righteousness." "Is there anything more sacred than serving faithfully at the altar of our Holy Efficiency?"[32]

Dyspepsia and neurasthenia were American diseases; constipation was an American delirium. "There is no rule of health more important than this," Catharine Beecher wrote in 1855: *"Take all proper methods to prevent constipation."* The American supplement to the *Encyclopaedia Britannica* in 1886 blamed meat-eating for our preoccupation with the bowels, noting that in carnivores constipation was the rule. Others blamed corsets, or sedentary living, or an American shyness about bodily functions, or pastries and fine flour. They might more astutely have blamed the heavy and complex costumes of women, which made any evacuation an awkward, time-consuming and oft-delayed task; or the absence of sufficient outhouses and toilets in slums; or the increasing use of opiates in patent and prescription medicines and baby foods.[33]

Even so, it is hard to show that constipation in 1900 was any more prevalent than in 1800. It is easier to show that constipation was more publicly worrisome in 1900 and that it was more closely associated with gluttony and overweight. Fat people had earlier been thought to have especially smooth digestive systems; now they would be seen as chronically constipated. Fletcherism appealed not just because it reduced weight but because it reduced, most literally, the waste.[34]

As American cities grew, they became dirtier and more congested. By the 1880s, it was time for "Municipal Housekeeping." Caroline Bartlett Crane of Kalamazoo billed herself as a municipal housekeeper and sanitary expert, skilled at getting cities to clean up their streets and alleys. A 1905 ad for Sapolio cleanser pictured giant women scouring skyscrapers; the slogan: "No Dirt Beyond Its Reach." Across the country, city residents were encouraged to produce less garbage. The Municipal Order League of Chicago in the 1890s sent out twenty thousand cards as kitchen reminders about better garbage disposal. Mary McDowell became known as the "Garbage Lady" for her efforts culminating in the establishment of the Chicago City Waste Commission in 1913. In New York City, street-cleaning commissioner Col. George E. Waring, Jr., formed Junior Street Cleaning Leagues, dressed his adult streetcleaners in white and put them all on parade.[35]

After it was swept up or stuffed into ashcans—that 120.7 lbs of garbage and 630.7 lbs of rubbish per capita per annum (in 1912 in Chicago for native-born Americans)—waste was still a problem. What should be done with it? The Columbian Exposition featured an incinerator, but large incinerators were costly and foul-smelling. Sanitary landfills spread too quickly over too much valuable real estate. People on the seacoast did not relish swimming through old mattresses or ashes dumped in the ocean and carried back to shore on the tides. The answer, according to Col. Waring in 1898, was extraction. Using digesters or cooking tanks holding 5 tons of garbage,

New York's Barren Island Works cooked garbage six to ten hours, then sent it through a series of presses, dryers, fume destroyers, condensers and screens to extract ammonia, glue and grease and to disintegrate the rest.[36]

Here was Fletcherism writ large, and Fletcher indulged the analogy. In 1912 he wrote to his friend John Harvey Kellogg, "I am working down among the drainage pipes where people of squeamish sensibilities do not come to molest me. I can live luxuriously in the midst of the most complex civilization on a dollar a day, all told, and dress like an angel, caring not how others may do." Like Kellogg and like Mrs. Rorer in her later years, Fletcher dressed in white. Sewers could not bother a man so pure.[37]

They did bother almost everyone else. With more paved roads and more flushing of streets, with more indoor plumbing for bathtubs and then for toilets, waste waters and organic wastes were overflowing from city cesspools and surface drains. Between 1890 and 1909, the number of miles of sewers in the larger towns and cities quadrupled, which meant that traffic congestion above ground (automobiles now as well as horses and carriages) would seem even worse as civic engineers struggled to reduce congestion below. And the more sewerage within a city, the more arguments between cities up and downstream of one another: Who should filter what waste, and how?[38]

Constipation (congestion) and waste were thus as much public concerns as problems of personal hygiene. "Hygiene" itself became a catchword for reformers, moralists, advertisers and politicians. It was applied as a salve against insanity, prostitution, venereal diseases, body odor and political corruption. The Reverend Charles H. Parkhurst, president of the Society for the Prevention of Crime, was to call his fight with Tammany Hall in New York City an exercise in "municipal sewerage."[39]

So widespread was the concern with sewers and cesspools that these images were turned back onto the body. Christine Frederick in her *Household Engineering* (1919), discussing overweight, compared constipation to the backing up of a sewer; she advised bowel movements thrice daily. Sir William Arbuthnot Lane, the English surgeon, was even more specific: "Any interference with the effluent of the main sewer of a town is followed by trouble in the drains of every house which discharges its sewage into it." Constipation was never local; blockage down *there* spread poisons everywhere.[40]

This was known as autointoxication, or self-poisoning. Too

much matter in the colon led to fermentation and an explosion of bacteria. The tachyphagia or hasty eating of modern carnivores left so much undigested food in the system that ptomaines formed from the putrefying meat in the intestinal tract. Gluttons who treated the body as a dump would suffer "intestinal septicemia." One had to be very careful: "Man is constantly standing, as it were, on the brink of a precipice; he is continually on the threshold of disease. Every moment he runs the risk of being overpowered by poisons generated within his system." The digestive canal, like the common sewer, was "a veritable putrefactive apparatus" filled with ammonia, bile and alkaloids. The extract of only twenty-five grams of putrefied meat was enough to kill. The stomach should therefore be distended for the shortest time possible.[41]

Essentially a European theory,[42] autointoxication seemed to be building directly toward Fletcherism. Dr. Ernest H. Van Someren made that point in the *British Medical Journal* in 1901. Complete mastication prevented the entrance of toxins; microorganisms in the lower intestine died out because they had nothing to feed on. The internal system was clean, neat, unoppressed. Stout Van Someren became Fletcher's thin son-in-law, and the two of them made "internal antisepsis" the widely accepted theory behind the practice of slow chewing. Druggists took this antisepsis seriously and sold new laxatives. Writers on popular health discovered constipation behind the common cold, obesity and fevers.[43]

Sometimes, argued surgeon Arbuthnot Lane, there was such chronic intestinal stasis (constipation) that the autointoxication would be fatal unless something drastic were done. In 1901 he undertook the first of hundreds of colectomies, having concluded that the entire large intestine was an evolutionary vestige like the appendix (for which, at the same time, the appendectomy had become popular in America). Lane excised the colon without a qualm. Functionless, it had become a foul cesspool dragging down the viscera. No matter that there was the poorest of evidence for such a thing as intestinal toxemia, or that his operations had a 24 percent mortality rate, or that the sole part of the colon involved in feelings of constipation (the sigmoid) was the sole part that Lane did not remove.[44]

Lane took to one unlovely extreme that common concern with constipation which had been taken to another more fanciful extreme by Californians at the Columbian Exposition. They had erected a statue of a medieval knight on horseback made entirely of prunes.[45] We may blanch at such purgative chivalry, but gastritis was listed as the third leading cause of death in the United States in 1900.[46] Gastritis was a blanket term for most intestinal ills, but we need not trust the diagnosis to appreciate how seriously constipation was taken at the turn of the century.

It followed that the causes of constipation—overeating, lack of exercise, hasty eating, poor hygiene—would be of grave consequence. The abstemious, athletic, bradyphagic, white-suited Fletcher, an optimist, a mind-cure pedagogue, a millionaire, was as perfect an American saint as one could ask for. His metabolism was to become the model for a physiological *novum organum*.

Counting Calories

"When Mr. Fletcher arrived in New Haven, I saw a man about fifty-five years of age, rather plump than otherwise, who certainly showed no signs of being undernourished, full of vitality and hyperenthusiastic over his newly acquired physical well-being." Prof. Russell H. Chittenden, director of the Sheffield Scientific School at Yale, had invited Fletcher to participate in a series of tests to determine "the smallest amount of food that will serve to keep the body in a state of high efficiency." Fletcher arrived in 1902 with hundreds of menu cards listing the appropriate numbers of chews for each food. Chittenden, who had been impressed by the Van Someren article on Fletcher, was still more favorably impressed by Fletcher in the flesh, by how strong he was and how little he ate. Fletcher in turn was impressed enough by Chittenden to help fund his further experiments on university athletes and on men from the Army Hospital Corps. By the time Fletcher returned in 1906 to surpass at the age of fifty-seven (and 177 lbs) the records of most of the young men in other Yale trials, Chittenden had published his *Physiological Economy in Nutrition*.[47]

Professor Carl von Voit, the "short, squat, plump, short-necked, well-fed" German physiologist, had established nutritional standards based on observations of a lab assistant and a manual laborer. Voit's already-high protein requirements were then adjusted further upward by Wilbur Atwater. Now the thin Chittenden, who had dieted himself down from a lean 143 lbs to a leaner 127 lbs in 1903, recommended cutting the protein requirements in half. For most purposes, 60 grams of protein daily (or 0.85 g/kg body weight) would suffice for the average man.[48]

Aside from the general threat of intestinal putrefaction from too much food, excess protein threatened to poison the body with its residue of uric acid, thought to cause gout, rheumatism and migraine headaches. Popular and medical worries about uric acid belonged to an old tradition in which acids were the scapegraces of nutrition, but they reflected also a more recent worry about fatigue. In Taylor's industrial world of high-speed machinery and in Fletcher's commercial world of telegraphs and typewriters, metal stress, mental stress and muscular stress were all being treated as problems of fatigue. Physiologically, the more work, the more muscle tissue was broken down. The more decomposed muscle, the more decomposed protein, and more uric acid floated into the bloodstream. "A tired person is literally and actually a poisoned person," wrote Josephine Goldmark of the National Consumers League, "poisoned by his own waste products."[49]

Of course, the more fat or "dead weight" one carried, the more unnecessary work one had to do, and so the more fatigue and the more poison. Chittenden's reduction of protein requirements was part of a proposal for an all-round reduction of energy intake. Stout men would lose weight but not strength under a Chittenden regime, while thin men might gain weight because they were eating the proper mix of nutrients. Best of all, by eliminating a heavy breakfast, most bread and much meat, and by substituting vegetables, fruit and milk, physiological economy would turn out to be fiscal economy and "might well amount to enough to constitute the difference between pauperism and affluence."[50]

Not everyone believed that less could be more, but by the 1920s Chittenden's standards would supplant those of Atwater and Voit in most American textbooks and tables. Even the physiologist Francis G. Benedict, long a skeptic, changed his mind. Benedict had studied the prolonged fasting of the Italian hunger artist Agostino Levanzin in Boston in 1912. He upset the proud artist by demanding that he end his distilled-water fast at 31 days 16 hours, much before Agostino had regained his "natural hunger." By 1918, Benedict had come to agree that the normal person's "natural hunger" did not demand all those Atwater proteins or Atwater calories.[51]

Those calories had been acceptable as long as the guiding principle of nutrition was Justus von Liebig's forceful distinction between protein as an exclusively "plastic" or tissue-repairing material, fats and carbohydrates as exclusively "respiratory" materials or fuel. But in 1849–50, the experimental chemist Claude Bernard had shown in France that meats, like starches, were converted into glucose by the liver. The implication was that protein too could be burnt as a fuel to provide body heat, and that excess protein could be stored, like excess carbohydrates, as fat in the body. Liebig himself had been among the first to argue that carbohydrates could become body fats; now it seemed that the body could turn practically anything into fat. Carl von Voit demonstrated the formation of fat from protein in 1869, but this idea was so incredible, making the digestive system into such a powerful alembic for the transformation of foods, that many physicians continued for decades to operate on the older principle of the exclusivity of protein and fat. As late as 1910, an international authority on obesity, Dr. E. Heinrich Kisch of the Marienbad spa, claimed that the question about whether protein could lead to fat was still under dispute.[52]

The only major diet to oppose the Liebig theory had gone so far in the other direction as to seem perverse. In the 1880s, Wilhelm Ebstein, physician at the Göttingen University clinic, believed that proteins alone could create body fat, that carbohydrates served simply as catalysts in the process, and that food fats in proper proportion were innocent victims of prejudice. He laid out a low-carbohydrate diet with normal dollops of protein and fat, reasoning that a reducing regimen should guard against the catalyst while ensuring protein strength and the satisfied appetite that was the specialty of fat.[53]

To Russell Chittenden and many other Americans after the turn of the century, fat was fat, and any food could end up as fat. The German physiologist Max Rubner in the 1880s and then Wilbur Atwater in the 1890s had shown that 1 gram of fat had more than twice as much energy (*in vivo*) as a gram of protein or carbohydrate. In other words, it took twice as much effort to burn off fat.[54] Fat had staying power. Excess was therefore doubly dangerous, whether it started out as broiled minced beef or tapioca pudding. The hunger artists and masticators had dramatized quantities and essences; now physiologists and physicians would take the hint.

Why not govern intake by energy rather than by instinct or appetite? asked Chittenden in 1907.[55] Was not nutrition really a problem of energy equilibrium? Working forward from Atwater's tables, Chittenden was leaning toward an entirely new dietary: eating ac-

cording to calories. Although Atwater had earlier given caloric values for different foods, he had still framed diets in terms of weight—
grams of protein, fat, carbohydrate; ounces of liquid. The calorie
was something else again: the amount of heat required to raise the
temperature of one gram of water one degree centigrade. This "calorie" was rather the marker of a process than the statement of a condition; it did not describe what food was so much as what it could
do, how long it would burn. When Americans began to count calories, they would not be doing simple addition or subtraction. Counting calories was like compounding interest. It assumed an appreciation of promises and futures— how long a walk it would take to
burn off a chunk of chocolate, how many flights of stairs to climb
off a piece of pie.

Chittenden welcomed a "new method of indicating food values"
based on standard portions of 100 kilocalories (the large Calorie,
which is the calorie in common parlance and henceforth the calorie
in this book). The method had been introduced in 1906 by another
of Horace Fletcher's friends at Yale, Irving Fisher. An economist,
Fisher drew a parallel between laws of thermodynamic equilibrium
in mechanics and chemistry and notions of market equilibrium.
Capital was no longer a "stock of wealth at a point of time" but a
"flow of services . . . through a period of time." An avid home gym-
nast, Fisher drew upon a similarly dynamic model of physiological
equilibrium to redefine nutrition as a flow of equal units of energy
into and out of the body. If this harked back to scientific management and time-and-motion studies, no one would have been more
pleased than Fisher himself, who had read about Taylor's life and
felt "throughout as though I were reading my own biography."[56]

We are almost full circle. Domestic and industrial engineers
chased fat around as it became awkward, embarrassing, wasteful
and finally ghoulish. The Fletcherites and hunger artists have led us
as far from fat as we dare go. Too far, perhaps. Henry James after
five years of devotedly slow chewing had nearly been done to death
"through the daily more marked increase of a strange and most persistent and depressing stomachic crisis: the condition of more and
more sickishly *loathing* food." Mrs. Cora Blanche Parkhurst, a
wealthy but squat widow in Los Angeles, died of a heart attack in
the offices of the Normal Life Company in 1912; she had been fasting for fifty-six days to reduce her 250 lbs to a weight more acceptable to her fiancé.[57]

Adjusting the Metabolism

The calorie was as intangible and compelling as any spirit medium or efficiency expert might have wished for: pure energy temporarily immured in flesh and fat. Youth, strength and lightness should have been but a flame away, now that the calorie promised precision and essence in the same breath. It should have been as easy to put the body in order as it was to put the books in order for a factory.

But bodies in 1900 did not seem to balance their figures the same way business did. Metabolism—the process of energy exchange in the body—seemed quirky. A fat person might eat like Mollie Fancher or chew like Horace Fletcher and still gain pound after pound. It would therefore be another generation before the calorie would truly conquer. The problem of metabolism stood in its way.

The calorie was an offshoot of the study of animal heat. The stomach had early been thought a kind of furnace acting mechanically on food to release warmth into the body. Beginning in the 1770s, the French scientists Lavoisier and Séguin had identified the lungs as the site of a slow combustion; animal heat was not an intermittent mechanical (digestive) process but a continuous chemical (respiratory) process. Granted this consistency, Lavoisier and the mathematician Laplace then began to establish basal metabolic values. That is, they calculated the total energy (the heat) expended by a living body at rest. In 1862, Max von Pettenkofer, Professor of Hygiene at Munich, was the first to design an insulated chamber by which to assess in fine the heat given off by an adult human body. Collaborating with the physiologist Voit in 1866, Pettenkofer studied the resting metabolic rate of a fasting man inside his "respiration calorimeter" in order to calculate as closely as possible the energy lost, as it were, just by living. Voit, the son of the architect of the Munich Glass Palace, and Pettenkofer, who designed the first modern drainage system for Munich, used both architecture and plumbing to take Santorio Santorio into industrial times. By measuring the increased temperature and flow of water circulating in tubes around the insulated chamber, and by measuring the perspiration given off by the subject within the chamber (the latent heat of evaporation), Voit and Pettenkofer could make decent estimates of standard basal metabolic rates and also of the extra caloric demands of such work as standing, walking or writing. Wilbur Atwater had seen a Pettenkofer chamber in use in Munich in 1882–83, fourteen years before he had his own chamber built at the Agricultural Experiment Station in Middlebury, Connecticut. His experiments, later refined by Francis Benedict at Harvard, continued the German charting of energy expended at different physical tasks. On the basis of those charts, compiled almost exclusively from studies of adult males and then extrapolated by fiat to women and children, the first standard daily calorie requirements were issued.[58]

Unfortunately, the basal metabolic rate varied according to body size, sex, age, and physical condition. The variance was so great that calorie specifications could seem almost senseless. Fat people were fat because they appeared to burn their food more slowly and more thoroughly. They could eat small meals and grow heavier while their thin tablemates ate ravenously. It was the thin person who was violating the laws of the conservation of energy. European physiologists, befuddled, came up with a Veblenesque theory of conspicuous consumption, or *luxuskonsumption*: The bodies of thin people directly oxidized superfluous food, especially extra protein. Instead of storing the extra as fat, the body blithely burned it off.[59]

Americans were generally uncomfortable with a theory that made the thin seem wasteful. They tended to shift the burden of explanation onto fat bodies. There were, most everyone agreed, two kinds of obesity, the exogenous and the endogenous. The first resulted from a misguided appetite; fat accumulated because so much was taken in from outside. The second resulted from an "unhealthy" metabolism; fat accumulated because the internal fires burned so low. The exogenous (or plethoric or alimentary) fat man was the former Big Man, happy but no longer go-lucky, threatened in later life by apoplexy and arteriosclerosis. The endogenous (or anemic or constitutional) fat woman was the former Invalid, now stuffed with sweets and likely to die of lung congestion or the complications of diabetes.[60]

A complex and potent set of associations was at work. The aggressive, glutted consumer took on the exogenous form of obesity, while the fearful, inundated consumer took on the endogenous form. The two types represented the double-edged threat of economic abundance: the exogenous fat man was the figure of overproduction, gluttony lured on by an economy run wild; the endogenous fat woman was the figure of underconsumption, domestic inefficiency in the midst of a floodtide of goods. In each case, abundance led to fatness but not to satisfaction. The fat man could never get

TABLE ONE
THE TWO KINDS OF OBESITY IN 1900

	Exogenous	Endogenous
Other names	sthenic plethoric alimentary	asthenic anemic constitutional
Seen most in	men	women
Due to	overeating	deficient metabolism
Location of fat	stomach	abdomen, breasts, hips
Distribution	symmetrical	asymmetrical
Texture	solid	flabby
General health	good	poor
Disposition	cheerful	sad or sour
Appearance	ruddy	pale, bloated
Appetite	keen	capricious
Skin	soft, smooth	wrinkled, pimpled
Muscles	firm	flaccid (atonic)
Heart	vigorous	feeble
Blood	full, rich	thin, poor
Blood pressure	high	low
Temperature	normal	abnormal
Pathologies	heart problems	diabetes
Remedies	reduced diet exercise laxatives	electrotherapy massage thyroid drugs
Prognosis	good when young	poor at all times

enough, the fat woman could never use enough. The one packed away more than there was call for, the other could not handle what she had and so, for the time being, packed it away.

The exogenous fat man, cheerful and responsive, was easier to treat. He was a familiar figure, a companionable creature of the sensuous moment, and his diet could be abbreviated without fearing for his health. Reducing his weight was a matter of will, conviction, and the restraint of impetuosity. Prescribe lean beef, laxatives and golf.

The endogenous fat woman was much harder to treat. She was haunted by history. She could not be held fully responsible for an inherently weak metabolism.[61] Her plight was depressing. Indeed, in 1892 F. X. Dercum of Jefferson Medical College gave a new name to the most extreme cases: *adiposis dolorosa*, sorrowful or painful obesity. Dercum's disease usually affected middle-aged women whose appetites were not excessive but whose fatigue and soreness were. They had nodules of fat on their limbs, painful fatty swellings which no one could explain.[62]

No one ever did explain them. *Adiposis dolorosa* remained a predominantly American and turn-of-the-century diagnosis which made of fatigue a special pathological category. Dercum did the same in 1898 with neurasthenia, calling it a "fatigue neurosis."[63] The term *adiposis dolorosa* would linger on in textbooks for sixty years until lost in the folds of normal, undifferentiated obesity. But it was a peculiarly apt term for the consternation of male physicians dealing with fat women.

Adiposis dolorosa lingered on for so long because Dercum suspected that it was associated with thyroid inactivity. That alone was enough to keep the disease in the books, for once linked to the rising stars of the endocrine system, almost any diagnosis had a good chance of popular success. The endocrines were to metabolism what efficiency experts were to industrial production or domestic economists to housework. They managed the internal flow of work. If there was one cure for obesity most synchronous with the new kinaesthetic of balance and flow, that was the use of thyroid substances to adjust the metabolic flame. And it was what we have been looking for: something truly new.

Well, almost new. Iodine had been discovered in 1811, isolated and named in 1813, prescribed for goiter in 1820 (in toxic amounts, so abandoned), applied against scrofula by 1829 and against obesity by the 1840s. Not conclusively linked to the thyroid gland until the 1890s, iodine was nonetheless recommended in the 1850s for treatment of glandular disorders, on the supposition that its cleansing or oxidizing action might be reproduced internally. In the form of *fucus vesiculosus* (bladderwrack, brown seaweed, the common tangle), the French physician Duchesne-Duparc in 1859 tried iodine against psoriasis but was charmed instead by its side effect. It rapidly thinned fat patients. He announced this as a discovery, although fucus had long been used as a face powder and may also have been a folk remedy for corpulence. From 1859, fucus appeared in formal medical literature as an obesity cure or adjuvant, effective either as a solvent, a lymphatic stimulant, or an antiplastic drug, constricting the cells. In 1880, fucus entered the standard pharmaceutical trade in the United States through Parke, Davis & Co. of

Detroit, selling at $1.35 a pound. It was already the secret ingredient in one of the most widely advertised patent medicines against corpulence, Allan's Anti-Fat.[64]

In 1883, the Swiss surgeons Reverdin and Kocher described how the use of fresh thyroid gland from sheep improved the condition of a patient after a complete thyroidectomy. They too noted the side effect of loss of weight. In 1891, thyroid extract was used successfully as a remedy for myxoedema, a condition of thickened skin, puffy eyelids and blunted senses first described in 1873 and associated with retarded thyroid activity. By parallel to the slow motions and bloated appearance of those with myxoedema, thyroid extract was first used as an obesity treatment in 1893. Three years later, when iodine was shown to be a significant constituent of thyroxine, the thyroid hormone regulating metabolic rate, everything seemed to come together: glands, hormones, metabolism, fat.[65]

Iodine (or fucus) had been effective against fat because it substituted for missing thyroxine. Endogenous obesity—obesity resistant to treatment by dieting—was the result of a defect in the internal regulatory system of the body; there was insufficient thyroxine to keep the body metabolizing at a normal rate. Thyroid extract could be introduced into the body to turn up the metabolic furnace and burn off the unwanted fat.

This was an enduringly popular theory with physicians and laypeople alike. One physician in 1911 was convinced, like many others, "that a large number of people whom I would formerly have unhesitatingly labelled obese are in reality suffering from a minor degree of thyroid inadequacy."[66] Francis W. Crowninshield of *Vanity Fair*, satirizing metropolitan manners in 1908, noted that "Banting has almost done away with the ancient custom of eating, but thyroid tablets and lemon juice are, of course, permitted."[67] American and French actresses took fucus or "thyroidine" to keep their "youth, lightness and elegance." Over the counter or through the mails, men and women could obtain Frank J. Kellogg's Safe Fat Reducer, Dr. Bertha C. Day's Fort Wayne prescriptions, or Marmola, Newman's Obesity Cure, Corpulin, Elimiton, Phy-thy-rin, San-Gri-Na and Trilene Tablets, all with fucus or thyroid extract.[68]

Thyroid preparations would remain popular despite early warnings against such side effects as glycosuria, extreme nervousness and tachycardia. To protect the heart, physicians often served up a cocktail of arsenic, digitalis or strychnine with the thyroid extract. Others prescribed small doses or intermittent short courses of the drug, realizing that a sped-up metabolism did not restrict itself to the burning of body fat but consumed muscle tissue as well. While fucus, iodine or thyroid extract appeared in unregulated dosages in patent medicines, regular physicians usually insisted on careful supervision of such therapy, lest the cure be worse than the complaint.[69]

This supervision was part of the appeal of thyroid treatment. The metabolic approach to obesity sidestepped all issues of appetite and will power. One could reform the inefficient body by fine adjustments within the endocrine system. The threat of a runaway gland put a fine whip in the hands of doctors, who had traditionally griped about uncooperative fat women. For the fat women themselves, glandular therapy awarded each a distinctive metabolic rate, personalizing and excusing a fatness all too often condemned as a general sloth. For both physicians and fat women, the recourse to slow metabolism was a welcome escape from a bitter battle of wills. Then, too, thyroid treatments promised an escape from the hereditary curse of that slow metabolism, relieving doctors of exasperation and fat women of despair. The glands were, almost, islands of refuge.

Treasonable Fat

World War I, the Great War, was not about fatness, but from the start it was about food and soon enough about fats. In 1914 Herbert Hoover of the Committee for the Relief of Belgium was organizing the delivery of five million tons of food. He consulted the nutrition authorities, including Horace Fletcher, and he decided on a minimum daily calorie requirement based on Chittenden's standards. In 1917 Hoover became the head of the U.S. Food Administration and set an example by counting his own calories, explaining, "I'm an engineer, and I'm not using my body. An engineer does not stoke the engine unless there is a considerable amount of power to be exerted. So, I eat as little as I can to get along." He mounted a propaganda campaign to persuade the rest of the country to do the same.[70]

"Food Will Win the War" was the overarching slogan, but there were others: "Do Not Help The Hun At Meal Time," "U-Boats and Wastefulness are Twin Enemies," "Conservation, Concentration, and Consecration." There was the "Gospel of the Clean Plate" and another gospel of the "empty American garbage pail." Good manners now required tipping the soup plate to get the last drop, sopping up gravy with bread, and taking home uneaten food from restaurants. "Have a 1620 Thanksgiving in 1917," the Food Administration implored, and Irving Fisher, by now the founder of the Life Extension Institute, asked Vassar students if they could not "get a New England conscience" behind their diet. While women suffragists went on hunger strikes, women in New Orleans marched in a food conservation parade. As Gandhi began his first political fast in India, W. E. B. DuBois was promoting food conservation as an opportunity for black Americans to learn better food habits. Food messages appeared on railroad cars, on the back of sheet music, inside chewing gum wrappers. Open a telephone bill or go to a movie, you would see "Cornbread, Crust and Crumbs" or "Food is sacred. To waste it is sinful."[71]

The foods worst to waste were fats and sugar, of which there were terrible European shortages. Much fat had been diverted to use as glycerine in the manufacture of explosives, much sugar consigned to military rations as quick energy for going over the top. Civilian populations had to rely on American exports. If Hoover announced wheatless, porkless and meatless days, there were to be months of skim milk, molasses and margarine. Scientists were called upon to revise downward the daily requirements for sugar and fat and to explain how vegetable fats were as nutritious as animal fats. "Hooverizing" meant more fruits, vegetables, and corn (or rye, or Graham) flour, less meat, fat and sugar. A woman overweight by 40 lbs was to be accounted as hoarding 60 lbs of sugar in her excess flesh.[72]

Nutrition took on a military cast. Twelve young New York City policemen became the Diet Squad, living on one meat meal a day. Physiologists like Francis Benedict at Harvard finally accepted Chittenden's lower calorie and protein standards, at least for adult civilians in wartime. Dieticians were admitted to the kitchens of Army hospitals and war plant cafeterias. New foods were advertised as congenial with the national interest and food conservation. HEBE combined "the healthful properties of evaporated skimmed milk with the nutritious fat of the cocoanut," while overseas the French accused Germans of rounding up tins of condensed milk and using them as hand grenades.[73]

In such an atmosphere, reducing weight became civil defense. Gordon Lusk, Professor of Physiology at Cornell, later one of the American representatives to the 1918 Interallied Scientific Food Commission, announced, "There are probably a good many million

people in the United States whose most patriotic act would be to get
thin gradually and gracefully and then to stay thin." New Yorkers
alone carried 10,000,000 lbs of excess fat that would have been better used as rations for soldiers in trenches. "Indeed," wrote Francis
Benedict, "it may become a serious question as to whether a patriot
should be permitted in times of stress to carry excess body-weight,
for the expense of carrying it around calls for calories that other people need." It was not just the initial gluttony but the subsequent
waste of energy that made fatness a nearly treasonable condition.
Fatness was as selfish as it was uneconomical, and the Germans,
wrote Gordon Lusk, were relying on American selfishness. Selfless-
ness was a matter of self-control, generosity a matter of (mild) abstinence. The war was building character as it reduced weight, noted
the *Woman's Home Companion*: "Men and women who, for years,
have never risen from the table without a feeling of surfeit, are consciously holding their appetites a little in check." With the money
they saved from eating lighter meals, they could invest in Liberty
Bonds.[74]

"Any healthy, normal individual, who is now getting fat is unpatriotic," Dr. Luella E. Axtell told a Milwaukee medical convention
in 1919. Twice president of the Wisconsin Medical Women's Association, Dr. Axtell was perhaps the first woman doctor in the United
States to open an obesity clinic. With her husband Eugene, a physician specializing in x-ray diagnosis and electrotherapy, she practiced
as a homeopath in Marinette from 1900 until at least 1921. She accepted the idea that fat was the end result of a failure of internal
combustion, but she had learned to distrust both drugs and the slow,
long hunger of diets. Herself once obese (5 feet, 2½ inches, 203 lbs),
she would have no truck with "soft, seductive, roly-poly plumpness." Beginning in 1913, she attacked it with exercise, electricity,
massage and a short-term very-low-calorie but bulky diet. She told
the convention that even endogenous obesity could be treated
healthfully, that "inherited tendencies are not irrevocable sentences,
but . . . demand unusual precautions and constant watchfulness."
This was Maginot Line language, the rhetoric of vigilance. Long
ago Epictetus had warned the philosopher that he must "mount
guard, and lie in constant ambush against himself." A well-worn
quote in the literature on obesity, mounting guard on fat became
part of a wider literature on nutrition and good health. *Eternal energy is the price of leanness!*" exclaimed a physician just before the
war began. The other price of leanness, of course, was eternal vigilance.[75]

Fatness was careless, selfish, wasteful, treacherous and un-American. During the prewar era, for the first time, fatness had been specifically associated with immigrant groups, especially with Jews and Italians, and most especially with Jewish women prone to diabetes. Americanization began to imply an actual physical change toward uniform American (Yankee) features. Led by Frances Kellor, a partisan of industrial efficiency and national planning, American-izers during the war shifted from the policy of nurturing a rich stew of cultures to the stirring of a "Melting Pot" (from Israel Zangwill's play in 1908) and the management of a "sausage factory" (from Dickens by way of the president of the National Municipal League in 1909). This 100 percent Americanism meant a change in food habits from the ethnic to the homogenized. Assimilation was not enough. The new watchword was that of the new sanitary ideal: absorption.[76]

Fatness was messy, dirty, poisonous. "Auto-Intoxication More Deadly Than Warfare," claimed one patent medicine ad in 1918.[77] Fatness suffered by unspoken association with the constipation of the war itself, the fatigue and anxiety of the trenches, the gas warfare. Most of the heroes of battle fought in the skies, deft and light and solo; most of the victims were crowded down below, slogging heavily through mud or holed up underground. Aside from the dynamic flying aces, the war seemed as sluggish, wasteful and blundering as a fat man. Or a fat woman: *adiposis dolorosa*.

The war itself did not create the fashions, passions, or rations for leanness. It did not even strip women of the protective disguise of the corset. During the war, women were encouraged to wear corsets for support, now that they were working outside the house in jobs demanding physical strength according to an industrial schedule.[78] The war effort was not responsible for a new kinaesthetic or a new sense of physical beauty. Rather, the war confirmed efficiency and economy, balance and flow, lean strength and central command—sometimes by direct propaganda, sometimes by painfully contrary example. The Great War was not the turning point in attitudes toward fatness but the outlying arm of that spiral away from fatness that had begun after the Civil War.

Nor did the war effort revolutionize dieting. It transformed gluttony into treason, but it did not set in motion a new program for weight loss. The most influential dieting expert of the war era was Susanna Cocroft, who claimed in 1919 to have had requests for help from more than 600,000 women, and in 1920 to have reduced the weight of 40,000 of them. Like Luella Axtell, Susanna Cocroft was a Wisconsin woman, but she was a physical culturist rather than a physician. While Axtell had studied at Hahnemann Medical College in Chicago and then moved to Burlington, Wisconsin, and thence to Marinette, Cocroft was born in Burlington, graduated from nearby Rochester Seminary, took scattered courses in literature, language, algebra and aesthetics at the University of Wisconsin, then moved to Chicago, where she married a successful banker. Luella Axtell was born just after the Civil War, Susanna Cocroft during the War. In 1919, testifying before the Committee on Military Affairs of the House of Representatives, Susanna Cocroft was a poised and elegant fifty-seven.[79]

She was poised because she practiced True Functional Harmony. Good posture and proper exercise brought her "Equilibrium, equanimity, and equity." She was elegant because her figure was trim but not angular, her movements strong and economical, her breathing full and unlabored. Since 1902 she had been conducting a mail-order beauty business which consisted essentially of a series of booklets explaining poise, carriage, diet, exercise and positive thinking. Thin women could establish themselves as rounded and healthy, stout women could shed fat without losing vitality. By 1916 Cocroft was talking about physical culture as "preparedness" and concentrating less on the thin women than on the stout: "a woman overburdened with flesh, untidy in outline, suggesting physical overindulgence, in a neat, tidy, attractive, artistic home, is like a cheap chromo in an expensive handwrought frame." What was crucial was not the clean wall or the dusted table but self-respect and individuality. The "woman worth while" was present "not to beautify the spectacle, but to strengthen the cast."[80]

Cocroft was testifying on behalf of the U.S. Training Corps for Women. In 1918 the War Department had asked her help in keeping women office workers healthy. That summer and fall she led 3,500 women in daily exercises and drill on the Ellipse in Washington, D.C. Now she wanted to extend that program into private life: "We do not wish it said of America that she looks after the health of her citizens simply for war." Endorsed by the General Federation of Women's Clubs and by the Surgeon General, she was requesting land and equipment for five camps for renewing America's rundown women. At a demonstration camp during the summer of 1919, she had shown how 127 office workers, teachers and housewives could be revitalized—and often reduced—with sit-ups, swimming, rub-downs, calisthenics, and a diet limited in fats and carbohydrates. She now projected a national movement putting half a million women through two-week sessions.[81]

The next year, Cocroft was presenting herself as a "nationally recognized authority on conditioning women as our training camps have conditioned men." One of her advertisements in the *Woman's Home Companion* began, "Be Well Why Not? Be free from nagging ailments as our soldiers are free! Weigh what you should weigh! Have a perfect figure! Be happy. *Enjoy* life!" And in boldface appeared the promise, **"You Can Weigh Exactly What You *Should*."**[82]

It was very important now to know your weight. Your weight said something about your health, your physical appeal, and your state of mind. Weight had personal significance, social meaning and national bearing for both women and men. Physical, numerical weight. No more euphemisms. Hard numbers instead: **"You Can Weigh Exactly What You Should."**

But how much *should* you weigh?

CHAPTER SIX

The Measured Body

The culture of slimming became a weight-watching culture as people began to accept the notion that the body when weighed told the truth about the self. Once gluttony had been linked to fatness and fatness to heaviness, heaviness had still to be regularly identified by numbers on a scale rather than by vague and subjective sensations. When criminologists began to use weight to index character, when life insurance companies began to use weight to index mortality, and when fashions began to consider weight as an index to beauty, scales became an integral part of the culture of slimming. The penny public scale, the bathroom scale and the kitchen food scale were instruments by which the narrowing tolerances for the healthy body were given force and a substantial numerical presence. The Roaring Twenties were also the calculating, calorie-controlled, ounce-conscious Grim Twenties.

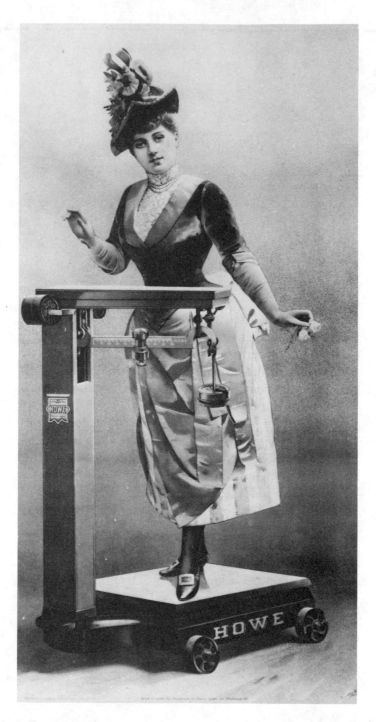

Actress Lillian Russell as a young woman posing on a Howe platform scale, from a late 19th-century company trade card. Courtesy of Special Collections, University of Vermont Library

Bodies and Minds

"**G**ENTLEMAN OF HIGH social and university position desires correspondence (acquaintance not necessary) with young educated woman of high social and financial position. No agents; no triflers; must give detailed account of life; references required."

Case Two was twenty-two years old, 5 feet, 5 inches tall, 117 lbs. "I suppose you would like some description of me," she wrote, "but I am sure I can't describe myself, though I can give you some cold facts that you might turn into an algebraic equation if you are very clever: $A = wt$, $B = ht$, $C = yrs$ $A \times B \times C = x$. Oh, I suppose that is all wrong, but never mind."[1]

Arthur MacDonald did not mind. He was after all a scientist of applied ethics and a specialist for the Bureau of Education. He believed in direct correlations between physical appearance, insanity and criminality. Since love itself had been called an obsession, an emotive delirium, a psychical neurasthenia, and an episodic symptom of hereditary degeneracy, MacDonald had placed personals in several Eastern newspapers in the early 1890s. He was offering himself as bait in this study of "abnormal women." When women re-

149

plied, he made arrangements to measure their bodies, their reflexes, and their sensitivity to changes in pressure and temperature.[2]

"Study me all you will," wrote Case Eight. "I am not trained scientifically in the method of psychology, but nothing has interested me in life so much as the human entity. I know the human heart and I warn fairly from the start, that if you study me . . . , I *will make you pay* for the privilege."[3]

Pay he did. He was fired in 1902. He seemed to be something of a crank, if not also a lascivious fool. His personals had been answered by poor housewives and society belles, by daughters of bankers and farmers. They all confided in him. He measured and weighed them. A woman in the doldrums wrote, "The outside day asserts itself again; it is raining cats, dogs, and *demons*! An indigo atmosphere surrounds me!! I am literally being wiped out! I am drowned!!!!! Chaos." He remained distant, addressing his letters, "My dear miss—madam—or what not."[4]

Son of an assistant district attorney in New York, MacDonald had studied at the University of Rochester and the Union Theological Seminary before setting sail for Europe, where he became familiar with the work of the Italian criminologist Cesare Lombroso. The problem for Lombroso and other investigators of abnormal psychology was that criminals, lunatics, degenerates (and lovers?) shared a special pathology: they lied. Either they lied in order to deceive or, because they were confused and overwrought, they mistook the unreal for the real. Willful or no, they could be trusted neither to speak the truth nor to act so that their gestures were true to their inner state. How to tell then if a criminal were feigning insanity in an attempt to avoid serious punishment, or if a manic patient were actually improving under therapy?

The answer was to key the reading of character to those aspects of the person least open to ruse. Palmists, physiognomists and phrenologists had done so in a rather static manner, relying on skin and bone structure. They might be accurate, even prophetic, but in general theirs was a science of slow motions. Palms, faces, skulls do not of themselves change their basic configurations overnight. For this very reason, police at the turn of the century could rely on the Bertillon system of anthropometric indexing and the Henry fingerprint system to keep track of criminals. A structural reading of the body might show that someone was a criminal type, but not that she or he was this very moment lying to you.

Mind-readers would seem to do that trick, but the psychometry of such as Mollie Fancher was too slippery a method, too dependent on the moods and the "nervauric impulses" of reader and subject.[5] Mind-reading compounded the problem of trust since it was so vulnerable to charges of complicity, especially in sideshow tents across from freaks and magicians.

In fact, the most successful mentalist acts relied upon the reading of subtle physical cues given adeptly by a helper or unconsciously by chumps in the audience.[6] Pickpockets, gamblers, confidence men and ladies of the night had for ages been expert in reading body movement, but their skill was dearly bought and, of course, criminal. Boxers and wrestlers, dancers and skaters had a similar skill, sensing the feint and the attack, the disguised preparation and the sudden leap, but it was hard to codify what it was they saw or felt or knew.[7]

Lombroso and the wayward MacDonald were in cold pursuit of instrumental measurements of body truth, some devices above suspicion and beyond intuition. They embraced psychophysics, a science delineated in 1860 by the German experimentalist Gustav Theodor Fechner. In his youth Fechner had written a satirical *Comparative Anatomy of Angels*, then studied physics, become a professor and suffered a prolonged nervous breakdown. During his convalescence he had a vision of the souls of flowers and was convinced of the principles of panpsychism, a philosophy equating matter and mind and making psyche all. When he turned in middle age to the study of stimulus and sensation, he was trying to determine the exact fit between matter and mind, expressed mathematically as the limits of discrimination between stimuli. From one person to the next there were measurable differences in the minimum intensity of stimulus required to provoke a response. The least sound, the least light, the least pressure (or weight) sensible to one person might be silence, darkness and absence to another.[8]

Those boundaries of perception were affected by inner or psychic stress. After years of experiments with reflex and reaction times, pressure and temperature sensitivity tests, psychophysicists built up a pattern of correlations between the strengths of these boundaries and the kinds of personalities. Since an individual's own perceptual boundaries also varied according to inner state, one could use such variances to decide the truthfulness of statements. The more a person's reaction times, for example, varied from his or her typical pattern, the more likely his confessions or her denials were false. Truth was steady because bodies at peace were true.[9]

So at least went the assumptions of the William James–Carl Georg Lange theory proposed in the 1880s. In the terms to which this theory was reduced by such as Lombroso and MacDonald, the body could not lie because the autonomous vasomotor system of the body essentially created emotions. If we could willfully inspire or terrify ourselves into the bodily expression of awe or fear, then there was little use in measuring any bodily function to get at the truth. Fortunately, it was the other way around. The nerves and circulatory system lay behind fear, tears, perhaps passion.[10]

Fortunately, too, it was becoming easier than ever to keep track of the vasomotor system. Lombroso's countryman Scipione Riva-Rocci perfected the mercury sphygmomanometer with pneumatic cuff in 1896; after that, taking blood pressure became common enough that adequate statistics could be furnished on the range of normal readings.[11] There were similar advances in the recording of nervous impulses and slight muscular motions. At last, in the 1920s, Leonarde Keeler and John Augustus Larson, American criminologists, developed the modern polygraph or lie detector. It recorded blood pressure and pulse from two parts of the body as well as changes in rates of respiration. The polygraph was the culmination of sixty years of psychophysical work to prove that "when people do not confess with their mouths, then they confess with their body."[12]

One other instrument was central to this array of lie detectors. The scale. Lombroso in the 1860s had used weight changes as the major criterion by which to distinguish the insane from impostors. It had been earlier observed that maniacs tended toward emaciation, and that if weight returned as mania subsided, the prognosis was good. Conversely, if the patient fattened while mania stubbornly grew, the prognosis was poor. Weight changes were indexes to mental condition, and weight, unlike behavior, could not be simulated or much disguised. If patients appeared to improve without gaining weight, or if patients gained considerable weight without any change in mental condition, there was a *prima facie* case for fraud.[13]

So the scale told the truth about the inner state of human beings. Weight was a guide to the mind—and, believed Lombroso, to moral stature. Thieves, murderers and whores were overweight. Following Lombroso, American investigators found adult criminals generally heavy. Frances Kellor, the Americanizer, compared white female students to white female criminals; the latter were shorter and heavier. Such statistics accommodated Yankee fears of being inundated by the stockier immigrants from Southeastern Europe. As aesthetic models became insistently slender, criminologists tended to identify male overweight specifically with rape and sexual assault, female overweight with cheap promiscuity and infanticide. If fat was the enemy of beauty, then it might well be the confederate of an ugly lust.[14]

Given the persuasiveness of the new kinaesthetic ideal of dynamic balance, it was particularly fitting that the scale should become the prime lie detector of the new century. As the body was reconceived in terms of flow, economy and efficiency, so character itself—the inner person—would come to be defined vis-à-vis the weighing machine.

Charting the Body

Braced by the truth-telling powers of the scale, weight began to carry with it a moral imperative. Overweight was less variation than deviation. Early height-weight charts had been constructed on the basis of select population averages; the charts implied that the average weight was a good weight, a healthy weight. Gradually, the charts were reconstrued to reflect not a mean but an ideal. Like the scales on which they were posted, the charts would become oracular.

The charts were promulgated by insurance companies. At the end of 1874, some 850,000 insurance policies were in force in the United States. Fifty years later, there were 92,000,000 policies in force. Premium receipts in 1874 totaled $92,500,000; in 1924, $2,250,000,000. All these zeroes made life insurance big business, big enough to account for many of the skyscrapers on the American skyline.[15]

Life insurance had reached the middle class during the Civil War, when the number of insured lives quadrupled. Insurance agents then went after the working poor, presenting themselves first as angels of mercy, next as emissaries of a lost community in an unfeeling world, finally as hard-nosed ministers from the Church of Thrift. But the Evil Eye hung over the poor, who suspected any anticipation of death. Putting aside something in a communal funeral fund, common to immigrant groups and fraternal chapters, was quite different from betting against one's own precarious life.[16]

By the 1920s, however, many American workers had been touched by insurance, whether through group life insurance plans, group health insurance or workmen's compensation laws and accident/sickness policies at the workplace. Personal health insurance was in its infancy, nursed extravagantly by the Metropolitan Life Insurance Company of New York, which by 1924 had distributed over 300,000,000 pieces of public health literature, including a popular pamphlet on overweight.[17]

Being touched by insurance meant in many cases being examined. During the 1920s, at least half of the larger American firms required medical examinations of prospective employees, and 10 percent required periodic examinations of present employees. Unions had protested that such examinations by company doctors would be used to intimidate workers, and the American Medical Association had resented this competition with private medicine, but after the Great War the medical scrutiny of ostensibly healthy people was solidly entrenched in the workaday world. Irving Fisher's Life Extension Institute provided exams in clinics and factories across the country, Metropolitan Life offered free check-ups to its policyholders, and the AMA pushed for yearly visits to private physicians. The physicals administered to draftees in assembly-line fashion during the war had led to a surge in life insurance applications; during peacetime, as one layman argued, physicals were good for doctors, since in three out of four cases a check-up would reveal some condition in need of medical help.[18]

With more than forty million life insurance policyholders and millions of others in jobs requiring medical certificates, with more than a million young men who had been run through the draft and millions of older immigrants who had been run through Ellis Island, the majority of adult Americans in 1925 were likely to have gone through a physical examination in which far more than health had been at stake. At its scantest, the exam consisted of rushing baggage-laden immigrants up and down steps in order to detect heart lesions and lung trouble, then a rapid glance at eyes and scalp to detect glaucoma and skin disease. At its most elaborate and time-consuming, the exam would have consisted of a detailed family history, urinalysis, the taking of pulse and blood pressure, the use of stethoscope and otoscope, measurement of the chest, girth and height, temperature and weight. Already in 1882 a physician had grumbled at such assault-and-battery: "Time was when the blank to be filled by the medical examiner was a model of conciseness, directness and simplicity. There was no genealogical catechism, reaching back to the third and fourth generations, no multiplied biographical cross-questioning, no remorseless vivisection, no experimentum crucis. No lantern of Diogenes." By the 1920s, whether the exam took the industrial average of six to eleven minutes or the full hour of the premium inspection, every examiner had a lantern of Diogenes, and that lantern was a scale.[19]

Whatever else might be omitted, standing on a scale had to be part of the exam. The picture of a patient on a scale, nurse or doctor hovering by the balance beam, became *the* popular icon of an exam. Not the blood pressure cuff, not the thermometer, not the reflex hammer, not even the stethoscope approached in power or in glory the role of the scale. No one compared the x-ray machine or the new electrocardiograph to anything Diogenetic or heavenly, but the *Saturday Evening Post* could refer to the scale as a Recording Angel without seeming in the least impious.[20]

Here anew was the ancient image of the Scale of Righteousness in which so often the heart was weighed against a feather. Mortality and virtue again seemed to ride on the knife-edge of the balance. Between 1901 and 1941, overweight would be statistically implicated with death, the range of variation in acceptable weight would be narrowed, and the typical weight gains of middle age would be declared unsafe. Obesity became an assassin, a sharpshooter with an eye for numbers. The pound markings on the scale assumed an earthly power they never had before.

As late as 1899, an insurance examiner bewailed the absence of statistics on how dangerous obesity really was. That same year, George R. Shepherd, president of the Association of Life Insurance Medical Directors of America, discussed some preliminary data from a number of insurance companies, all of which suggested that "from our mortality records the overweights are clearly less desirable than either the normal or the underweights." Two years later, Dr. Oscar H. Rogers of the New York Life Insurance Company reported the results of his analysis of the insured lives of 1553 men who were 30 percent or more overweight. They had an excess mortality of 34.5%. That is, a group of normal men of the same ages would have experienced one-third fewer deaths in the same period. Despite the care taken by insurance carriers to accept only the healthiest of overweight candidates, these men had died sooner than they should have. Moreover, the older the fat man, the more likely his premature death. By age sixty-five, fat men had a mortality 75 percent in excess of normal.[21]

Between 1912 and 1914, the Actuarial Society of America and the Association of Life Insurance Medical Directors published five volumes of studies summing up insurance experience, 1885–1908. On the basis of more than 700,000 insured male lives, they found that the more overweight a man was, the shorter his life, and that overweight was deadlier than a corresponding degree of underweight. Men 5 to 10 lbs overweight were slightly better risks to the age of thirty-five, then underweight was far preferable. Considerable overweight was to be discouraged at any age.[22]

This study, confirmed by others in 1919, 1923, 1929, 1932 and 1937,[23] was remarkable for its refusal to accept average weight as the healthiest weight at any age beyond adolescence. It was equally remarkable for its dismissal of underweight as an important threat. The study marked the subsidence of tuberculosis, the primary reason to dread thinness throughout the 19th century, and the rise to prominence of the chronic diseases of later life, including obesity. No matter that its weight data were unreliable, that nearly half of the weights before 1900 had been estimated by either examiners or applicants, and that most actual weighing had been done in street clothes whose bulk varied from season to season. No matter that its subject population was skewed toward the white urban Protestant and sedentary middle class. No matter that its data on women were particularly poor—since women resented intimate examinations by male physicians, wore more "disguises" (corsets, cosmetics) and an unpredictable number of layers of clothing—and yet its conclusions about overweight men were quickly applied to overweight women.[24]

What mattered was that the report lent its authority to the model of lean strength promoted on so many other fronts. Like the new kinaesthetic ideal, the report made no concessions to maturity. Before, people had expected to put on flesh as they advanced through their middle years, and extra flesh had not been medically worrisome until weight was 20–30 percent above average. The 1912–14 study saw no reason for any weight gain whatsoever after the age of thirty-five; above forty even the average weight was deemed excessive.[25]

Between World War I and World War II, height–weight–age tables were subtly adjusted downward from the average toward an "ideal weight," a term coined by the Life Extension Institute in 1923. First, a tighter noose of healthy variation was drawn around the average weight. Next, table-makers stopped adding pounds in and began subtracting pounds from the "acceptable" weights of older people. Finally, at the special promptings of statistician Louis Dublin of Metropolitan Life, table-makers began to list only "desirable" weights.[26]

This spurning of averages was encouraged by fasters, Fletcherites, physical culturists and fashion illustrators, all of whom inclined toward the lither, lighter run of bodies. Specialists in the treatment of obesity, like Dr. Luella Axtell, approved of studies showing that "the desirable weight from the standpoint of longevity is much below that which even physicians have until recently considered normal." In 1924, on the basis of the new health charts with their disrespect for averages, it could be claimed that more than half of all Americans over the age of thirty-five were overweight.[27]

The intolerance of overweight was growing faster than bodies themselves. American college students, for example, had grown 1 inch and 3 lbs in fifty years, according to R. Tait McKenzie in the *American Physical Education Review* in 1913. College gym instructors like Amherst's Edward Hitchcock (son of that earlier Hitchcock of the eupeptic millennium) and Harvard's Dudley Sargent had been among the first to keep thorough records of heights and weights. The Amherst entering class in 1861 measured 5 feet 7 inches and 134 lbs; at graduation the average was 5 feet 8 inches and 141 lbs. At Yale the entering class in 1883 averaged about 5 feet 8 inches and 138 lbs; in 1923 it was 5 feet 9 inches and 141½ lbs. In less patrician environments, the young men were slightly shorter, and in the South and Midwest, slightly heavier. Young women during the same general period grew from 5 feet 2 inches and 115 lbs (1875) to 5 feet 3 inches and 114 lbs (1893) to 5 feet 4 inches and 121 lbs (1933). Two inches and 6 lbs in sixty years.[28]

For army recruits and inductees, a population with a mean age in its mid-twenties, the Civil War's 5 feet 7 inches and 147½ lbs became World War I's 5 feet 7½ inches and 141½ lbs (or 5 feet 8 inches and 144 lbs for white troops alone), but this loss of weight reflected in part the younger mean age and different racial mix of 1918 draftees, who at 5 feet 10 inches were 4 lbs heavier than those of a similar age and height in the Union Army. This did not mean, to say the least, that young American men had become fat. The Selective Service physicians, who allowed 15 percent leeway either side of the average weight, rejected as entirely too obese less than 0.5 percent of all candidates and put 5 percent in "too-fat-to-fight" Army jobs during World War I. (They found an equal number too thin to fight.) By World War II, white soldiers in their twenties were up to 5 feet 8 inches and 148 lbs—1 inch taller and ½ lb heavier than the Union soldiers. For equivalent ages and heights, they were as much as 7 lbs heavier—after eighty years.[29]

For older Americans, and especially for older uninsured women, the statistics were cloudier. At New England fairs in 1859, men of all ages taken together had averaged 146 to 152 lbs, women of all ages 124 to 126 lbs; at a fair in Philadelphia in 1875, nearly sixteen thousand men yielded an average weight of 150 lbs, while more than seventeen thousand women stood at 129 lbs; at the Century of Progress Exposition in Chicago in 1933–34, men from twenty-five to sixty ranged in weight from 153 to 171 lbs, while women ranged from 123 to 136½ lbs. Both sexes had gained perhaps 2 inches and put on perhaps 10 lbs in seventy years.[30]

Whatever fan dance we may do with the figures, there is little disguising the bare fact that concerns about overweight had nothing to do with a newly heavy society. One might argue that those middle-aged and prosperous people who most desired insurance were the heaviest Americans, so that insurance companies had a terribly skewed picture of the population, but it seems to have been just the opposite. The 1912–14 records on insured men over thirty showed average weights that were extraordinarily *low* in comparison with other data.[31]

"Concerning obesity," commented one physician in 1927, "the amount of scientific information which we have regarding it is in marked contrast to the large amount of public opinion on this subject." People believed that Americans were overweight long before any good data had come in. By 1926, more than twenty thousand women had written to the *Delineator* asking the editors of that popular magazine for advice about their weight, while physicians admitted that they had no reliable standard weights for adult women of any age or height. At the Adult Weight Conference called in 1926 by the AMA to deal with just this statistical lapse, no reliable standards were promulgated. Nonetheless, in his address at the conference, Dr. L. F. Barker of Johns Hopkins could praise girls for reduc-

ing because "they are exhibiting a willingness to curb their natural
appetites for food and candy and for the fattening things of life for
the sake of an ideal."[32]

That ideal was enshrined by Metropolitan Life in new tables issued in 1942–43. Five years earlier, the company had published a
dramatic paper on "Girth and Death," revealing excess mortalities
ranging from 30 to 60 percent for successive levels of overweight.
The paper concluded with the motto, "The longer the belt line, the
shorter the life line." That motto went directly into the veins of public health (and patent medicine) advertising. "Shorten Your Belt,
Lengthen Your Life" read one Metropolitan Life ad in 1937, offering a weight-reducing booklet, *Overweight and Underweight*, for
which some one hundred thousand requests were received. In 1941,
the company followed up with an attack on Old King Cole. "We
Hate to Disagree with Mother Goose," the company sighed from its
tall, thin tower at One Madison Avenue, but "it isn't very likely that
anyone burdened with such excess poundage would actually live to
be *old*" or, indeed, merry. In 1942, the company produced its "Ideal
Weights for Women" and in 1943 its "Ideal Weights for Men." Both
charts were part of a patriotic wartime fairy tale. A person at the
ideal weight, like a soldier in the ideal army, would have the lowest
mortality. The best weight to keep for all of one's adult life was the
ideal weight of, say, a captain twenty-five years old. And overweight was as inexcusable among the young as it was in basic training. There was no room any more, coming out of the Depression, for
a comfortable cushion of fat at any age. "Overweight," the company announced with the stridency of a drill sergeant in 1942, "is so
common that it constitutes a national health problem of the first
order."[33]

The Problem of Fit

It was, rather, a problem of the second order: not of what was, but
of what should be. The nation had not grown suddenly heavier;
rather, the tolerances had narrowed. What had been acceptable before was no longer acceptable. The body had to be perfectly honest
with its mortal self. As Brenda Ueland wrote for the *Saturday Evening Post* in 1930, "those women who are now trying so desperately
to get thin are perfectionists. . . . They have taught themselves not
to edit their figures when they look in the mirror. . . . [T]hey want

to look actually slim—slim, long, sinewy, panther-like"—and Ueland admired them. She herself had been "fat and woggling" in her youth in the 1890s, dismayed by "the curtailed action, the disgusting hard-shell matronly appearance, the beetling hips" of her obesity. Her biography, *Me*, was an account of one battle after another to find a body and a career that would fit the tolerances of a perfectionist century.[34]

The success of ready-made fashions and standard sizings made the problem of fit that much more important. Ready-made clothiers polled by Edward Atkinson in 1887 thought American men were growing larger; they were being obliged to adopt a larger scale of sizes "and many more extra sizes in width as well as length, than were required ten years ago." Atkinson—who had made his wealth in the fire insurance business and then invented the Aladdin slow-cooking stove to improve domestic economy, who would finance the Scientific Eating movement and work with Atwater on nutrition and Fletcher on chewing—took this demand for larger sizes as evidence to rebut European slander that white men across the Atlantic were degenerating. Atkinson was proud to reveal that American men were growing stouter, their waists wider. His sartorial chauvinism, however, obscured the issue: Did a change in demand imply a change in proportions?[35]

The demand had more to do with questions of fit than of physique. Though Americans were indeed growing, their bodies were moving up as fast as they were moving out. What the ready-made clothiers were experiencing was a demand for sizes to fit those whose proportions did not follow those of the perfect man. This did not mean that there were more overweight (or underweight) men than before, but that fatter men (and thinner men) wanted clothes that would keep to a minimum all signs of deviation from the physical standard—no bulges, no unnecessary material, no obviously forced stitching, no awkward flapping or goring. In the days of personal tailoring, trousers had required exact measurements and had met a fashion for tightness that ended around the time of the Civil War. By the end of the century, fashionable trousers were somewhat looser but creased to present as long a vertical line as possible down from the shoulders of the square coat now in style. If, at work, blue collars and loose overalls finally distinguished laboring men from the white collars and tailored suits of men in offices, on the promenades the classes had the same fashion lines in mind. The difference was that the poorer men, buying ready-made clothes, were constantly brought up against standard models of the body based on

Civil War measurements of relatively youthful soldiers, while the richer men could retain the traditional tailor and an individual, aging form. Ready-made extra-large clothing in the 1880s came in response not to greater gluttony but to a greater self-consciousness about a standard, youthful male body.[36]

In women's fashions, "Stylish Stouts" and "Full Form Suits" appeared in ready-made clothing around the time of President Taft's administration (1909–13) as M. Gross & Co. established the Stout House of Philadelphia and Lane Bryant began to manufacture clothes for "nearly forty percent of all women who were larger in some or all of their dimensions than the perfect 36 figure." Again, this did not mean that women had grown heavier or rounder. Again, it was a question of fit. In a world of bicycles and then of self-starting automobiles, of snapshots and then of motion pictures, of flexible dress-forms and then of flesh-and-blood women modeling clothes in public, those who felt overweight could no longer rely on presence, drapery and posture to compensate for mass. Nor could they rely on tight-lacing; corsetry was slowly turning toward lighter, more elastic materials rather than fully girded forms. Underwear became more closely fitted as bulky underskirts vanished. New sanitary pads and disposable sanitary napkins freed underwear of other obligations. With shorter hair, fewer layers of clothing and higher skirts, the body was forced to be honest or, at least, subtler in its own disguise.[37]

By 1919, for the first time in more than a century, the summer clothing of a woman would on average weigh less than that of a man. For women whose bodies plainly did not conform to the youthful silhouettes of ready-made fashions, the relative freedom from undergirdings and superstructure was a mixed blessing. Now the outer dress itself would have to do what had been done before by half a dozen artfully managed layers. Thus the renewed interest in the techniques of optical illusion: how to appear to have a longer waist, a thinner body, a lighter frame. "Stout people, to look well, must study how to appear as slender as possible." The more they studied, the more they would wear navy blue or black with vertical lines, slender jewelry, soft collars and noiseless materials. No large or glaring patterns, no jangling trim, no noisy taffeta or satin, no striking colors. The clothing designed for the Stylish Stout was clothing designed to be inconspicuous, to fit in.[38]

Fat women were therefore to be especially clean, dry, odorless. As if, almost, they would leave no trail. Their perfumes must be light, their corporeality unpresuming. Deodorants, advertised since the 1870s, would become more desirable after the turn of the century as fatness and heaviness were implicated with other unpleasant aspects of the body: sweat, bad breath, body odor. Neutraline, Mum, Odorono, Ever Sweet were intended for anyone who had ever danced in a crowded ballroom, but they would hold a special attraction for women (and men) who had been made to feel heavy and obtrusive.[39]

In any era, there are problems for those whose bodies do not come close to what is fashionable. But now the tolerances were finer, the standards harsher. Women had less clothing to manipulate or hide behind. The mode for almond-shaped eyes and shorter hair made cosmetic disguise more difficult; wrinkled foreheads and fat necks lay open to view. Men no longer had beards to cover up double chins, and tight belts were slowly replacing expansive suspenders. There was more athleticism to recreation, more leggy dancing, more physical examination as a matter of course. And better eyesight.

The Body Seen More Clearly

The body measured more obsessively, charted more precisely and fitted more closely was also being observed with greater clarity. The eye troubles that forced the young Frederick W. Taylor and Simon Patten to withdraw from study were common in the late 19th century. Students and neurasthenics complained of blurred eyesight, garment workers and telephone operators of eye strain. Diseases of the eye, "eminently diseases of the poor" according to an 1828 Boston report, were in 1898 the occupational hazards of tobacco workers, of women shellacking pencils using wood alcohol, of steelworkers and machinists laboring under arc lights, of grinders and polishers exposed to fine metal particles. One-third of two thousand college women examined at the turn of the century had defective eyesight. Nearly one-fifth of the first million draftees in World War I were rejected for defective vision. Children contracted corneal infections during measles epidemics, got lesions on the eye from chicken pox, or suffered gross vitamin deficiencies and lost distance or night vision. Treated with opium eyedrops, potato poultices, eyewashes of zinc, witch hazel, golden seal or eyebright, their vision would remain dim.[40]

Fashion did not help matters. The more extensive use of eye makeup and commercial face powders led to eye infections from impure chemicals in cosmetics, from small particles of alum lodging in the eyes, or from the hairs of brushes used as applicators. Fashion also frowned on eyeglasses. Even Teddy Roosevelt in his thick glasses was scorned at first by the Rough Riders.[41]

Glasses were a particular problem. Myopia and presbyopia could be corrected by concave and convex lenses which had been available commercially since the 16th century, but more often than not the degree of lens curvature had been haphazardly matched to the wearer. By trial and error, one picked one's glasses from a heap in a stall or at an oculist's. With the invention of the ophthalmoscope in 1850 and the Snellen sight test in 1862, the fitting of glasses for near- and far-sightedness improved considerably. Indeed, the ophthalmoscope was used as a lie detector against those who feigned myopia in order to avoid being drafted; the scope enabled physicians to determined the degree of optical distortion by consulting the retina itself. Like other lie detectors, it relied upon the body— and not the devious words of nervous young men—for the truth.[42]

Correcting for distance vision (and for fraud) was a small part of the problem. The greater problem was to correct for distortion along the vertical or horizontal axis. Aside from an astronomer and a mathematician or two, people had long been unaware of their own astigmatism. Not until the publication of a seminal work by the Dutchman Frans Cornelis Donders in 1864 did physicians begin to realize the extent of this visual distortion among the general populace, and it was years before symptoms of astigmatism were dissociated from mental exhaustion or neurasthenia. S. Weir Mitchell noted in 1892 that many a case of headache and vertigo (like Taylor's) could be handled by the simple prescription of a pair of glasses. At century's end, just as the necessary cylindrical lenses became easily available in the United States, astigmatism was the most commonly diagnosed of visual defects.[43]

By the 1920s, there were goggles for workers in heavy industry, electric lights and windows for garment workers, silver nitrate for the eyes of infants, vitamin A and sunshine for children, safer cosmetics for women, and fitted glasses for anyone with myopia, presbyopia or astigmatism. Stimulated in part by the visual demands of early motion pictures, sales of optical goods (primarily eyeglasses) increased thirtyfold between 1880 and 1929. This meant that the visual blur with which millions of Americans had lived was no longer acceptable. If Brenda Ueland's "perfectionist" women had taught themselves not to edit their figures when they observed themselves in mirrors, this was in good measure because they could no longer count on an accommodating blur in the public eye.[44]

Public Weighing: Penny Scales

The finer the tolerances, the greater the anxiety for a good fit. The more important one's precise weight as an index to character and mortality, the more elusive the "ideal" weight and the more often one had to weigh oneself. The occasional curious step onto a fairground scale would not be enough.

Fairground scales were heavy platform scales designed for commerce, agriculture and industry. "Hemp fever" in Vermont in 1829 had led farmers to expect fortunes from the raising of hemp, but they needed a means to weigh hemp by the wagonload. The traditional steelyard scale was inadequate; it could take nearly twenty minutes to weigh a single load, and bulky loads were difficult. Thaddeus and Erastus Fairbanks, given the contract to manufacture hemp-dressing machines at their foundry, in 1831 also patented a platform scale with a mechanical advantage of 112 to 1, which solved the problem of heavy loads while making the weighing procedure much simpler. The platform scale placed most of the weighing apparatus *beneath* the load. By means of knife-edge pivots at the tip of A-shaped levers, the platform transmitted the weight to an easily balanced beam with a small counterpoise. Bulky wagons, railroad cars, even canal barges could be weighed by extending the length of the platform. In 1857, the Howe Scale Company, also of Vermont, began to manufacture platform scales whose knife-edges were protected by the interposition of ballbearings between platform and pivot. The ballbearings absorbed shocks and vibrations, reducing the wear on the pivots and improving the long-term accuracy of the scale.[45]

Between the Fairbanks and the Howe companies, most fairs were provided with public weighing machines whose design and function had little to do with human bodies. The companies encouraged personal weighing at fairs as good publicity for the accuracy and convenience of platform scales in stores, farms and factories. Posters and trade cards often showed a man, a woman or a child on these scales, always dwarfed by them or posed so daintily above them that their cast-iron solidity overwhelmed any impressions of human weight. At Philadelphia's Centennial Exhibition in

1876, the Howe Scale Company gave people printed cards with their weight inscribed to the quarter pound as evidence of the precision of the mechanism and the new visibility of the balance beam markings, but the shape of the scale remained disproportionate to the human form, as it would also be when ex-President Grant was weighed on a Howe scale at the Paris Exhibition in 1878 or when the folks of Charleston received weight certificates in 1880 after stepping off a Howe "monster platform scale."[46]

By 1891, the Fairbanks Scale Company had redesigned one platform scale for human loads of 300 lbs or less. It looked much like the commercial platform scale in shape, but it had cherrywood trim and was portable enough for hotels, clubs, racecourses and athletic facilities. It was meant as well for doctors' offices and insurance examiners, whose forms had begun to insist on exact weights.[47]

If the examiner did not own a scale (cost: $70–$100), he was advised to take applicants to the nearest grocery or drug store.[48] There, by 1900, they would find a new scale designed from the very start for the shape and the weight of an adult human body. It was the penny scale, and almost from the beginning it boasted a height-weight chart and a mirror.

Coin-operated scales had been patented as early as 1870, but the first working penny scales in this country were lugged over from Germany in 1885. They weighed 600 lbs, had mahogany cabinets, and were modeled after grandfather clocks. In 1887 the first American penny scale was created by Blauvelt Joy & Blauvelt, who cast an exquisite monument to foundrywork rather than to commerce. In 1888 the Watling Manufacturing Company of Chicago began the production of more businesslike penny scales. Over the next fifty years Watling would be joined by a dozen other prominent companies and a hundred smaller firms. Together they would put at least half a million penny scales in railroad stations, subways, pharmacies and groceries, then in bus stations, restaurants and five-and-dimes, then in movie theaters, banks and office buildings. The Commissioner of Health for Chicago put a scale in the lobby of the City Hall in 1922. There were lines in front of it all day long.[49]

At first, penny scales had the large, round public face of a clock; gradually that clock face shrank or was replaced by a peephole on a pedestal or by a printed ticket with date and weight. At first, penny scales were loud, ringing as they weighed, chiming the Anvil Chorus or "Oh Promise Me," or speaking the weight by means of a hidden phonograph record; later they were quiet. The shift from publicity to privacy, from the sociable to the personal, was a semantic shift from the third person to the second person and from the declarative to the subjunctive—from *what this person weighs* to *what you should weigh* and *what you could be.* There were plaques on the columns of scales: "Your Doctor Says Weigh Yourself Daily" and "Did You Weigh Yourself To-Day?" By the late 1920s, penny scales gave your fortune and the portrait of an aviator or a movie star: *what you could be.* As the scales departed in shape from the grandfather clock, stolid and paternal, they departed from the passive present tense and entered the realm of the active ideal: the sleek silhouette of a woman in evening dress, the streamlined thrust of a skyscraper.[50]

Weighing on a penny scale was less a search for information than a search for fit. You would weigh yourself several times a day to check daily diurnal variations, small personal changes. You would weigh yourself on scales set side by side, or try different scales in different places, or try the same scale three times in a row, searching for the number that best fitted your own sense of what you should weigh. A scale with a coat rack was a big success; you could divest yourself of that extra, wrong weight. Guess-Your-Weight scales, which returned your penny for the accurate preplacement of an inset pointer, were the finest embodiment of the notion of fit. Manufactured since 1904, their popularity in the 1920s and 1930s reflected a growing belief that you should know your exact weight. These scales had stingy, almost impossible tolerances of half a pound (what you would gain by drinking a glass of water), several degrees more rigorous than the "ideal weight" charts printed alongside the pointer.[51]

By definition the penny scale was a slot machine, and you gambled against it. There were scales with three slots at the top, testing your intuition. (All the slots actually fed to the same channel, and a penny would return on the *fourth* try, regardless of slot.) There were yet other scales which returned a penny every so often as "your share of the profits." But this gamble (or this sporting capitalism) was ultimately less important than the gamble on your weight, which the insurance companies insisted was as much a gamble with death as with beauty. You played the scales with a poker face, and surreptitiously: "I am sure that many of you have meekly slipped off the scales, as I have, scarcely waiting long enough to see what weight was actually registered, praying meanwhile that no one saw where the arrow pointed." And you knew that the scale would always call your bluff: "I was fat as fat, or else the machine had lied. And as between me and that machine, I could pick the liar at the first pick."[52]

As a business proposition, the penny scale was not much of a gamble. In 1927, 500,000,000 weights were registered by some 40,000 penny scales. Most of that $5 million was net profit to split between the distributor (the Peerless Scale Company, the Mills Novelty Company) and the daily operator, the grocer, the druggist, the theater manager who changed the date on the printing wheel or simply kept the machine spotless. A chain of five-and-dimes in 1926 had $500,000 in profits off its penny scales, $600,000 in 1929. A single scale could hold from 8,000 to 30,000 pennies and might take in as much as $20,000 over its lifetime. At an initial investment of less than $150, a penny scale could pay for itself in months if only ten people an hour tried their luck. A bystander watching one scale in the New York subway in 1928 counted twenty people an hour, or one every three minutes. In less busy parts of the world, as for example a Virginia town of 3,500, two scales accounted for 500 weighings each per month. "It's like tapping a gold mine," exclaimed the Mills Novelty Company brochure which gave these figures around 1932. At the 1933 Chicago Century of Progress Exposition, the largest return on any investment came from the Guess-Your-Weight scales.[53]

The Peerless Scale Company, major distributor of penny scales, was worth $50 million in 1929 and did not suffer much during the Depression. The penny scale was the machine of the times, honest and yet prophetic, giving as good as it got. It was so widely used that a national conference of weights-and-measures officials in 1932 proposed a code to keep the scales honest. Even banks put penny scales in their lobbies. Their scales issued tickets which had, instead of fortunes, penny receipts of deposit good for opening an account.[54]

So the most plebeian and yet most oracular of vending machines would not fare badly during the Depression. People saved their weight cards, which were at once a personal medical record and a set of promises about what lay ahead—marriage, fame, money, children, good health, the end of troubles. Penny scales, like the new Bally pinball machines, offered the right balance of skill and luck, fit and fortune. The scales shared too in the success of that revolution in merchandising which had begun in the 1890s with coin-operated gum machines and by the 1930s included automats, laundromats, public telephones, subway turnstiles, and mechanical dispensers of sanitary napkins and condoms.[55]

If the penny scale had a failing, it was immodesty. The penny scale was a public lie detector that could not truly do its work because its patrons were too modest. As doctors and diet experts continually reminded people, the best weight records were those taken on the same scale at the same time every day in the nude. Even patent medicines sold by mail requested information on "disrobed weight."[56] A high number on a penny scale could too easily be excused as the weight of the nickels in one's pocket or the heavy brogans on one's feet or. . . . How far could one disrobe in public?

Private Weighing: Bathroom Scales

The finer the tolerances, the more naked the body had at last to be. The drive for fit brought the act of weighing into the most personal of arenas, the bathroom and bedroom. One-fifth of American households had indoor flush toilets in 1920; one-half had them in 1930. While the bathroom was being drawn inside the house and the "master" bedroom was being set farther apart, the scale entered each as if to confirm the privacy of both.

Scale companies had begun to respond to a demand for bathroom scales at the turn of the century. This was a small market, and the first private scales were no different in shape or principle from platform scales in doctors' offices. They cost half as much ($18–$36), accepted a lower maximum weight (250 lbs), were enameled in a more delicate color (pale blue), and had a slightly taller pillar for the easier reading of the balance beam by the person standing on the platform. The first picture of such a scale actually in a bathroom dates from a 1918 advertisement by a company that sold plumbing fixtures. By this time, the scale had been slenderized and domesticated, but it had the old round face of the public scale.[57]

Another, more private bathroom scale had appeared in Germany. It was featured in Chicago in 1913 in Marshall Field's new household utilities department. The Jarasco scale was essentially a counter scale converted to a floor scale to fit human feet and support a human body, but its dial was still placed as if it were to be read at waist level. So awkward was this placement that the scale came with a mirror canted at the proper angle to permit a standing person to see the dial far below. Despite the awkwardness, the scale was a success at under $10, and Marshall Field did well with it until World War I.[58]

Their supply cut off by the war, buyers for the department store turned to the local Chicago Scale Company, where they found an engineer who had the first American patent (1916) on a bathroom scale. Mathias Weber's invention differed in two principal respects from the German model: its weighing mechanism and its dial. The Jarasco worked as a typical knife-edge ballbearing-protected platform scale; Weber's worked on the Roberval or parallelogram principle, with spring suspension. One vertical arm of the parallelogram was stationary, the other was movable, attached to the platform above and a spring below. A person standing on the platform depressed the movable arm and so compressed the spring that the properly calibrated weight was registered according to the tension of the spring. Such a design was advantageous to a small scale that would be banged, shoved, hoisted up and slammed down in bathrooms early in the morning or late at night. But no blurry-eyed consumer would notice the technical ingenuity beneath the cast-iron exterior of this 1917 Madaco scale. What consumers would see, happily, was a dial mounted just below and ahead of the scale platform, a dial designed in explicit imitation of the speedometer on the dashboard of a car.[59]

Through his barber, Mathias Weber found two investors to help him establish an independent firm for the production of his bathroom scale: Alfred Hutchinson, an engineer, and Alfred's brother Irving, who was in pursuit of an investment prospect to match the excitement of his Stutz Bearcat. In early 1919 this barbershop trio founded the Continental Scale Works to manufacture and sell one thing: the Health-O-Meter bathroom scale, 8 inches high, painted white, list price $16 and guaranteed accurate within 1 lb.[60]

In 1921, the Jacobs Brothers of Brooklyn, who had been supplying pushcart peddlers and butchers with commercial scales, entered the bathroom scale business. By 1925 they claimed that their Detecto scale was "used by over 1,000,000 people." Whether or not they meant that they had *sold* a million bathroom scales, business was good enough to encourage yet another company to market a low-profile bathroom scale, the Hanson Weigh-Master, in 1926.[61]

All scale manufacturers used weight charts and medical opinion to bolster sales, but bathroom scale advertising was intent on investing the scale with a lifelong universal gravity. "From the cradle to the grave," read a Fairbanks Health Scale brochure in 1922, "the personal weight of every human being is an almost infallible indicator to his or her state of health." The brochure pictured the Health

Scale (a platform scale of the old design) in the living room as well as the bathroom. The Jacobs Brothers took their Detecto across generations "From Grandchild to Grandfather," and from the playroom to the bedroom. The personal scale was to be with you from birth to death and in nearly every room of your house, a constant companion bringing you "Health, Wealth and Happiness."[62]

A constant, truthful, snow-white companion, the bathroom scale was the perfect scale for "the long pull" of dieting. Hanson and Continental issued their own diet books to promote their bathroom scales, which made daily weighing so much easier and so much more rigorous. "Beauty is here today and gone tomorrow unless it is under the guiding hand that never errs," read a Continental brochure in the 1920s. The company insisted on the narrow tolerances of beauty: "A few pounds underweight and the delectable curves give place to ugly angles. A few pounds overweight and the graceful contour of youth has become heavy and unpleasant." The weight charts alongside the Health-O-Meter were all based on weighing in the nude.[63]

With the appearance of the personal or bathroom scale, weighing became newly intimate, newly sensual. Weighing was intimate now not only because it was private but also because it shared with the bathroom and bedroom mirrors the daily rituals of personal scrutiny. The Detecto was the Detecto, after all, because "It Detects." And weighing was sensual now not only because it demanded nudity but also because it demanded the close alignment of two bodies. The 19th-century advertisements for platform scales showed beautifully dressed young women on toe-point, floating over the cast iron with nary a glance toward the weight marked on the balance beam. Advertisements for the smaller bathroom scales in the 1920s showed women in towels, slips, girdles or bathrobes bending over toward the dial in provocative balance. With the scale platform 8 to 12 inches high and the scale itself liable to tip over if one stood off center, the act of weighing was literally a balancing act, excellent allegory for the daily concourse of Beauty and Truth.

Beauty stood here above the Truth. The low-profile bathroom scale drew the eyes groundward to read the weight, as if weight were something that kept one down. The industrial platform scale, the doctor's scale and the public penny scale presented the weight at waist level or above. The bathroom scale presented the weight at one's feet. In the 1930s, as profiles were streamlined and brought even closer to the ground, the bathroom scale would seem to draw its powers far less from a celestial justice than from an earthly retribution. When Beauty set foot on Truth, she became Persephone enticed by the bloom of the narcissus, carried off for a time to the underworld. If the Detecto scale was "a practical gift that is true and forever remembered," it could be no less than mythic and not a little daemonic, like other detectives of the age: Batman in his cave, the Green Hornet in his abandoned building, and of course the Shadow, who knew what evil lurked in the hearts of men, and of women.[64]

Weighing Food: Kitchen Scales

Forty years before the Detecto entered bathrooms and bedrooms, the Little Detective had entered kitchens. Sold by the Chicago Scale Company in the 1880s, the Little Detective was not the first kitchen scale, as the Detecto was not the first bathroom scale, but its name, like that of the Detecto, caught best the meaning of its presence. "No one is so poor that he should not have a scale of some size under his own control," read an 1874 catalogue from the Jones Scale Works of Binghamton, New York. "Every family can save the price of a scale by reweighing after their Grocer or Butcher. Not that they are necessarily dishonest, but when it is known that you have a scale, they are less liable to make mistakes." This scale, called a family scale, was on the family's side, a detective in the employ of consumers at a time when the weighing of commodities must have seemed unusually suspicious. During the late 19th century, businessmen and physicists alike were clamoring for the standardization of weights and measures; muckrakers were protesting the adulteration and short-weighing of ingredients; grocers and butchers were beginning to change over from the familiar pan balance to strangely automatic self-indicating computing scales. In the midst of a new world of chiming cash registers, clicking adding machines and clacking typewriters, scales too had gone a bit berserk. How comforting to have a simple scale of one's own, with weights one could trust.[65]

After the creation of the National Bureau of Standards in 1901, the passage of the Pure Food and Drug Act in 1906, the addition of a Net Weight Act in 1913 to assure proper marking of packaged goods, and the stiffer inspection of public and commercial scales, the kitchen scale came to be used less defensively. Cookbooks which had scorned or ignored weights, listing most ingredients by volume, began to recognize the virtues of a scale accurate to the ounce. Recipes demanded precise weighing of food, with little tolerance for pinches and snippets. The Woman's City Club of Chicago in 1912 mailed out ten thousand postcards urging housewives to buy not by volume but by weight. Now volume was deceptive, weight honest.[66]

In the 1920s, the kitchen scale became as central to dieting as the personal scale. This was a significant switch from a century before, when even Grahamites generally refused to teach "that we should weigh our food, and limit ourselves to *so many ounces*, and watch over ourselves constantly, for fear something will go wrong, till we actually make ourselves sick by it." In 1871 the prospect of weighing out one's food appeared speculative, almost utopian, to the neurologist George Beard: "If the time ever arrives when physiological chemistry is an exact science, so that by a mathematical computation of the changes of tissue that take place in the body, we can determine precisely the amount of nutriment that the system demands at each meal, it may be possible to apportion our meals by the scales, as is done with prisoners and paupers." Not long after, in 1888, a professor of hygiene at New York Medical College was willing to advocate "the unusual feature of letting the scales determine the amount of food to be taken," and within a generation American doctors were recommending that their obesity patients in particular have all their food weighed out carefully. During the 1920s, physicians would give patients short courses in weighing food, training them toward such sensitivity that they would eventually become human extensions of the kitchen scale, able to measure by eye the weight of portions of food.[67]

Atwater and the physiological chemists were partly responsible for the eminence of the kitchen scale. They had come up with the tables about which Beard had merely speculated. But it was one thing to publish charts of nutrients, ounces, and daily requirements, quite another to weigh out food at every meal in daily life. Doctors, nutritionists and wardens might rely on kitchen scales in hospitals, prisons and insane asylums, but living by the kitchen scale in one's own home . . .?

The avant garde were the diabetics. Diabetes mellitus was an ancient disease, common in India by the 2nd century but uncommon in the West until the late 18th century. Von Fehling's chemical test for sugar in the urine, devised in 1849, made the diagnosis of diabetes simpler and the awareness of diabetes more widespread, but there would be no adequate medical treatment until Banting and

Best isolated insulin in 1921. Meanwhile the therapy was dietetic, often resembling the diets prescribed against corpulence, with which diabetes was (and still is) frequently linked. On a low-carbohydrate and high-protein diet, the typical diabetic would live less than five years from the time of diagnosis. (On a high-fat diet, much less.) Surely a new approach was necessary, especially as the incidence of diabetes was rising markedly. Between 1860 and 1900, the diabetic population increased 150 percent; the death rate from diabetes nearly doubled between 1900 and 1915.[68]

In 1914 Dr. Frederick M. Allen of the Rockefeller Institute Hospital in New York introduced a program of modified starvation for hospitalized diabetics, with a follow-through program of weighed foods for diabetics at home. He was seeking explicitly to reduce those who were overweight. Patients were to calculate food intake by grams and to remain on a low-calorie diet. Widely adopted, this new diet added more than a year to the lives of adult diabetics, who were provided with tables of carbohydrates, protein, fat and calories. Of necessity, they had to own and to use kitchen scales. Daily. At every meal. On penalty of death.[69]

In 1921 Dr. Elliott P. Joslin of Boston, America's authority on diabetes epidemiology and himself a man of 300 lbs, reported on his study of more than one thousand diabetics. Forty percent had been obese before the onset of diabetes in middle age. He thought diabetes therefore "largely a penalty of obesity, and the greater the obesity, the more likely is Nature to enforce it." He approved of the current fashion models "whose sylphlike figures are models of weight and height—nay, more, they are invariably a trifle below the standard weight and so might bear the legend: 'immune to diabetes.'"[70]

So closely tied were obesity and diabetes by 1921 that when Banting and Best isolated insulin, they prescribed with it a low-calorie, low-carbohydrate, low-fat diet that required the weighing of foods. For the next decade at least, the insulin syringe and the food scale would be inseparable. Scale manufacturers (Hanson, Chatillon, Jacobs Brothers, Pelouze) began to market small "diet" or "dietetic" scales measuring in grams up to a kilogram. While public penny scales proclaimed their honesty in bold, sociable letters across their faces, diet scales were to be known for their intimate, scientific accuracy. You could banter and gamble with the penny scale, but you bought the diet scale because you could not afford to guess.[71]

Scales, Pounds and Calories

It was a small transition from the diabetic use of the weighed diet to the popular use of the weighed diet to ward off incipient diabetes. If, as Dr. Joslin said, the obese were two to forty times more likely to get diabetes then reducing their weight before any symptoms of diabetes appeared would make sense, and the weighed diet would also make sense. Though in 1933 Joslin noticed fewer fat diabetics, that did not mean the country could scrap either the bathroom scale or the kitchen scale. There were thrice as many deaths from diabetes among doctors themselves in 1932 as in 1902, and 1938 estimates of the number of diabetics in the United States ranged from half a million to more than two million. Many, still, fat.[72]

As the logic for the weighed diet worked backward from the avant garde of diabetics, it also worked forward from the Hooverizing of the Great War, during which many healthy people had become accustomed to the notion of calories. Sarah Tyson Rorer's cooking school courses in 1892 had made no reference to calories, but by 1917 her *Key to Simple Cookery* specified daily caloric requirements. During the war, calories represented power: The power in food was the power in fuel was the power in explosives was the power to win the war.[73]

The first popular weight-reducing diets geared to calorie-counting appeared just before the war: Gustav Gaertner's *Reducing Weight Comfortably* and Vance Thompson's *Eat and Grow Thin*. Gaertner, a Viennese physician, had reduced more than 1,600 obese patients by instituting a low-calorie, high-anxiety diet. Since calories were proportionate to the weight and not to the volume of food, kitchen scales were absolutely essential. Gaertner himself invented two such scales. "*Without scales*," Gaertner wrote more than once, "*no cure.*" In comparison, Vance Thompson's "Mahdah Diets" were a relaxed presentation of calorie-counting as based on dietary charts prepared by the U.S. Department of Agriculture in 1911. Thompson, married to actress Lilian Spencer, was a Princeton graduate, a playwright, and founder of *M'lle New York* magazine. His menu suggestions were expensive and glamorous. Still in vogue in the 1920s, reaching its 112th printing in 1931, *Eat and Grow Thin* associated beauty with the Orient and the panther, fatness with illness and embezzling.[74]

Bonded as they must be to the food scale or to the practiced eye, calorie-counting diets were from the start encumbered with the rhetoric of law and justice. The "scientific" accuracy of the diet scale did not free the personal scale from its obligation to judgment. When Dr. Robert H. Rose wrote *Eat Your Way to Health* in 1916, he called calorie-counting "a scientific system of weight control" and obesity "Criminal Negligence." Of course, one could cheat on any diet, but images of "sinful" foods, of crime and punishment, would most prevail where the two sorts of scales were most in tandem. If, as Christine Terhune Herrick wrote in her *Lose Weight and Be Well*, the bathroom scale was "a sort of materialized conscience," then the diet scale was the guard at the gate.[75]

Near the end of the war, in 1918, appeared the first edition of *Diet and Health, With Key to the Calories*, dedicated (by permission) to Herbert Hoover. The book would reach its sixteenth edition by 1922 and remain in print for the next twenty years. The first weight-reducing manual to become an American bestseller, *Diet and Health* stands yet on the all-time lists with 800,000 hardback copies sold. The title itself was in imitation of another sort of bestseller, Mary Baker Eddy's *Science and Health, With Key to the Scriptures*—though now calories had become the sacred numerology.[76]

Lulu Hunt Peters, author of *Diet and Health*, was an overweight Episcopalian, born in Maine but at home in California, where she got her M.D. in 1909. During the 1920s she became "undoubtedly the best known and best loved woman physician in America" through her syndicated newspaper health columns, where she emphasized that three out of four adults in this country were disgracefully overweight. Unlike her Midwestern contemporaries like Susanna Cocroft who gave as much advice on how to get plump as how to get thin, Peters was not interested in helping anyone gain weight, "for I cannot get your point of view. How anyone can want to be anything but thin is beyond my intelligence." This signaled a change in attitude more permanent than any wartime passions against fat people as traitors hoarding food. Calorie-counting diets, like the scales they depended upon, would have low tolerances for any excess, any kind of fatness; they had more in common with sackcloth and ashes than with banting. Indeed, Peters's weight-reducing program began with a fast ("to show you are master of your body"), then continued with a low-calorie diet and Fletcherism. She worked with the 100-calorie portions proposed by Irving Fisher in 1906, with the Chittenden standards of (lower) protein and calorie requirements, and with weekly personal weight charts. Weight-reducing began with a starvation boot camp, then basic training on 1,200 calories a day, then a lifelong tour of duty called the Maintenance Diet, with constant calorie-counting. Always? "Will they always have to keep it up? . . . Yes!"—just as people must always be neat, kind, tender and loving. So the counting of calories would become a quality of personality, akin to vigilance or devotion. Like early Christian Science, caloric science demanded only faith and fortitude to be effective. Peters supplied forms for writing testimonials on behalf of her diet.[77]

Calorie-counting in the 1920s became part of the menus of the Childs restaurant chain, each plate identified by its caloric value. Calories were part of fashion advertising: "Rounded Slimness is the subtle part of every smart ENSEMBLE. . . . We must glow with health while we grope with calories!" Metropolitan Life used 100-calorie portions as the centerprice of its own Home Office reducing program. Neither cookbooks nor dieticians could shake the 100-calorie habit. Irving Fisher's *How to Live*, which sold half a million copies and was in its eighteenth edition by 1929, spent pages on how to count calories. In 1931, army doctors were advised to maintain "an obesity consciousness," and army dieters were to "think of all foods in terms of carbohydrate, proteins, and fat, and know that each gram of carbohydrate furnishes four calories; each gram of protein four calories, and each gram of fat nine calories." Pocket-sized calorie calculators (paper) began to appear. With all this counting going on around him, one wag suggested, "Why not at polite dinners a tastefully engraved invitation with calories listed?"[78]

A calorie-counting dinner would be a low-calorie affair. The tendency of calorie-counting was toward less food for everyone. Where fat was "a physical crime," when there could be "no alibi for fat," when the formerly globular citizen Samuel G. Blythe could conceive of a balanced diet on a thousand calories a day, the old energy requirements of three to four thousand calories would seem exorbitant if not fatal for all but lumberjacks. Calorie-counters tended to reduce the standard to 2,500 calories for those who were acceptably slim. For the overweight, the tolerances were even finer. An innocent switch from boiled to fried potatoes would yield 14,508 extra calories over six months; three extra pats of butter a day would produce 25 lbs of fat in a year. The numbers mounted up if you did not watch them with the eyes of a hawk. That old pathfinder, Hawkeye himself, would have been astonished.[79]

The apogee (or the nadir) of calorie-counting was the very-low-calorie diet (600–750 cals) instituted in medical circles around 1928 for severe cases of obesity. By 1938 this diet was down as far as 400 calories daily. (By comparison, the Banting, Oertel and Salisbury diets had been between 1,200 and 1,600 calories daily—not counting Banting's cordials and grog.) The interim success of such radical diets was used to prove that it was food, not metabolism, which accounted for overweight, and that one's glands were rarely an excuse for obesity. There could be no escaping the calorie.[80]

The Grim Twenties

The calorie was a figment, as invisible to the naked eye as the stars being counted by patient women at Harvard's observatory around 1900, and as much a cultural invention as the waist being measured on bathing beauties in the Miss America contests of the 1920s. There *were* calories, and distant stars, and waists, but one found them by extrapolation from scales, spectra and tables of symmetry.[81] Calorie-counting became "second nature" because calories belonged to a different order of nature from food, just as ideal weight was of a different order from actual weight. As a habit of seeing through and beyond food, calorie-counting gave dieters a power which no scale could equal. Scales measured immediate bodies and dispensed random fortunes, but dieters could truly anticipate the future: so many extra, invisible calories would mean so much extra, visible fat.

The counting of calories was a visionary act. The finer the tolerances, the more one had to shift from portraiture to prophecy, from an intolerable present to an invocable presence. That same desire for a reconciliation of body and spirit which had informed Spiritualism now informed dieting. The body was recast in terms of units of energy. The ideal person on the Other Side was a person become (the pun was there) light.

This system of beliefs held for fabric and flesh as well as for foods. While one counted the invisible calories, one shaped one's body with as invisible a presence as possible. Women's corsets between 1913 and 1930 were further elasticized, lightened and softened until they turned into corselettes, wraparounds, scanties. The Lady of France corset appealed because "You can wear it invisibly!"

Brassieres were now designed to fit distinct breast sizes and shapes. Corsets were designed over live, moving models. Girdles, once worn over a chemise, were snug against a (deodorized) skin. Elastic panels maintained body lines without boning or steels, as if the body could be left without artifice. In 1931 latex thread made it possible to weave low-cost, lightweight, two-way-stretch fabrics to shape and hold irregular bodies, while smaller zippers promised nearly seamless garments. In 1936, when corset manufacturer S. H. Camp sponsored the national tour of the "Transparent Woman," the connection between "scientific" supporting garments and the desire for invisibility could not have been clearer.[82]

Stronger, thicker, heavier garments became specifically reducing devices, catering to the "short stout," the "stubby stout," the "long stout" who were most difficult to fit. Sheet rubber union suits (for men as well as women), rubber girdles and bras took on svelte style lines of their own, lighter and more chic in the midst of all that perspiration. The old-fashioned Dowager Corset for stout figures became the "Flatter-U" foundation and the "Flatter-U" brassiere of the Kabo Company, which published its own booklet on dieting in 1922. Though the Scott Hip Form had been advertised in 1905 as "Form-fitting, invisible, reversible, light in weight and thoroughly ventilated," those promises were better met as ready-to-wear sizings in the 1920s expanded to incorporate the ten million women who were heavy and the tens of millions of others who were normal but misshapen.[83]

For those who felt desperately fat, who could not abide or would not be held by any arrangement of elastic panels and gussets, there was a more drastic approach to the invisible. That it should be popularly recognized in the 1920s as a treatment for obesity was further proof of the narrowing tolerances for overweight.

The surgical removal of fat from the abdomen dates back to Roman, Talmudic Jewish and Byzantine times, if we can trust scattered stories of great men submitting to heroic excisions. The first modern abdominal lipectomy was reported in 1889 by Howard A. Kelly, a professor of gynecology at Johns Hopkins who sliced layers of fat from the pendulous abdomens of obese women (and men) in hospital for other surgery. Over the next thirty years, there were sporadic notices of similar operations abroad (France, Germany, Russia) and across the United States, enough so that by 1920 the idea of plastic surgery for severe obesity was accepted with equanimity by Drs. William S. Sadler and Lena Kellogg in their popular book,

How to Reduce and How to Gain. In 1922 Dr. Max Thorek of Chicago began recommending what he called "adipectomies" for less severe cases. Adipose tissue, he argued, was a serious ailment affecting mental poise and vigor as well as health; plastic surgery was a responsible way to deal with fat, especially for those whose professions were handicapped by their overweight. He had operated on a young dancer, a young singer, a young nurse, and a thirty-year-old housewife. The operation was simple; one only had need of "artistic genius" to leave behind as little evidence of the operation as possible. By 1926, Dr. Joseph C. Bloodgood (*sic*) was warning the audience at the Adult Weight Conference that the all-too-frequent beauty operations could lead to complications, but from the other side of the same podium he noted the dangers of excessive fat during many surgical procedures. Tolerant of fat as an aesthetician, he was intolerant of it as a technician. In 1932, when a procedure was devised to create a new or false umbilicus after removing skin and fat from a drooping abdomen, both the aesthetician and the technician could rest easy. As the perfection of technique was invisibility, so the preservation of beauty (and efficiency) must be handled invisibly: "vanishing" creams, calories, scalpels.[84]

There was an eventual grimness to these Gay Twenties, as there usually is to tales of the invisible. The decade had begun with a good-humored "Jack Sprat" debate sponsored by the National Press Club on the topic, "Resolved, that it is more noble to be fat than lean." In the affirmative were two plump Republicans from the House, in the negative were two rangy Democrats from the Senate. Jasper Napoleon "Poland" Tincher, Representative from Kansas, argued for an amendment to the Book of Deuteronomy, such that "Thou shalt have no other gods before me" would read "Blessed is the fat man, for he shall be in the Kingdom of Heaven." "I can prove by the actuary of any insurance department in the world," said Tincher, "that the fat men are closer to Heaven than the lean men." To this there was no rebuttal by Senator Pat Byron Harrison of Mississippi, for indeed Tincher had lost his case in the making of it. Instead, Harrison (distant relation of the presidents Harrison and once a semiprofessional baseball player) made cruel fun of his "old, fat, reactionary" opponents: Tincher, appropriately, raised "a lot of big, fat hogs"; Sam Winslow (Republican of Massachusetts) was a roller skate magnate, "and I am not unmindful of the fact that he slips away from Congress sometimes and goes up in his planes to New England and on his roller skates he glides around like a camel and with all the grace of an elephant." Sam Winslow in (his own) defense was curiously confessional and diplomatic. He admitted to having been fat all his life, to having performed at the age of twelve as James the Fat Boy and having been called Jumbo on the baseball field. The fat man after all is "a cheerful critter," popular, a "master of sentiment," and did not fat men rule the world?

Senator Henry Ashurst of Arizona had the last word. A tall man, range rider and lumberjack in his youth, now customarily dressed in splendid black-braided coat and striped trousers, Ashurst was less genial and more to the point than the others. "To think of a man being fat and noble," said Ashurst, "is like thinking of an iron balloon, of lazy lightning. . . . Nothing fat ever enlightened the world." Fat men were neither intellectual nor spiritual, neither heroic nor industrious. How ludicrous it would be to associate nobility with "some hill of tallow, whose legs are giant columns of flesh, whose torso has the capacity of a hogshead, who has a dewlap like an old jersey cow, whose nose is red and bulbous, whose jowls are the jowls of a Berkshire, who has three double chins on the back of his neck."

The Speaker of the House, moderating the debate, called for a voice vote of ayes and nays from the audience, then declared the question still in doubt. Speaker Gillett, however, was a Republican, and his hearing on that evening may have been less than acute. Keith's Theater was crowded for the debate and, as the *New York Times* noted, "the event marked the first time that all the Ambassadors and Ministers of the diplomatic corps had turned out in force for an extra-official occasion." Before such an assembly, at a time of famine in Russia and Central Europe, with Herbert Hoover a national figure and Prohibition on the books, it is difficult to believe that the Senators did not have the edge. They had made fat men out to be animals and anachronisms, clumsy and dull, and their opponents had merely been jocular and good-natured, more apologetic than defiant.[85]

The decade closed in 1930 with a short, quiet afterthought on the aims of reducing, which were "to make the patient feel better, to make him look better, and to enable him to carry on with increased vigor and pleasure. I mention these aims first," Dr. William M. Ballinger wrote from the nation's capital, "because, strange as it may seem, we sometimes are so gratified by the reduction of weight that we fail to inquire how the patient is feeling."[86]

Where then, between the stern straits of penny scales, bathroom scales and diet scales, were the flappers, fast cars, bathtub gin, Charles Atlas, Hollywood vamps and all that jazz?

The flappers were chewing gum and smoking cigarettes. Silph Chewing Gum or Slends Fat Reducing Chewing Gum or Elfin Fat Reducing Gum Drops. Lucky Strike Cigarettes. The gum had laxatives, sugar and wintergreen. Lucky Strike had class. Aviatrix Amelia Earhart, actresses Constance Talmadge and Alla Nazimova knew enough to "reach for a Lucky instead of a sweet." (Men too: Al Jolson, actor John Gilbert, Lt.-Gen. Robert L. Bullard.) It was the "Modern way to diet! Light a *Lucky* when fattening sweets tempt you. . . . The delicately toasted flame of *Luckies* is more than a substitute for fattening sweets—it satisfies the appetite without harming the digestion." Smoke might get in your eyes, but it had no calories.[87]

Fast cars were in the hands of those who made and sold bathroom scales. The first of the Health-O-Meters had a dial modeled after a car speedometer. The chief salesman for the Jacobs Brothers scales raced against an airplane around the track of the Indy 500. George Borg, "Mr. Clutch," who made his fortune from the automatic clutch, went into the bathroom scale business in 1936.[88]

Nearby, the bathtub was full to overflowing with Every Woman's Flesh Reducer (Epsom salt, alum, camphor, baking soda and citric acid), Lesser Slim-Figure-Bath (cornstarch, baking soda, borax and sensational advertising), Florazona (baking soda, iodides, perfume and $20,000 annual gross), Fayro bath salts (Epsom salt, table salt, perfume and 1.5 million packages sold by 1931), the Slenmar Reducing Brush and La-mar reducing soap (potassium iodide, sassafras, bathroom soap and 200 to 300 orders daily). Once the tub was empty, there would be Tumminello bathtub exercises, pulling against the faucet.[89]

Angelo Siciliano had sand kicked in his face on the beach at Coney Island in 1909. He stood in front of the lion's cage at Brooklyn's Prospect Park Zoo in 1910 and discovered the natural leonine principle of pitting one muscle against the other to achieve strength and symmetry. By 1916 he was a famous strongman and a model. He became the "Dawn of Glory" in Prospect Park, "Patriotism" at the Elks' National Headquarters in Chicago, Alexander Hamilton in front of the U.S. Treasury Building, and George Washington in Manhattan's Washington Square. In 1922 Bernarr Macfadden named Angelo the World's Most Beautiful Man; in 1922 Angelo renamed himself Charles Atlas. He began a mail-order business almost immediately, but not until 1928 did his most famous dynamic tension ads begin to appear in such magazines as *True Detective*,

Popular Science, and *Moon Man.* When a 90-lb weakling sent away for the Atlas course, the return mail would bring isotonic exercises, homilies on cleanliness, a low-fat and moderate diet, a recipe for a Salisbury morning drink of warm water and lemon juice, and instructions on fletcherizing food, including the chewing of water and milk. The Atlas program was fully compatible with the finer tolerances of the 1920s and with the most popular of the exercise diet books, Frederick A. Hornibrook's *Culture of the Abdomen* (1922, 18th ed. 1952). Atlas's sense of physical beauty was as classical as that of Elizabeth Arden's in the same era, and like the Arden beauty salons, his course worked strenuously on posture, grooming and complexion. The Atlas course would reduce fat as well as build muscle, more effectively than the Battle Creek Health Builder which vibrated the chewing-gum mogul William Wrigley, Jr., or the electromechanical horse that rocked Calvin Coolidge in the White House.[90]

Across the country, Hollywood vamps were being pummeled by Sylvia. The unwanted child of an opera singer, she studied massage in Copenhagen then emigrated to Chicago, where she headed a large health institute during and after the First World War. She made friends in Hollywood and was soon working on a much overweight Marie Dressler. By 1925 Sylvia was ensconced in Hollywood, 4 feet, 8 inches and a bit under 100 lbs but massaging with such intensity that "fat comes out through the pores like mashed potato through a colander." She reduced Jean Harlow's waistline and Norma Shearer's legs, kept Mae Murray in trim, tailored Gloria Swanson and Ina Claire. Her tolerances for the body were so narrow that it was said she would find something wrong with anybody, even the Queen of Sheba. Shape and build concerned her more than weight, but she believed that "You should have scales in your bathroom just to put the fear of God in you." With each mauling she delivered a blow for a low-fat diet, lecturing on the value of spinach, liver, whole wheat toast and steamed vegetables.[91]

For the stargazers, there would be the Hollywood eighteen-day 585-calorie diet of grapefruit, oranges, Melba Toast, green vegetables and hard-boiled eggs. Sylvia of Hollywood gave diet advice in *Photoplay*, while Constance Talmadge testified on behalf of the thyroid drug Marmola, advertised in *Motion Picture*. Fanny Hurst began dieting according to "that strange branch of lower mathematics, the counting of calories," in 1931. There were rumors of Hollywood deaths by dieting all through the Twenties, brought out again by the collapse of Louis Wollheim in 1931 after he lost 25 lbs in one month to keep the part of the managing editor in that sprinter's play, "The Front Page."[92]

As for all that jazz, the "King of Jazz," Paul Whiteman, had lost 113 lbs in one year to sue for the hand of his beloved Margaret, who then wrote a diet book, *Whiteman's Burden* (1933), dedicated "to the 24,000,000 fat people in the world generally." Her book began with a new version of an old favorite:

> Just you, dear, and me
> To share a calorie
> Moonlight, spinach, and you!

A Retrospect

"Reducing has become a national pastime . . . . a craze, a national fanaticism, a frenzy," wrote one journalist in 1925. "People now converse in pounds, ounces, and calories." The national hero was Charles Lindbergh, nicknamed Slim. In 1931 Francis G. Benedict, now director of the Carnegie Institute's Nutrition Laboratory, thought the weight reduction wave may have receded a bit, "yet even to-day the interest in weight reduction is so great that the lecturer on physiology, medicine or nutrition has but to introduce the words 'weight reduction' at any part of his discourse to change a quiet, sleepy group into an eager, agitated, expectant band of zealots."[93]

If we seem to have arrived prematurely at a passion so much more commonly associated with our own times, it will be good to review the path we have taken. We shall have as our guide a short, quick steam engine of a man, born in 1852 and still going full throttle in the 1920s. He was a surgeon and an inventor, an editor and a cook, father to forty-two waifs, guardian angel all in white and probably a millionaire.[94] We have met him in passing at the start of the Civil War and again as a friend of Horace Fletcher. We meet his brother every day in the aisles of supermarkets or across the breakfast table. Kellogg is not an unfamiliar name.

John Harvey Kellogg began to work at the Seventh-Day Adventist press in Battle Creek, Michigan, in 1864 at the age of twelve. He set type for the Adventist magazine *The Health Reformer*, read the works of Sylvester Graham and Dio Lewis, and stayed often with the prophetic leader of the Seventh-Day Adventists, Ellen G. White. White's own experiences at the Dansville Water Cure led the young Kellogg to study at the Hygieo-Therapeutic College in New Jersey. From there Kellogg went on to medical study at the University of Michigan, an M.D. at Bellevue Hospital Medical College in New York City, and in 1876 to the directorship of the Adventist sanitarium in Battle Creek. A busy and popular man, he would seem thereafter to be doing an impossible number of things at once, but we shall follow his career as if he lived out the chapters of this book in clean sequence.[95]

GRAHAMISM

Around 1863, James Caleb Jackson of the Dansville Water Cure baked Graham flour and water in thin sheets until the mixture was hard and brittle, ground it up, baked it again, ground it up again, and baked it again. He called this first successful cold breakfast cereal Granula. Kellogg, convinced that American dyspepsia was due to hasty eating of improper foods, wanted a healthy predigested food to serve patients at his sanitarium. In 1877 he baked up his own version of Jackson's cereal, stirring in several different grains and calling the result Granola. He was not satisfied. He was looking for the ultimate Grahamite process: turning each flake of grain into a flake of toothsome toast. The secret was a tempering process he came upon in 1893. Pleased, the doctor added these Granose Flakes to his Sanitas Company line of diabetic, dietetic and infant foods. Will Kellogg, John Harvey's younger brother, put some sugar in with the malt and corn of one of the flaked cereals. Corn Flakes by 1906 was doing so well that the brothers created a separate company for that product alone. Because Frank J. Kellogg, no relation but also of Battle Creek, was taking in cash hand over belly on national advertisements for obesity cures, and because 108 different brands of corn flakes were being packaged in Battle Creek after the Kelloggs lost their patent on the process, Will Kellogg began signing his own name across the front of the boxes of Kellogg cereals in proprietary self-defense. Fifty million packages of Corn Flakes would be sold under Will's name by 1929. Corn Flakes were Sylvester Graham's greatest (indirect) legacy to the American public, a food that was at once a medicine and a comfort, each flake meant to be as pure, digestible and wholesome as home-baked bread.[96]

THE BUOYANT BODY

The Battle Creek Sanitarium was the chief water cure center in America from the 1880s on, and John Harvey Kellogg the most influential hydrotherapist. His annual health almanacs sold as many as 200,000 copies each year. His magnum opus, *Rational Hydrotherapy* (1st ed. 1900) sold 15,000 copies despite its encyclopedic technical account of every faucet of water cure. His popular works had pages on medicated baths and many more pages directed against Sunday dinners, desserts and gluttony. His water cures for obesity involved cold rain douches, sweating packs, cold dripping sheets, short plunge baths, electric arc light baths, sunbaths. Though still worried about indigestion, he shifted gluttony away from dyspepsia toward obesity, whose treatment he distinguished from neurasthenia by the low-fat, lean-meat, green vegetable and pure water diet he prescribed for fat patients.[97]

THE BALANCED BODY

Partisans of the Kellogg regimen and visitors to the Battle Creek Sanitarium included dancer Ruth St. Denis, economist Irving Fisher, scientific forest manager Gifford Pinchot, and physical culturist Joseph H. Patterson, founder of the National Cash Register Company. Kellogg's operating principles were fully compatible with the new kinaesthetic ideal promoted by dancers, efficiency experts and home economists. With his wife Ella, Kellogg established a School of Domestic Economy in 1880 and a School of Health and Home Economics in 1904. Meanwhile, he was applying the principles of economy and efficiency to the treatment of overweight. He had studied electrotherapy with George Beard, had been impressed by the display of Gustaf Zander's exercise machines at the Centennial Exhibition in 1876, had visited Zander's Mechanico-Therapeutical Institution in Stockholm in 1883. That year he began teaching massage for women and invented a vibrating chair to stimulate abdominal organs. The next year he discovered a means for using high-frequency oscillating (sinusoidal) current as a form of passive exercise, though such ergotherapy would be credited later to the French physician Bergonié. By 1896, Kellogg's Sanitarium had vibrating chairs and platforms, trunk rollers, chest beaters and stomach beaters for exercising and massaging fat people, who were coming to be the mainstay of the place. At the Sanitarium, fat people would be trimmed, energized and rebalanced.[98]

THE REGULATED BODY

Kellogg was a gifted surgeon, quick and neat. His specialty was the repair of the sphincter. As he restored muscle control to the bowels, he sought to extend "sensitive colon conscience" to the habits of daily living. People should wear soft white flannel from ankles to neck to keep the pores—those "2,000,000 little sewers"— open. The worst of germs were bacteria in the intestine, which caused putrefaction and, yes, autointoxication. Rather than excising the offending colon, Kellogg promoted bran and Fletcherism, the bran to scrub the intestines and the slow chewing to limit bacterial opportunities. The Kellogg Food Company began selling sterilized bran in 1908; during the 1920s Kellogg's All-Bran became part of reducing diets, adding bulk and iron for satisfaction and health during weight loss. Dietician Margaret Sawyer in 1927, frustrated by the uphill battle for healthy eating, identified the history of dietetics first and foremost with the campaign for the use of bran: "Woman who is trained a dietitian is born to trouble as the food goes downward. She rises up with her spinach and bran only to be smacked firmly and put in her place. . . . To the consuming fire we consign thee—BRAN. Ten thousand dietitians have wept over thee in vain." But she was overstating her case. It was fat that was burning up and bran that would remain.[99]

Kellogg introduced "fletcherizing" as a verb in his magazine *Good Health*. Converted to Fletcherism in 1903, Kellogg helped Fletcher organize the Health and Efficiency League of America. At the Sanitarium, the staff sang Fletcher's chewing song which began, "I choose to chew because I wish to do / The sort of thing that Nature had in view." The motto "Fletcherize" was cut into the arch above the entry to the Grand Dining Room. The family at home, Kellogg said, could save as much as a dollar a day in food costs by chewing well. With such prospects of health through economy, was it any wonder that financier C. W. Barron and U.S. Treasurer W. A. Julian were frequent visitors to Battle Creek? Or that the Sanitarium attracted the great volume merchandisers of the times: John D. Rockefeller, J. C. Penney, Montgomery Ward, Mrs. Walgreen, S. S. Kresge? Kellogg's program, like the business strategy of many of his guests, was intended to keep the body (the corporation) flowing and regular.[100]

THE MEASURED BODY

Kellogg used a plethysmograph, an ergograph and a pneumograph to measure muscle work and lung power. True health could be told by machines sensitive to the body's strength and energy. Kellogg's own strength was considerable, but his calculated energy intake was half that of the average American; if he with his ferocious schedule required only 2,500 calories daily, then those confined in state hospitals, prisons and asylums needed even less. He persuaded the State of Michigan to reduce its daily institutional ration from 5,000 to 2,000 calories. At his Sanitarium, every portion of food was weighed out on kitchen scales in the serving pantry. From 1904, the caloric values of portions were shown on the menu, inspiring Irving Fisher's 100-calorie standard portion.[101]

As the Sanitarium came to handle more than seven thousand patients a year during the 1920s, Kellogg's reducing regime of a low-calorie, high-bulk, moderate-protein diet with daily baths and exercise would be spread throughout a wide network of the national elite. The Naval Academy would adopt his exercises. By 1935, 300,000 people had been to Battle Creek as patients; millions of others, less wealthy, had read his books, tracts and magazines. In 1943, while Kellogg lay dying, teachers would order 142,000 copies of the Kellogg Company booklet, *Health from Day to Day*.[102]

John Harvey Kellogg was born within six months of the death of Sylvester Graham. He has taken us, as a sort of coda, from the end of the world to "A Kellogg's Good Morning," from crackers to flakes, from bread to bran, from vital economy to Pep, the new cereal of the 1930s. He has taken us from dyspepsia to obesity and from the water cure to calorie-counting. For him, as for society at large, overweight became more and more disturbing, more and more the mainstay of the $135,000 annual profit of the Sanitarium. Even the Sweetheart figure on packages of Kellogg cereals would soon be slenderized.[103] Kellogg's parents had been abolitionists; now he was seeking to free the body from another sort of slavery.

CHAPTER SEVEN

Hearts of Darkness, Bodies of Woe

During and after the Depression, fat began to seem more stubborn and more dangerous than ever because more centrally fixed—to the heart. Metaphorically, fatness was linked to an inestimable sadness and a hunger that could never be satisfied. So appeared the amphetamines, liquid formulas and group dieting meant to limit that hunger and appease that sadness. Physiologically, fatness was linked to arteriosclerosis and heart attacks. The cure here was exercise, to deal with a newly energetic fat, invasive and (it seemed) purposeful. Given a new moral architecture of the body that typed people according to build as endomorphic, mesomorphic, or ectomorphic, fat people (endomorphs) were further isolated by their own unfortunate but hereditary frames. Dieting had then to be lifelong, a constant vigil over oneself.

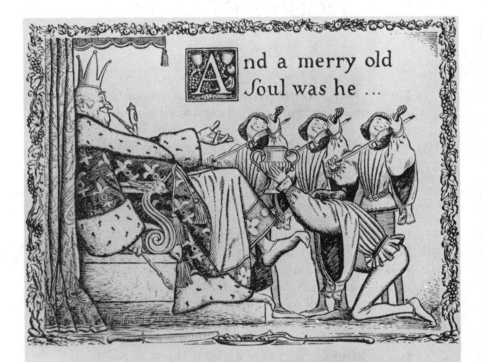

Banner and cartoon from a 1941 Metropolitan Life Insurance Company
advertisement which argued that Old King Cole could hardly have been
merry when he was so fat. Courtesy Metropolitan Life Insurance Company

Depression Dieting

DINITROPHENOL is a derivative of benzene. It was a common agent in the synthesis of those aniline dyes—mauve, bright yellow, shocking pink—which appeared in women's fashions after 1856. It was the main constituent of certain explosives used during the Great War. In 1936, perhaps 100,000 people were taking it to reduce their weight.

At low dosages dinitrophenol speeds up metabolism by as much as one-half. Dieters on dinitrophenol could lose 2 to 3 lbs a week more assuredly than on any laxative or thyroid compound. Like its contemporary, sulfanilimide, dinitrophenol promised to be a miracle drug.

Dieters taking dinitrophenol felt warm. They perspired. They noticed rashes forming on their skin. Some lost their sense of taste. Some went blind from cataracts. A few died. Whether they had bought Corpu-lean, Formula 37 or Slim, they were taking poison.

Dinitrophenol had been noted as an industrial toxin since 1889. It had poisoned workers in munitions factories during the Great War. Absorbed through the skin or inhaled as a dust or fume, dinitrophenol is not neutralized by the body, nor is it easily washed out of the system by liquids. The higher the concentration in the body, the faster the metabolic rate. Eventually there is a fatal hyperpyremia. That is, the body succumbs to an extraordinarily high fever. It burns itself up.[1]

Physicians who experimented with dinitrophenol as a reducing agent had in mind a controlled burn. It seemed possible in 1933 to light as careful a fire under a depressed metabolism as the New Deal meant to light under a depressed economy. The *New Republic* explored this analogy while heralding dinitrophenol as a possible wonder drug. If dinitrophenol were truly safe and effective, then an economic revolution would follow. "Those who now suffer from obesity will be able to work harder and be more productive than before, and will probably thereby come into conflict with future interpretations of the Industrial Recovery Act." Perhaps the drug should be suppressed for the national good?[2]

By 1938 dinitrophenol had been suppressed. Even in low dosages it was very dangerous to diabetics. Further, dieters tended to exceed the recommended dosages on the principle that twice as much of a miracle drug would produce twice as great a miracle. The result, of course, was hyperpyremia.

The more recalcitrant fat seemed to be, the more entrenched was the culture of slimming and the more drastic the drugs and diets. Dinitrophenol was but the harbinger of a new attack on fat which was meant to be stringent and thoroughgoing. The Depression did not put a stop to the national "frenzy" for reducing. Indeed, as one diet author wrote in 1935, the word "reducing" now referred to salaries, dividends, wages, budgets, credit and the gold content of the dollar as well as to weight. The Depression could prove a blessing in disguise: "If the truth were known, there are probably many people . . . 'reducing' during this depression period in order to take a slice off the food bill." A single radio broadcast on reducing could bring 35,000 letters. When Victor Lindlahr, a diet personality, held a radio "reducing party" in 1936, he had 26,000 people nationwide joining him. The diet book he wrote sold close to half a million copies.[3]

Rather than curtailing dieting, the Depression decisively shifted the emphasis in dieting from production to consumption, from metabolism to appetite, from glands to calories. Throughout the 1920s, calorie-counters had had to contend with arguments that no matter how little they ate, their glands would manage to lay away some fat. In the 1930s, the theory of endogenous obesity among adults was put on the back burner as dinitrophenol took its toll. Just as New Deal economists denied that the Depression was a symptom of internal contradictions within the capitalist mode of production, so leading American physiologists denied that obesity was a symptom of internal contradictions within the human metabolism. The issue for both the New Deal economists and 1930s physiologists was consumption. Appetite.[4]

As a result of lengthy experiments with basal metabolic rates, exogenous–endogenous distinctions between types of obesity had become so blurred that by 1933 Dr. Russell M. Wilder of the Mayo Clinic would "confess" his "inability to distinguish between the so-called glandular forms of obesity and those of exogenous origin." The consensus among biomedical researchers was that there could be no *luxuskonsumption*, that the obese did not have a systematically lower metabolic rate, that obesity was not a problem of metabolism for any but the rare few with true thyroid deficiencies, and that if something on the inside was wrong, it was not the glands but the mind. "Many obese patients sincerely believe that they are not large eaters and mention with hope and longing some gland trouble," reported Dr. Frank Evans of Pittsburgh, pioneer of the very-low-calorie diet. Such patients, he advised, should be reminded of the law of conservation of energy and given to understand that "the weight is made up of tangible material, and that there is no gland with an aperture through which it can be introduced. It may be observed that the material is not rubbed through the skin, does not enter the eyes as views, nor through the ears as sound." Fat might be insidious, even (as calories) invisible, but it was not insubstantial. Glands could not make something out of nothing.[5]

Plainly, fat people were fat because they ate too much. But why did they overeat? As dieting during the Depression shifted from a concern with production (metabolism) to a concern with consumption (appetite), theories about the causes of obesity shifted from the biological to the psychological.

Broken Hearts: Fatness and Sadness

Hunger by itself was not to blame. Physiologist Walter Cannon in 1911 had shown that hunger was associated with gastric contractions. This was an ancient idea, but it seemed newly confirmed by x-ray studies and stomach tube experiments. Anton J. Carlson in

1916 supposed that gastric contractions might be prompted by blood sugar levels, and others looked for some homeostatic (glucostatic) mechanism in the central nervous system. For the next forty years, hunger would be defined as an unconscious and primitive physiological phenomenon. Because unconscious and primitive, it could be trusted. Hunger was honest.[6]

Herbert Hoover should have known better than to question such hunger. After all, he had been the world's expert on hunger during and after the Great War. But in 1930 his administration hovered between production and consumption, pushing for greater manufacture but advising thrift. The dams he so loved were his economic model: energy and profit through industry and restraint. When basic hunger appeared, he was unwilling to disrupt the budget for relief measures. That would be "squandering ourselves into prosperity." People turned their empty pockets inside out, called them "Hoover flags," and went hungry.[7]

Appetite was another thing altogether—deceptive, conscious, physiologically diffuse, stricken by emotions and fixed by habits. It had to do with desire and nostalgia rather than with need. Pavlov had shown that the appetites of dogs could be stimulated entirely apart from hunger, and American farmers had begun to use self-feeders to fatten their stock "because it lies in the nature of the beast to get fat." In modern human society, appetite also overrode hunger. If nutritionist Clara M. Davis at Berkeley in the 1930s could prove that infants would choose the right kinds and amounts of food when left to themselves, she was helpless to prevent their natural hunger from being swamped by the appetites of modern civilization. It was in this sense that *Fortune* in 1936 could take up the old Grahamite claim that "the stomach is a liar. It pretends to be concerned with the digestive system, whereas in reality it is in the pay of the nervous system."[8]

In reality, the stomach was under contract to the mother. As "Mrs. Consumer," as "The Nervous Housewife," as chief cook and bottlefeeder, the mother was responsible for appetite. Whether isolated in the private and increasingly suburban homes of the 1920s, or segregated in relatively low-paying service jobs, or surrounded by children and chores on the tenuous small farm, women were seen as gatekeepers. In the house they managed the flow of food and love; on the job they made telephone connections, arranged appointments, took inventories, carried out doctors' instructions. They were middlewomen, brokers of desire. They handled the things of a middle world: perfumes, flavorings, aromas, drugs, cosmetics, messages. Where they entered higher echelons, they entered the worlds of fashion or advertising. Realms of appetite.[9]

During the Depression, as food became a special concern, and again during World War II, as food was rationed, the role of the mother as the mistress of appetite came under close scrutiny. Between behaviorists on the right and Freudians on the left, the mother was caught in the middle of an impossible situation. Since women's jobs were often more Depression-proof than men's, women could become the primary breadwinners for their families, but then they would be charged with taking jobs away from working men and neglecting wifely duties. Children would develop bad food habits in their mothers' absences, overeating to compensate for missing love. If women stayed home, focused on germs, meals and children, they would tend to express their frustrations and their love through indulgent foodgiving. Their children would be fed too much or would of themselves overeat as an assurance of love to an insecure, isolated mother. It was a narrow strait between the sheer rock of uncaring and the turbulent whirlpool of "maternal overprotection," a phrase made popular by psychiatrist David Levy in 1938.[10]

In such circumstances, fat people could not possibly be jolly. However cheerful they seemed on the outside, their appetites and their overeating had to be symptoms of an inner emptiness. Fat people were paradoxically incomplete people, fearful of sex, adulthood, independence. Psychologists and psychiatrists gave examples from their casebooks of fat women who saw their fat as a fetus, of fat men who substituted food for sex. Fat protected a fragile self. Too distant or too close, the mother had not bequeathed these children security or autonomy, and so they were cautious, anxious, and depressed, or angry, bored and lonely. As more women after World War II were shunted from industry and college to early marriages, maternal investments in children became even fiercer, and the mother loomed even larger in the sad café of obesity. Generations later she remains there still, an Albee-like antagonist in the slow ballad of *b*oredom, *a*nger, *l*oneliness, *l*ethargy, *a*nxiety, and *d*epression.[11]

Abraham Myerson, the same doctor earlier worried about nervous housewives, was the first to try to reduce the disturbed appetites of their fat children by prescribing amphetamines. Benzedrine, synthesized in 1887, had been taken up again in 1927 by a pharmacologist looking for a synthetic substitute for expensive ephedrine, a drug used in the relief of asthma. (Asthma itself had long been associated with fatness—the fat person, like the asthmatic, is often short of breath—and in the 1930s the "smothering" mother would become as much a fixture in the discussion of asthma as of obesity.)[12] Put on the market in 1932 as a nasal inhalant, benzedrine was soon adopted by college students to keep themselves awake while studying. Physicians prescribed benzedrine to control narcolepsy, exhaustion and depression. Since loss of appetite and loss of weight were frequently noted as side effects, it occurred to Myerson and his colleague Mark F. Lesses to test benzedrine on a population that was at once lethargic, depressed and fat. These were people suffering from what Myerson and Lesses called "anhedonia," the inability to take pleasure from life. Such people ate to compensate for their emotional restlessness, but they could never be satisfied, and so they grew fat.[13]

Myerson and Lesses published their results in 1938, just as dinitrophenol was fading from the scene and thyroid drugs were losing professional favor. Benzedrine almost *had* to work, and work it did. No one understood quite how, but this was hardly important. Depression America had been waiting for something that would forestall fatigue, melancholy, appetite and fat. Something honest and powerful, like the new comic book hero, himself an orphan, Superman. And here it was, counteragent to the overprotective mother whose cover had been broken the same year.

Amphetamines (benzedrine, then methedrine and dexedrine) took on a masculine cast. Other reducing drugs (especially diuretics, cathartic teas and bath salts) appealed primarily to women. Their advertisements appeared in women's magazines, their packages and tablets arrived in pastels, their logos featured luxuriantly thin Venuses. When men secretly tried such drugs, they regularly abandoned them in favor of abdominal belts, fasting, chewing, calorie-counting, exercise, and massage. Though endogenous–exogenous distinctions were disappearing from the medical literature, they continued on in popular practice: soft internal organs were women's domain; men occupied themselves with what was visible and tough. Amphetamines fitted this male mode. They promised alertness and vigor, promises fixed during World War II when 180,000,000 amphetamine tablets were dispensed *ad libitum* to U.S. troops, most notably to fighter pilots maintaining combat readiness over long hours. After the war, returning soldiers stuck with amphetamines, obtained by prescription or under the counter. As truck drivers, they used them on long hauls; as railroad engineers they took them on the

night express; as lotharios they grabbed a "fistful of 'hearts'" to jit-
terbug from dusk 'til dawn. Girls learned about them from boy-
friends, wives from husbands. By 1952 and the practical end of the
Korean War, more than sixty thousand pounds of amphetamines
were being produced annually in the United States, enough for
nearly three billion 10-milligram tablets. By the summer of 1970
and the peak of the war in Vietnam, 8 percent of all prescriptions
written were for amphetamines: ten billion pills, not counting the
tremendous illegal traffic.[14]

At least two billion of those pills were for weight-reducing. The
AMA had issued a public disapproval of amphetamines for the treatment of obesity as early as 1943, but five years later physicians were
recommending dexedrine as the drug of choice for weight-reducing,
often adding a complementary prescription for barbiturates to calm
the dexedrine jitters. If the clean plate and the overprotective
mother were legacies of the Depression, so too were appetite
suppressants. When it was found that the amphetamine effects on
appetite wore off after six to ten weeks, pharmaceutical companies
began research on longer-acting or delayed-release anorectics,
which would become familiar as Tenuate, Preludin, Lucofen and
Didrex. "For the obese patient chained by the habit of overeating,"
Biphetamin and Ionamin would crush the links between appetite,
anxiety and fat. Advertisements in 1965 featured a fat man in coils
from shoulder to ankle, another sad victim of the Cold War and
mother love.[15]

Appetite suppression for men became appetite control for
women. The same amphetamines that freed overweight men from
the clutches of habit would render overweight women agreeable
and disciplined. Women, not men, starred in the promotion of
drugs called Appetrol and Obedrin. "Obesity need not be a frustrating problem," Strasenburgh Laboratories assured the readers of
Postgraduate Medicine. The defiant, pained, "diet-hard" overeater
glaring out at the doctor, her horned head turned away from the
balance beam of the platform scale, her red right hand anchored to
her broad hip, could be handled easily enough by Biphetmine-T.[16]

The use of amphetamines thus perpetuated the gender stereotyping inherent in the distinction between endogenous and exogenous
obesity. Men had only to be released from an external force to be re-
deemed of their fat, while women had to be taught an inner control.
Maternal overprotection evidently had a different effect on boys
from that on girls: boys became too docile and compliant; girls be-

came obsessive and aggressive in their orality.[17] So the pattern would repeat from one generation to the next. The devouring fat woman would marry yet another Mr. Wimple and stand guard over her children until they too could never be satisfied.

Amphetamines—"hearts"—could scarcely interrupt such a vicious circle. They could do little to set to rights an historical error— call it fixation or conditioning—which had put food squarely in the way of love. What was needed was something that could reconstrue the past—call this decathecting or deconditioning—as it soothed in the present.

Regression in the Service of the Scale

Enter, once again, the milk diet. While modern mothers were being persuaded to abandon the breast for the precise formula and the sterilized bottle, fat adults were asked to regress to a series of liquid diets, as if their unquenchable appetites and their ungovernable heartache might vanish in a ritual return to the source. The milk diet had been a fattening diet for neurasthenics, a thinning diet, then a calming, placating diet for those with ulcers. In 1934 it was once again a reducing diet. Dr. George A. Harrop found skim milk and bananas to be an ideal combination for a low-calorie menu with "high satiety." The United Fruit Company, delighted, publicized Harrop's work. Simple and cheap, the diet was a signature of the Depression itself, bland, infantilizing, monochromatic. It was the proletarian cousin of a new set of diet beverages that began as food powders in the 1930s and have returned in every decade since, in new cans, with new flavors, under new names. Dr. Stoll's Diet-Aid, sold through beauty parlors in 1932, contained milk chocolate, starch, and an extract of roasted whole wheat and bran. Mixed by the teaspoon into a cup of water, it was intended as a substitute for breakfast and lunch. Twenty years later, doctors at the Rockefeller Institute, studying metabolic changes, mixed together evaporated milk, corn oil, dextrose and water for another low-calorie formula diet whose balance of protein, fat and carbohydrate approximated that in breast milk. This became *Vogue*'s "peasant diet" and the *Ladies Home Journal*'s "fabulous formula." It was imitated in 1959 by Metrecal, a product of the Mead Johnson Company, known for half a century by its infant foods Dextri-Maltose and Pablum. Today

it is Carnation's Slender, marketed by Nestlé, controversial distributors of infant formulas worldwide.[18]

The formula diet was a regressive diet, tacitly and technically
derived from diets for infants, the infirm and the psychotic.[19] The
milk-and-banana menu, its successors and its heirs apparent were
meant from the start to be "filling," to satisfy the appetite even as
they deceived the body. Unlike the sheer neutral bulk of methylcel-
lulose,[20] liquid diets were to fill the hollow in the heart, not just the
small wrinkled bag called the stomach. They did so by a trick of
memory, by allusion to what *had been* filling, and perfect, and
pure.

For many, the prodigal return to the breast seemed incomplete
without a second, deeper regression. If Clara Davis's newly weaned
infants could recognize good food when they saw it, then the restoration of true appetite demanded a return to Mother Earth and un-
corrupted food. The Depression witnessed an upsurge of popular diets which insisted that only the pure (the natural, the primitive, the
raw) could satisfy. This was not a new idea. In one form or another
it had been defended by "Pythagoreans" (vegetarians), Grahamites,
naturopaths, home economists, the Kelloggs and pretty much anyone opposed to indigestion, heartburn and constipation.

What was new was a persnickety concern with food combinations. People had long been anxious about the balance of acids and
alkalis in their guts. The acids seemed too dangerous to be down
there as they ate away at beef jerky or salt pork. Indeed, it was not
clear to physiologists why, with all that hydrochloric acid, bile, and
pancreatic juice, the stomach and intestines did not digest themselves. The common use of the alkaline bicarbonate of soda as a digestive aid was founded on the fear that once the body dissolved its
dinner, it could begin to go after itself. Fears were aggravated by the
appearance of stomach ulcers as a notable medical problem after
the turn of the century, and by the "national, international, silent,
suppressed tussle" to keep the colon clean. With "36 Feet of Fear"
coiled up inside them, people had cause to worry about provoking
their personal anacondas with the wrong foods or the wrong combination of foods.[21]

During the 1920s, with so much talk of protein, fat, carbohydrate, calories, bran and vitamins, with food powders and infant
formulas, with vegetable margarines competing against lard and
butter, with near beer and home brews instead of the real thing, the

problem of food mixtures began to seem very important and very complicated. The Defensive Diet League of America took as its symbol a classical pan balance, "Acid 20 %" in one pan, "Alkaline 80 %" in the other: "The Weigh to Health." But should one mix fruit (acid) with bread (alkali, starch) at the same meal? The two together caused fermentation. And what about a sandwich of bread and meat? Carbohydrate (bread) was digested by fermentation in the stomach, while protein was digested by putrefaction in the intestines. Taking them in the same gulp would muddle the stomach and mystify the glands. Acids would spray out like blind assailants, fats would go unmolested, carbohydrates would find themselves in bad company.[22]

The Depression itself was a result of overindulgence, bad company and mongrel investments, was it not? "Making money," advised naturopath George H. Brinkler in 1932, "is fundamentally a problem of nutrition." Brinkler had his own profitable School of Eating in New York City and an institute in Miami for the dietary cure of cancer, diabetes and Bright's disease.[23] His advice was overshadowed by that of Dr. William Howard Hay of Pocono Hay-ven, Pennsylvania. Hay's "Medical Millennium," recognizable in 1981 as the Beverly Hills Diet, began in the 1920s with an overweight man who found by careful chewing and ever-so-careful food combining that he could lead a healthier, leaner life. With the help of a daily enema to keep the usually lazy colon free of poisons, the Hay dieter would stave off acidosis, the excess accumulation of acids in the body. Acidosis sapped vitality, opened one up to infections and gave the go-ahead sign to fat. It was strange that acids and fats should so easily coexist, but the crucial opposition here was between acid and alkali. The Hay dieter would eat starches separately from proteins and both separately from fruits—like Henry Ford, who ate only fruits at breakfast, only starches at lunch, and only proteins at dinner. The best diet was monotrophic—one food at a meal—and alkaline. A fat person could eat potatoes, butter, sugar, and cream without qualm, as long as the starches (potatoes, sugar) were taken separately from the proteins (butter, cream: dairy foods).[24]

That such a diet should attract millions of people during the Depression is not difficult to understand. It was a diet as suspicious of homeostatic mechanisms in the body as people were of such mechanisms in the economy. The body, like the economy after 1929, could not be trusted to regulate itself. Through careful chewing, colonic irrigations and strict rules governing the combination of foods, the

Hay canon gave dieters a sense of regulatory power without imposing any restraint on appetite itself. Not abstinence but timing—
what to eat when, in what company—was the real Depression skill.
One learned how to space foods for perfect digestion and least envy.
Only undigested foods made one fat or susceptible to the Evil Eye.

The Hay diet was, conveniently, a poverty diet. In modern industrial society, only the poorest of poor men and women had ever
settled for one food at a meal. In primitive societies, among those
"happy poor" so fervently sought out during the 1930s, people did
eat a single food at a meal—or so believed Hay advocates who
pointed, for example, to the long-lived, bright-toothed islanders of
Tristan da Cunha.[25]

Dentists, anthropologists and adventurers beating the bush, de-
scending into hidden valleys or climbing through distant mountain
passes during the 1930s were trying to go back in time. The farther
back they went, the more happiness they would find, as in James
Hilton's *Lost Horizon* of 1933, whose Shangri-La came to be upset
by modern appetites. The moral was always that one could be satisfied with very little if that little were pure and simple.[26]

Those most content with a single food at a single meal and with
the simplest foods for the longest periods were, of course, infants.
Trusting to mother and to Mother Earth, infants had no urge for
spices or acids. They had floated pleasantly in the alkaline fluid of
the fetal sac for nine months, and they would feed pleasantly on
whole milk for months thereafter. Their colons were active, their
food liquefied, and their systems clean. They were, if left alone,
perfect Hay devotees.

The Hay diet convened the infant and the primitive, mother and
Mother Earth, at the same timeless, trusting table. "Nature never
lies to us, she never kids us," Hay wrote. "Nature struggles continually to bring us back to the ideal in stature, weight, blood pressure,
health, efficiency, and everything else." We were fools to resist her.[27]

If the Hay diet worked for health or weight-reduction, as it must
have for some, it did not work because it was "natural." There are
few foods that in and of themselves are not already combinations of
protein and starch, that do not in and of themselves mix acid and alkali. Under normal conditions, in fact, the stomach fluid is generally more acidic than alkaline. Not physiology but psychology was
crucial to the success of the Hay diet. A behaviorist would say that
the rigors of food combination upset old food habits and created
new ones which resisted random nibbling and indiscriminate gorg-

ing. A Freudian would say that monotrophism was regression in the service of the ego, bringing into play a new mother, stern but nurturant, who allowed for what another diet book would call "sylph-determination."[28]

Group Therapies

Beyond the biochemistry of amphetamines, the emotional comforts of formula diets and the nutritional primitivism of monotrophic meals lay psychotherapy. Psychotherapy was an obvious and yet a delayed consequence of the Depression shift of emphasis from metabolism to appetite. Despite Dr. Hilde Bruch's seminal studies of obesity in family context, 1939–41, psychologists and psychiatrists had little *specific* to offer the fat person until the late 1940s.[29] Since oral gratification was an issue in the establishment of anyone's habits early in life, behaviorists and Freudians alike would deal with the obese person as with any other anxious, lonely, angry, depressed person. They had no strategy geared specifically to the frustrations of fat people. Because so general, so diffuse and so slow, psychotherapy was seen as an adjunct to appetite suppressants and low-calorie diets, not as a substitute for them.[30]

Classical Freudian theory associated overeating with introjection, the absorbing into oneself of the traits of another person. In the case of obesity, introjection meant the fully "cannibalistic incorporation" of the mother or the maternal breast. The overprotective mother, invasive and narcissistic, became by fierce synecdoche the fat deposited throughout the body, and the appetite behind it. Fat people ate to satisfy a devouring mother now inside them. Counting calories was but to trifle with a higher power, especially when the "word 'diet' is as battered and bruised as the word 'love.'" Long and harrowing was the analytic surgery necessary to excise the hungering mother.[31]

Gestalt psychology put introjection into a more social, more immediate context. The gestalt school had begun in Germany with the study of visual perception, arguing that what we see is conditioned by the totality of our experience rather than by the literal operation of our optical apparatus. This argument was then generalized: What we take in from our environment affects and is affected by the totality of our being. None of our senses is independent of memory, habit or emotional state. Neither is appetite. Consider overeating, therefore, a mistaken relationship between the world and the self.

As Frederick Perls defined it during the late 1940s, introjection was a problem of assimilation. All things taken into the self must be "de-structured" and transformed to be used appropriately in an individual's life. Introjects are those things swallowed whole and never properly chewed or digested, "food which 'rests heavy on the stomach.'" Fat people gulped without tasting, as if they did not really want to eat at all, as if they had been forced to eat and had taught themselves how to clean their plates while repressing disgust. Now, like alcoholics, they consumed but did not assimilate. The fat person was a congeries of "thousands of unassimilated odds and ends."[32]

How familiar this sounds. Perhaps we should credit Horace Fletcher rather than Frederick Perls with the gestalt approach to overeating. Perls himself set up a number of introjection "experiments" which were Fletcherism redux: intense concentration on one's food, biting food off "by clean, efficient action of the front teeth," savoring the flavor, chewing a single morsel until it was entirely liquefied. And he explicitly affirmed the fit between the physiology of digestion and the psychology of assimilation. As one chewed one's food to a pulp, one "de-structured" those things taken into the self; the less gulping, the less indigestion/introjection. He was impressed that of all his gestalt experiments, those devoted to thorough chewing were the most resented by his subjects. Surely that proved his case. Slow, careful chewing restored a proper disgust for forced feeding, brought back to immediate experience the feelings of guilt and anger that underlay habits of self-compromise.

Gluttony in this context was a peculiarly selfless selfishness. Those who overate had learned how to conform to the demands of the world without having learned to make sense of those demands. They ate, as it were, without eating. Their fatness was not so much a part of them as it was apart from them. Gestalt psychology, assimilated in bits and pieces to the commonplaces of therapy during the 1950s, hoped to restore a thoughtful sociability to eating and to the rest of life. The therapy for the person who was fat was in many ways a model for reaching wholeness and integrity. Physicians could thus get "a good deal of pleasure watching the *real self* emerge from the fatty shell."[33]

We might take such an image as an allusion to the birth of Venus, but it bore far greater reference to escape and rebirth. As essayist Cyril Connolly had it in *The Unquiet Grave* (1945), "Imprisoned in every fat man a thin one is wildly signalling to be let out."[34] Still the most frequently quoted and misquoted aphorism about obesity,

Connolly's observation was nicely consistent with the primitivism of the dieting literature. The true person was the thin person, lost and inaudible behind the mountainous mother but frantic to be seen.

Such an image was equally convenient to the literature of addiction, which depicted addicts as prisoners of themselves. "Almost without exception," wrote Bill W., "alcoholics are tortured by loneliness. Even before our drinking got bad and people began to cut us off, nearly all of us suffered the feeling that we didn't quite belong." The alcoholic needed outside help from friends and a Higher Power. William G. Wilson ("Bill W.") found a friend in a fellow alcoholic and a Higher Power through the Oxford Group Movement (Buchmanism, Moral Re-Armament) in the mid-1930s. By 1940, Bill W. had established a national organization, Alcoholics Anonymous, whose chapters met for fellowship, spiritual rebirth, mutual support and evangelism.[35]

In 1948, the message of A.A. reached Esther Manz in Milwaukee. She was addicted not to alcohol but to food. She began Take Off Pounds Sensibly (TOPS), the first of the national group dieting organizations, followed in 1960 by Overeaters Anonymous (OA), in 1961–63 by Weight Watchers, and in 1965 by Diet Workshop, Inc. As businesses, Weight Watchers and Diet Workshop belong in the next chapter; as modes of therapy they belong here with TOPS and OA as legatees of the Depression shift of emphasis from metabolism to appetite.

Much earlier, in 1912, Mrs. Ernest L. Prann and Mrs. James H. Messenger of Deep River, Connecticut, had mobilized a women's walking club for weight-reducing. A dozen women competed in two groups against each other. Those who lost the least would give a dinner for the better losers. (Was this reward or vengeance?) During the war, Lulu Hunt Peters suggested the formation of "Watch Your Weight Anti-Kaiser Classes" whose members would meet in patriotic assembly once a week to weigh themselves on an official scale. Those who had not lost weight each week would be fined. After the war, in October 1921, the Commissioner of Health for New York City sponsored a public fat-reducing contest. The press watched some sixty fat women in low shoes and bloomers exercising in Madison Square Garden, dog-trotting along Fifth Avenue to Central Park, and preparing meals dictated daily by the good Dr. Royal S. Copeland, Commissioner. "I am watching," Copeland warned his dieters. "I am having the co-operation of the police in this matter. I have interested the plain-clothes men and they are following you around, and each day I get a report and I know the ones who are cheating." When the month had passed, Copeland had received hundreds of desperate letters from across the country, while star contestant Sarah Strong had lost 31 lbs, down to 250 from 281.[36]

I cite these precedents to explain that it was not the idea of addiction *per se* which led to the idea of collective dieting. In those early instances, overeating was curtailed by that code of shame which only a group can enforce. While the scale stood as deity and judge, its powers were incomplete without social surveillance—a surveillance parodied by Copeland's (supposed) enlistment of plain-clothesmen. Shame, publicity and company were motive enough for dieters to come together. The notable difference in the later groups was the assumption that fat people were fundamentally lonely, frightened, sad. This assumption, as we have seen, had its roots in a psychology of appetite which attributed overeating to a paradoxically empty self. Although Esther Manz of TOPS and the organizers of OA took as their inspiration the work of Alcoholics Anonymous and Gamblers Anonymous, the impulse toward the modern dieting group had begun with the slow beat of the ballad of the fat café. It was not simply that dieting would be more companionable or competitive within a group, but that fat people, anxious and lonely, *needed* a group before they could conquer their appetites.

The notion that a group of itself can be therapeutic may seem commonsensical to us now, just as it must have seemed reasonable and exciting to those who stood in circles around tubs of mesmeric fluid in the late 18th century and to those who sat in circles, their fingers touching, at spiritualist séances in the late 19th century. But the idea came hard to psychologists and psychoanalysts accustomed to dealing with their subjects one at a time in controlled environments. Only in the 1930s and 1940s did group therapy make its appearance in the United States in any stable forms, first through the group marriage counseling of Hannah Stone, Abraham Stone and psychiatrist Lena Levine, then through the analytic group therapy of Samuel R. Slavson in work for the Jewish Board of Guardians in New York. During World War II, the shortage of trained therapists for distressed soldiers led of necessity to wider experience with group therapy. After the war, this experience was applied to a broad range of psychological problems. The more often obesity was described as a personality defect and the more vehemently it was designated a national concern, the more likely it was that group therapy would be brought forward.[37]

Something was happening to groups. Groups—small groups, peer groups—were beginning to seem more powerful, more intimately persuasive. Historians and philosophers were fascinated by the group dynamics of early Nazism, theologians and psychiatrists by the forces at work in the stalags of concentration camps. The "authoritarian personality" and "the lonely crowd" appeared in the same year, 1950, as images, ultimately, of the power of groups to shape character. Conspiracy surfaced in the rhetoric of McCarthyism, while the sociologist David Riesman worried about the consequences of a seismic change in American character from the inner-directed to the outer-directed. Inner-directed persons sought an internal consistency; their values had been implanted early enough and strongly enough to make the satisfaction of them the crux of self-worth. Outer-directed persons struggled to please others throughout their lives; their sense of self-worth depended upon a constant acknowledgment by peers. Inner-directed persons were producers, able to distinguish between work and play; outer-directed persons were consumers, whose obligations muddied all distinctions between work and play. *The Lonely Crowd* reached a large and well-disposed audience with a theory that pitted the autonomous individual against the stifling group in much the same way that psychological theory pitted the thin person against the overprotective mother. Fatness, as the fat person well knew, was anonymity.[38]

Perhaps the extraordinary power of the group could be turned inward in an extraordinary homeopathy. Could the group not restore what it had at other times forced people to surrender, especially in that most recalcitrant of social diseases, obesity? The director of the National Institutes of Health in 1952 had declared that obesity was the primary national health problem. Another physician, Dr. Edward L. Bortz, had used the language of McCarthyism to announce to the AMA convention that year, "We're going to have to take off the kid gloves in dealing with people who are wallowing in their own grease." Only if we appreciate the new power attributed to groups can we make sense of the popularity of group dieting as a means of handling such a tough problem as obesity.[39]

Even as TOPS got spinning between 1948 and 1952, interest in dieting groups came from an astonishing number of directions. Chic Beverly Hills naprapath, Gayelord Hauser, best selling author of *Diet Does It* and *Eat and Grow Beautiful*, started an Eaters Anonymous. Nutritionist Cecile A. Hoover wrote glowingly about a Fatties

Anonymous for the black readers of Tuskegee Institute's *Service* magazine. In suburban Newton, Massachusetts, was a Gluttons Anonymous. Group psychotherapy sessions for the overweight were held in university hospitals (Berkeley), public dispensaries (Boston), and private practices (Brookline, Massachusetts, and Alexandria, Virginia). In 1952 the Public Health Service convened a national conference on the Group Approach to Weight Control.[40]

By 1958, thirty thousand women had entered TOPS; by 1963, sixty thousand. Local chapters went by such names as Invisi-Belles, Inches Anonymous, Shrinking Violets, Thick 'N Tired. (Offshoots and imitators called themselves WADS: We Are Dieting Seriously, or SIRENS: Slenderness Is Right Endeavors Never Stop.) The playfulness of the names, the childishness and exhibitionism of TOPS rituals were meant as an antidote to the anonymity and sadness of the fat person. If TOPS worked by shame and competition, it also worked by group exuberance. The pig bibs, the pigpens, the piggy banks for fines, the pig song "We are plump little pigs / Who eat too much / Fat, Fat, Fat"—all this may seem forced and foolish, but it was therapy for that lonely crowd of the fat and forlorn. The light-heartedness of TOPS was strategic and balanced by its reverence for calories, scales and food diaries. The naked, blank-faced Venus called TOPSy, emblem of community, was no sillier than the "litter-bug" invented by the Keep America Beautiful campaign around 1953; calorie-counting games and cheers were no less fanciful than that "Bibbidi-Bobbidi-Boo" by which the fairy godmother transformed Cinderella from waif to starlet in the Walt Disney cartoon of 1949. TOPS was at once a celebration and a parody of "outer-directed," consuming America.[41]

TOPS made anxiety fun as it made fun of anxiety. OA would be grimmer, tougher, focused on eating as a deadly compulsion. While TOPS worked through carnival and the extravagant display of the self, OA worked through *psychomachia*, that inward battle for the soul which could be resolved only by a human admission of weakness: "It is weakness, not strength, that binds us to each other and to a higher power and somehow gives us an ability to do what we cannot do alone." The divine in TOPS was the Lady of Misrule, She who turned the world upside down one moment only to restore it in the next. "As I started to lose weight," said Mrs. Delphine Kobyl-czyk of East Detroit, "wonderful things began to happen. It was wonderful to wear a belt again; to kneel straight in church and to sleep on my side again." The divine in OA lifted the abstinent into a new world, made them daring and autonomous. A dancer grown fat and then lean left the stage for the business world and skydiving: "Throwing myself out into the sky for all I was worth was the ultimate moment of trust in God and myself!" TOPS promised a return to normal, whence the scales and the counting; OA promised an Eternal Gospel and an everlasting pilgrimage, whence the call to a personal inventory and acts of faith.[42]

Where TOPS stuck audaciously to the present and OA moved one day at a time into the future, Weight Watchers was curiously attached to the past. It worked through *anamnesis*, the calling to mind. "Wherever you are," wrote founder Jean Nidetch, "the best trick I can suggest is: Do not have a loss of memory." She who had compiled album after album of family memorabilia advised Weight Watchers to carry a "before" picture, a "fat" picture, with them *"at all times."* Lecturers at Weight Watchers meetings stood beside photographs of the way they were. Jean Slutsky Nidetch of Brooklyn, daughter of a manicurist and a cabdriver, F. F. H. (Formerly Fat Housewife), would try on her size 44 dresses each month for years after she had trimmed down to a size 12. "I pray that I'll never forget where I came from," she wrote. "I pray I'll never get to the point where I'll think I've always been thin, successful and at the end of the rainbow."[43]

Indeed, whatever the temptation to forget, a fat person was never free of the past: "I don't know of anybody who has been fat who ever feels totally safe again. We know we're not cured. We're merely arrested." Lecturers, exemplars of success, still had to weigh in every month. There would soon be a Maintenance Diet for the end of the rainbow. No migrant from the land of the fat to the land of the thin ever completely renounced the homeland. Without nostalgia, without the memory of sadness, there could be no true vigilance.[44]

OA shared some of this concern with memory, because it shared with Weight Watchers the notion of fatness as an addiction. But for Weight Watchers the past so beckoned that its diet program had to compensate for desire and insatiability, allowing "free" foods, drawing "legal" distinctions between good and bad foods. The use of the food scale was required, as Nidetch explained, not only to instill discipline and control but also to keep the weight watcher *full*: "The idea of the Weight Watchers program is that you must never be hungry." Where OA struggled with the power of appetite itself, Weight Watchers juggled hunger and desire, trying for a proper balance.

Where OA talked of abstinence, Weight Watchers talked of pounds and ounces, recipes and flavor. Where OA spoke of surrender to a higher power, Weight Watchers alluded to shame and crisis. The confessions and communion of OA allowed explicitly for absolution and amends; in Weight Watchers, confession and communion led to remembrances of things not entirely past. Before-and-after pictures were for OA (and for TOPS) proofs of what could be done, of possibility; for Weight Watchers they served as warnings of what could happen again, at any time, almost instantly.[45]

I have been bearing down hard on the contrasts, and I will bear down harder for a paragraph more, in order to make a point about a similarity that would not otherwise be obvious. It will be best, first, to lay out the contrasts schematically, as in Table 2. Each group had formed around different elements of that fundamental sadness which all acknowledged as the essential quality of the fat person. Because the core emotions in each group were different, the therapy and the direction of the cure also differed. Each group meant to fill the emptiness of the fat person in a different way because each had a different definition of appetite and a different sense of time.

In each group, however, the only middle figure between the fat person and the thin person was the dieter. Though the brochures of all groups counseled moderation, their systems were at root Manichaean, setting fat against thin. Only the dieter, escaping from a prison of fat, moved in the middle ground. The dieter was a woman.

TABLE TWO
DIETING GROUPS CONTRASTED

	WW	TOPS	OA
Center of time	past	present	future
Def. of appetite	desire	consumption	compulsion
Emotional focus	anxiety/ loneliness	boredom/ lethargy	anger/ depression
Healing method	anamnesis	carnival	psychomachia
Root metaphors:			
fat person as	military	biological	religious
	barbarian	animal	sinner
dieter as	crusader	shape-shifter	prodigal child
thin person as	civilian	human	devoted servant
Direction of cure:			
from	primitive	instinctive	dependent
to	civilized	rational	adult

There were good reasons for more women than men to be dieters in general. Food and figure tolerances were narrower for women than for men. Women were supposed to require fewer calories than men for the same work and to be by nature lighter eaters. Women also wore clothes that despite the "New Look" of the late 1940s were more revealing than men's clothes, with less protective coloring and less camouflaging fabrics. The new fiberglass mannequins in show windows would model lighter clothing with finer figures.[46] The definitions of a beautiful woman involved precise circumferences as well as weight, while the handsomeness of a man rarely depended upon numerical measurements of hips, waist and chest. Poor Marty, that thirty-four-year-old Italian butcher who was "just a fat little man . . . a fat ugly little man"—even he would find a plain, shy woman who for all her supposedly anonymous features had a thin waist. The realism of the 1955 Academy Award movie did not extend to matching actor Ernest Borgnine with an actress of corresponding weight. Indeed, not a single fat little woman was to be seen under the dome of the Starlight Ballroom.

If there were strong reasons for more women than men to be dieters, there were even stronger reasons for group dieting to be the special province of women. Fatness was more socially isolating for women than for men, precisely because of the narrower cultural tolerances allowed women's bodies. Fatness further trapped the housewife and further restricted the already difficult advancement of the career woman. Diet books talked again and again about keeping the diet a secret, as if a fat woman's diet should be as furtive as her eating. Her failures, like her shame, would be private.[47]

Dieting groups were to women of the 1950s and 1960s what water cures had been to women a century before: floating islands under their command, a middle ground by which to establish a sense of dominion and networks of sodality. Their inlets and elevations, their geography and topography, were fixed by women with long histories of social involvement and abiding desires for a place in the public world. It was hardly accidental that Rozanne S., founder of OA, had been a copywriter, adept at that language which mediates between intensely personal appetites and intently impersonal sales. Nor that her grandmother campaigned with Margaret Sanger for birth control and her mother was one of the country's first trained dieticians. Nor again that Jean Nidetch of Weight Watchers had been president of the North Hills League for Retarded Children and that "whatever organization I got into, I usually ended up heading it." Nor that Lois

Lindauer, founder of Diet Workshop, had been a Welcome Wagon hostess and then run her own small business selling wall plaques. Nor that she had studied with the psychologist Abraham H. Maslow at Brandeis University, embracing his ideas about self-actualization and living one's life to its potential. Nor that, when she left college, she was aiming to be the president of a company, just as, years earlier, "when other kids were playing house, I was playing office."[48]

These were all married women in their thirties when they began OA, Weight Watchers, and Diet Workshop. For them, losing weight meant taking charge of their lives *and* resuming an audience. The group was not incidental to the dieting, it was the crux. It made the act of dieting an empowering act. It gave substance to the newly slimmed body, a social significance apart from the thin fiberglass mannequins in shop windows. It was the group that made something of the body, endowed it with a new, comfortable presence. It was the group that, unlike the individual dieter after her thirty-ninth diet, could lay claims on the future and so talk boldly about maintenance programs and being "Thin Forever."[49] The group would go on, no matter what. In the group there was world enough and time to trust to small changes. Outside, everything moved by leaps and jerks, and you went crazy trying to leap and jerk along. Outside, no one would notice a loss of weight until you had crossed some sudden threshold. You went on panic diets for weddings and parties just to cross that threshold for a moment, knowing beforehand you would gain the pounds back days later. Or you starved yourself in public to make your dieting seem honest, then gorged in private. Inside the group, everything was steadier. People applauded the smallest decrements, the least sacrifice, the gradual succession of insights. The group maintained a slow but confident time during which you would grow as you lost.

Fat men too needed another rhythm, but they did not seem to need another world. Less isolated, or at least less sensitive to their isolation, they did not (and in general do not) seek out a middle ground. When Elmer Wheeler at 230 lbs reduced his weight in 1950 to become "Captain of My Soul," he recomposed time without changing his social geography. He allotted himself 1,500 calories a day but spread the counting across three days. That is, his unit of time was 72 hours and his diet in that time was 4,500 calories, eaten when and how he chose. Wheeler's *Fat Boy's Book: How Elmer Lost 40 Pounds in 80 Days*, serialized by the General Features newspaper syndicate, reached the attention of thirty million Americans, according to one Gallup poll. His book sold 112,000 copies the first year. More than three million letters came in response to his diet. Mills Music Company published "The Fat Boy Bounce," perhaps in retaliation for the 1947 "Too Fat Polka." Bering Cigars put out "The Fat Boy Cigar." Nearly 90,000 people sent away for his dieting slide rule offered by the *Chicago Daily News*.[50]

The slide rule represented caloric moralism at its peak. Human skeletons and unhappy lovers could live on 300 calories a day; barflies and somnambulists on 1,700 calories; models and bums on 2,100 calories; mothers of triplets and three-day poker players at 3,200; gluttons at 4,500 and grave diggers at 5,000. But Wheeler could not stick to his own three-day plan, and in 1952 he was on tour with a second diet book, *Fat Boy's Downfall and How Elmer Learned To Keep It Off*. This book began with a caloric thermometer based not on normal intake but on a dieter's program. The minimum was 900 calories a day, 1,200 was "No Fun," 1,500 was Safe Reducing. Beyond that, at 1,800, were Kitchen Sneaks, then at 2,100 Cheaters, 2,400 Backsliders, 2,700 Self-deceivers, 3,000 Fat Boys, 3,300 Gluttons, 3,600 Hopeless Cases. The new diet was itself nothing new. Elmer had just added in a few exercises—the Fanny Fandango, Tummy Bumps—and an F.B.I. (Fat Boy Institute) to supervise eating habits.[51]

In tone, the Fat Boy books bore a close resemblance to TOPS. There was the same childishness: the fat *boy*, the Fanny Fandango. The same self-mockery: "I got fat because my name's Elmer. Bill is slender." The same allusion to animality: Wheeler had learned about balanced diets, he claimed, by studying the labels on cans of dog food. There was the same joking familiarity with calories, the same free-wheeling attack on sadness.[52]

But this was a man's diet, a man dieting alone. It was, as Wheeler noted, a former newspaperman's diet, and "diet" was an anagram of "edit." Editing was what dieting was all about, taking the blue pencil to fat. Editing was a private job; one did not edit by committee. Fat men cramped in the seats of a DC-6 or fumbling with burst collars had social reasons for losing weight, but they would labor at it themselves. If Wheeler's diet did not approach the extreme unsociability of Fletcherites, it was clearly undercover, wherefore the invention of Wheeler's F.B.I. after first he fell from grace.[53]

The Depression legacy of sadness did not take the fat man as far toward confession as it took the fat woman, but the fat man was more inclined to diet than ever before. That was due only in part to the Depression shift of emphasis from metabolism to appetite. It was due also and literally to a change of heart. While fat women were the particular victims of the psyche, fat men would be the particular victims of physiology. Where fat took hold of a woman's metaphorical heart, it was clutching more tightly at the man's actual anatomical heart.

Bursting Hearts: Fat and Physiology

Thomas Parr, "The Olde, Olde, Very Olde Man," was sent to London to meet the King and his court in 1635. Snug in his village near Shrewsbury, Parr had lived for one hundred fifty-two years on cheese, milk and coarse bread. He was blind now and had a poor memory, but the Earl of Arundel brought him to the capital as "a piece of antiquity." After less than two months in the city, Parr died, a martyr to celebration and rich foods. He was entombed at Westminster Abbey as one of England's treasures.[54]

Parr might have graced the very first chapters of this book, for he was after Cornaro the most oft-cited example of the virtues of a simple, meager diet. I have reserved him for this point in the narrative because he was honored at his death with an autopsy by the great English surgeon William Harvey, who seven years earlier had proved the circulation of the blood through the heart. Harvey took a close look at Parr's heart, which he found completely covered with fat, with small clots in the right ventricle. Likewise the mesentery and colon were loaded with fat, and the kidneys too. "All the internal parts, in a word, appeared so healthy" that Harvey explained Parr's death as a result of breathing the foul air of London.[55]

In fact, Parr was not so very old. There had been a succession of Thomas Parrs in his village, not all of whom had been registered by birth or death in the parish books. This Thomas Parr was two or more generations of men bundled into one and thus endowed with a remarkably long life.[56]

Nor were Parr's innards so very healthy. This, however, is a modern diagnosis.[57] Neither Harvey nor any other surgeon of his time had much experience with fatty hearts or, indeed, fat bodies. Anatomists tended whenever possible to dissect the lean, whose bodies were more immediately revealing. Surgeons tended to avoid operations on the obese, considering them (as they still do) bad risks. Giovanni Maria Lancisi in 1707 was the first to explore in depth the anatomical relationship between apoplexy—the traditional cause of death for fat people—and clusters of fat in the body, but he saw no direct link between obesity and diseases of the heart. After several excavations of sad and querulous fat women who had died sudden deaths, Giovanni Battista Morgagni in 1760 was ready to hint at a connection between heart disease and obesity, but the English physician John Fothergill in 1779 was the first to propose weight (and fat) reduction as a specific remedy against angina pectoris and that set of symptoms leading to sudden death. The eminent English surgeon John Hunter did an autopsy on one of Fothergill's apoplectic patients, a corpulent man whose arteries turned out to be ossified. When Hunter himself, no scarecrow, died of apoplexy in 1793, medical interest was piqued. Over the next decades, researchers drew a tighter circle around arterial hardening, the fatty degeneration of the heart, angina pectoris and apoplexy or sudden death (what today we often call a heart attack).[58]

John Hunter had written, "I did not consider either the fat or the earth [the calcium] of bones, as part of the animal: they are not animal matter: they have no action within themselves: they have not the principle of life." For him, as for most others of his era, fat was inert. It was a cushion, a lubricant, an insulator. When overmuch, it was an impediment. It could weigh heavily on joints and organs, slow down the blood, immobilize the body. It was so inert that when animal life departed from the body, the corpse itself was reputed to resolve into fat. Fat was strangely foreign, the part of the body that was apart from the body. Like any foreigner, it could by its mere presence interfere with confidences and confessions, disguise symptoms, make examination awkward and unrewarding. In 1816 Dr. René Laennec found this to be too true. Trying the new technique of percussion on a fat young woman suspected of a diseased heart, he could hear nothing by tapping her on the back and chest. Her obesity became the mother of invention, for Laennec then devised the first stethoscope, a listening tube which could detect the beating heart and the hollows of the body beneath the alien presence of fat.[59]

But where did this foreigner, so inert and yet so diffused throughout the body, come from? Was fat deposited by sluggish blood? Did a gland secrete fat? Did the colon extract fat from fecal matter? The anatomist William Hunter, John's elder brother, proposed that fat was the product of a specific tissue, an adipose tissue. Sustained by Xavier Bichat and most 19th-century physiologists, the tissue theory gave fat a new position in the body. As a tissue, fat had some rights; it was not so much an alien as a denizen, a permanent boarder, and as such it had to be fed. Like other boarders, fat could be inconspicuous or obnoxious. The ideal boarder would be sociable but not intrusive, inoffensive and slow to take offense. In moderation, fat was the ideal boarder. It was congenial, pleasantly available as a connective tissue and quite insensitive to insult—you could cut it with a knife and it would not demur. But when fat became heavy and overbearing, it threatened the common board, endangered furniture, made passage down stairways and through hallways a troublesome risk. The mid-Victorian ambivalence toward the boarder extended to fat itself.[60]

Under the late-19th-century microscope and momentarily free of anthropomorphism, fat seemed to be a spongy substance, nerveless, threaded with capillaries. The more fat, the more blood vessels the blood had to reach, and the harder the heart had to work to pump the blood. While physicians became accustomed to looking for fatty hearts and arteriosclerosis as causes of death in obese individuals, evidence mounted that body fat could also strain the heart by its insatiable demand for blood. In lay terms, as several doctors wrote, 30 lbs of extra fat meant 25 miles of blood vessels added to the burden of the pumping heart. With the improvement of the sphygmomanometer and the development of a portable electrocardiograph machine during the first three decades of this century, physicians noted consistent correlations between high blood pressure (hypertension), heart arrythmias, heart disease, and excess fat. These correlations were in the public domain by 1921, when humorist Don Marquis, inventor of the phrase "girth control" and later of Archy the literary cockroach, described his own 55-lb weight loss. At the age of forty-two he had tipped the scales at 225 lbs and his blood pressure looked "like Babe Ruth's batting average." He was the sorry victim of "false angina pectoris," which was "some damned thing that takes hold of your heart and twists it, just as you take hold of a fountain pen that won't unscrew, and unscrew it *anyhow*." And his heart, he knew, was fat: "All the good, healthy heart muscle that I had inherited from generations of hard-praying, pessimistic Presbyterian ancestors had been turned into fat by my own careless life

of light and laughter." "Eat, drink and get fat," concluded Dr. K.
H. Beall of Fort Worth in the same vein in 1924, "And tomorrow
you will die."[61]

The suddenness of this death deserves remark. We have seen how
life insurance companies had come to figure fat people for shorter
lives. In a parallel set of studies between 1929 and 1959, actuaries
were at pains to demonstrate the risks of cardiovascular disease and
heart failure associated with overweight, most particularly for
men.[62] The seeming unpredictability of heart attacks made dieting
all the more urgent and weight-watching all the more perpetual.
Though obesity might statistically reduce length of life in the long
run, the heart struck suddenly. Obesity was being cuffed to mortality in two ways, as a syndrome in itself and as partner to the most
threatening adult disease of midcentury America. Heart disease
ranked fourth as a cause of death in the United States in 1900, just
behind gastritis. In 1960, gastritis had disappeared from the list and
heart disease was number one.[63]

As heart disease became the premier murderer, obesity became
the national "problem," fat the national "enemy." It would make a
kind of symbolic sense, then, for the stomach to be drawn closer to
the heart in the popular imagination and in medical imagery. The
position of the stomach, first revealed in the living person by x-rays,
was found to be not horizontal but vertical and literally closer to the
heart. The stomach, *Fortune* magazine explained in 1936, was located "on the left side between the second and fourth vest buttons
counting down, or in other words, where most people think their
heart is." In 1937 the Jacobs Brothers introduced "a very *different*
bathroom scale," Detecto No. 918. It was "a very perfect circle,
deftly and artfully broken by a low, gracefully tapering, triangular
dial housing, with dial subtly placed off center to lend rythmic balance to the entire design." What else could this be but the round
belly conjoined to the tapering, "rythmic" heart? The scale took on
weight with its stomach, registered the consequences above and off-
center through the heart.[64]

The closer the stomach to the tell-tale heart, the less likely it
could be that fat was simply inert. The heart after all was an energetic muscle; it would take some doing to surround it or crowd its
arteries. If, in the mechanics of industrial efficiency and home economy, fat was dead weight, "an absolute ballast," a "Dead Sea," bio-
chemically it was more engaged.[65]

Physiologist Claude Bernard had been the first to show how body fat could be metabolized as an energy source. From the mid-19th century, the common image of body fat as a bank account of energy relied upon the sense of fat as ready capital. There were times, indeed, when fat seemed amazingly volatile: the spontaneous combustion of fat alcoholics was a prize anecdote for Temperance lecturers. Even when spontaneous combustion was damped down to legend, fat was never far from the fire; it was "unburnt body-fuse," and the corpulent person lived "on the brink of a volcano."[66]

As a deposit, as a fuse, fat was passive. In the 1870s, with the competing work of several German scientists, fat began to appear more independent. From the histological perspective of Carl Toldt, adipose tissue was industrious. It removed fats from the blood and processed them. It had a close, active relationship with the vascular system. Fat might accumulate in passive connective tissue, but it had more positive roles to play than as a mere "water-pillow." From the cellular perspective of Rudolf Virchow and Walther Flemming, fat was invasive. It floated in on the blood, infiltrating cells, promoting fat production at the expense of protoplasm, causing the fatty degeneration of organs. Adipose tissue was connective tissue that had been transformed by an influx of fat.[67]

Over the next half century, Toldt was proved right. "Our whole attitude toward fat and its place and dignity in the body economy has undergone a positive revolution in the light of our new knowledge of nutrition," wrote Dr. Woods Hutchinson in 1924. Fat, called "by such polite and high-sounding titles as lipin, lecithin, palmitin, and even vitamin," had outgrown its supporting roles as "mere storage stuff" and "a blanket of blubber." Now it was adventurous: "It still renders yeoman service of highest value as a reserve and storehouse of the sinews of war, but instead of merely dozing peacefully in snug harbor, it is also in the thick of the fight all over the body. Wherever the vital spark burns brightest, there is fat to feed and protect the flame." Hutchinson was writing one of the rare articles of the 1920s in defense of fat men, so he cast fat in the very best of lights—"our very life stuff, protoplasm, is an emulsion or whipped cream of fats." This was not the whole truth—there were proteins and carbohydrates as well as lipids in the protoplasmic colloid—but Hutchinson is quoted here for the frothiest of contrasts with the older image of fat as something inert. In his eagerness to make the fat man seem once again vital, Hutchinson overstepped his bounds, but he also anticipated several decades of research which would show that adipose tissue was in constant motion, converting carbohydrates to fats and adjusting the energy balance of the body through "endless" exchanges.[68]

Physicians began to consider the gross pathology of the heart of less immediate importance than high blood pressure and arterial degeneration. They had found that fat near the heart was compatible with health and that fatty "infiltration" of the heart occurred as often among the thin as among the obese. It was the insidious, active spread of fat through the blood, not the slow, obvious mechanical thrust of fat around organs, which most menaced.[69]

The close relationship presumed between fatness, fat, blood and the heart was exploited by many reducing schemes. For a moment in 1941, bloodletting returned with Miss E. Millet of New Orleans, Anemic people, the Millet pamphlet argued, were thin people. Fat people who wanted to be thin should therefore let blood. More commonly, digitalis was added to thyroid preparations and diuretics, as if diet drugs had also to be drugs for the heart. Marketed before the 1938 Federal Food, Drug and Cosmetic Act, thyroid-digitalis and diuretic-digitalis combinations were exempt from new drug safety regulations until 1972. If thyroid-digitalis compounds were unwise, stimulating possibly weak hearts, diuretic-digitalis compounds could be lethal, since potassium loss from diuresis increased the sensitivity of the heart to digitalis. In 1966, just before her untimely death, Helen Bailey was taking a rainbow of diet tablets whose effects on her appetite were probably less great than their effects on her heart:

> white (digitalis)
>   red (digitalis and aloin, a purgative)
>   small yellow (barbiturate and amphetamine)
>   yellow (digitalis)
>   green (barbiturate and atropine)
>   lavender (niacin)
>   black (aloin and belladonna, a stimulant
>   and antispasmodic like atropine)

This was extreme. Perhaps only a quarter of a million people that year were on such a regime.[70]

Using digitalis was like kicking a horse because its rider was bound to be mean—a kind of prophylactic cruelty. Digitalis might "protect" the heart from the ill effects of the anti-fat drugs meant to save the heart. Far better to work on the rider than on the horse, on fat than on the heart. But could one change the personality of fat?

One could. French scientists in the 1820s had done careful chemistry to distinguish one fat from another. When body fat began to seem active and independent, those fats acquired personalities. The first to take on a real character was cholesterol, an aromatic fat originally isolated in 1823. By 1880, physicians had been advised to watch blood cholesterol levels in the obese, since cholesterol seemed the true culprit in the circulatory problems of fat people. In 1913 the Russian scientist Nikolai Anichkov fed rabbits a diet high in cholesterol and showed that their artieries were later lined with fatty plaques. From 1917 on, while reports confirmed a correlation between obesity, high blood pressure and arteriosclerosis, other reports confirmed the correlation between obesity and high blood cholesterol levels. For years, however, there were no proofs of a causal connection between high blood cholesterol in humans and arteriosclerosis—and the controversy continues. Nonetheless, cholesterol by the 1930s had acquired a reputation as a complex, important and dangerous fat. If Dr. Daniel Munro in his 1953 diet book could call cholesterol "death-dealing," it was because cholesterol was guilty by association. There was little evidence throughout the 1950s that reducing the cholesterol intake in daily diet would significantly reduce arteriosclerosis or heart disease.[71]

It would be disheartening to follow that "mysterious, yellowish, waxy substance" known as cholesterol through the many subsequent turns and twists of public pronouncement by the AMA, the Public Health Service, the National Heart and Lung Institute, and the American Heart Association, or to trace in detail the recent literature on low-density and high-density lipoproteins.[72] The point is that dieters became attentive to fats during the Depression and that by the late 1940s weight-reducing usually involved some attempt to change the character of the fats in the diet. It happened first with the blacklisting of cholesterol, next with saturated fats.

Saturated fats are fatty acids that do not have double carbon bonds. They are chiefly animal fats, "saturated" because their single bonds make it difficult for them to be broken down by other chemical agents. In the popular imagination, they are heavy, indigestible, calorie-laden, sluggish fats. While unsaturated fats carry the fat-soluble vitamins A, D, E and K and therefore seem lighter and livelier, saturated fats just hang around. They must be the ones responsible for heart attacks. The badmouthing of saturated fats began with the turn-of-the-century presumption that saturated fats could not be effectively absorbed by intestinal mucosa and so would end up as concretions of fat in the appendix and the intestines. Soon it was also presumed that saturated fats were harder to burn off, and so they became excuses for fat people who claimed to eat very little and yet gain weight. The Weight Watchers diet was the "Prudent Diet" devised in 1952 by Dr. Norman Jolliffe, director of New York City's Bureau of Nutrition, and the diet was prudent especially in regard to saturated fats. When Elmer Wheeler in 1963 went forth on his third diet and diet book, this time it would be *The Fat Boy Goes Polyunsaturated*. As with cholesterol, the evidence for a causal relationship between saturated fats in the diet (or in the body) and rates of heart disease among the obese was hardly impressive, but the characterization of saturated fats as bad fats had stuck. As with cholesterol, it would be pointless here to pursue saturated fats through a Thirty Years' War between the American Dairy Council, the National Research Council, the Department of Agriculture and the American Cancer Society, or to review new scientific data on short-, medium-, and long-chain triglycerides. The point is that dieting, as a result of its concern with the heart, had come to concern itself as much with fat as with weight. Where before one shed fat because it was dead weight, now one shed weight because it was dangerous fat.[73]

Beginning in the 1940s, some authorities wanted to substitute fat for weight as the criterion of obesity. Etymologically, obesity should refer to over-fatness, not to overweight. The physical examination of football players drafted during World War II clearly demonstrated the difference between adipose tissue and sheer poundage. Football players were, it was true, above standard acceptable weights, but they were not fat. The Navy medical staff proved this by determining the specific gravity of players who would otherwise have been rejected as obese. Since the specific gravity of fat is much less than that of water (the oil always floats atop the vinegar in my Italian dressing), a fat person can be told from a muscled person of the same height and weight by the amount of water each displaces when submerged in a tank. The fat person—the truly *fat* person— displaces less water. The fatter the body, the less water displaced.[74]

One could use such densitometry to create an age–height table that would reflect fatness rather than weightiness, but even Archimedes would not measure the amount of water overflowing from his tub every day, and accurate readings of specific gravity involve rather dedicated observers and sensitive instruments. Hardly practical, densitometry is unreliable for heavy smokers, whose diminished lung capacity affects their buoyancy. Separate tables must also be used for each racial grouping, since the healthy ratio of lean mass to body water varies from one group to another.[75]

Calipers were more practical. Proposed first in the 1880s, the skinfold test for fatness was brought forward again in the 1950s and 1960s. Calipers became a primary tool in physical anthropology and, soon, in national dietary studies. Exploited later on television and cereal boxes as "pinch an inch," the skinfold test took on a popular if casual authority.[76]

"A realistic appraisal of the nude body is often a more reliable guide for estimating obesity than body weight," the Public Health Service declared in 1966. "If sheer appearance fails to give a clear answer, there is the "pinch test'"—or the ruler balanced across the abdomen from ribs to pubis as one lies prone.[77] The Depression shift of emphasis from glands to heart entailed a slow shift away from tables of numerical weight to the visible and tangible features of the fat body. As adipose tissue became athletic and autonomous, as dietary fats assumed distinct personalities, fatness gained back a definite corporeality, which the scale had for a while not so much denied as disguised through a veil of numbers. Fat was still deadly, but it was no longer ghostly.

Builds

I am contradicting myself here. In the first part of this chapter I wrote of fat and fatness as increasingly impalpable conditions, rooted in emotional complexes and familial anxieties. And now I have just written of fat and fatness as increasingly palpable, corporeal. I have been led to this contradiction by design, by juxtaposing the metaphorical heart with the physiological heart. I have further complicated matters by taking seriously that confusion of stomach, heart and womb inherent in theories about "maternal overprotection" and by granting a promiscuous personhood to unassuming lipids.

Very well then, I contradict myself. Or rather, we contradict ourselves. No more than Whitman (the poet or the candy sampler in the heart-shaped box) have we made perfect peace between the soul and the solid, and this tension, so often stretched across the heart, is with us still. We tend to use the notion of structure to link spirit to body, and therefore our contradictions find their most extravagant expression in our understanding of the moral architecture of the body—what has been called "temperament" or "constitution" and what we now call "body type" or "build." It is not altogether remarkable, then, that as the Depression put at risk the union of body and soul, especially for those who were fat, structure should be reasserted and a new moral architecture of the body should be drawn up in hopes of bringing body and soul together again, one more foolhardy time.

In the language of medieval medicine, there were four types of people: the sanguine (plump, ruddy, cheerful, hot and moist), the choleric (thin, angry, hot and dry), the phlegmatic (fat, pale, stupid, cold and moist), and the melancholic (thin, shallow, sad, cold and dry). Such types accounted at once for physique, complexion, character and disposition to certain diseases. The sanguine person, for example, tended toward obesity in middle age, but this was a healthy, solid deposit of fat; if ill, a sanguine person suffered from hemorrhages and inflammations. The phlegmatic person, in contrast, carried about an unhealthy, sloppy fat and suffered from diseases of weak circulation. In the 19th century, the four types were shuffled around and recast, most often as the sanguine, bilious, lymphatic and nervous. We have already made the acquaintance of the sanguine and the phlegmatic/lymphatic under the guise of exogenous and endogenous obesity.[78]

When the exo-endo distinction faded, it was in part because of the Depression shift of emphasis from metabolism to appetite, but it was also because the underlying theory of temperaments had been changing. There was a new moral architecture of the body based not on the balance of four quadrants but on a linear continuum. The line ran from one extreme, the pyknic or endomorphic (short and round), to the other, the asthenic or ectomorphic (tall and thin), with the athletic or mesomorphic in the favorable middle (neither short nor tall nor round nor thin). Although the German researcher Ernst Kretschmer in the 1920s explained that no type was inherently better than any other, he found pyknics associated with enlarged thyroid glands and manic-depressive psychoses, asthenics with tuberculosis and schizophrenia, and athletics generally free of regular association with physical or mental illnesses.[79]

From then on, the fat person would seem far more isolated in the scheme of things. The quadrants had allowed for a correspondence of forms and characters. Types shared qualities. The sanguine and the phlegmatic were both moist, the sanguine and the choleric were both hot, the phlegmatic and the melancholic were both cold, and so on. No type was completely estranged from another. The linear continuum allowed the athletic type in the middle some negotiating room on either side, but pyknic and asthenic were as far apart as far could be. When actuaries, physicians and physical culturists began actively to prefer underweight to overweight in adults, the fat person would be left alone at the pyknic end of the spectrum while the athletic was crowded toward the asthenic on the other, "healthier" end.

This was not a simple isolation by body shape (somatotype). As Dr. William H. Sheldon of Harvard would make eminently clear in his influential books on varieties of physique and of temperament (1940, 1942), it was an isolation by character as well. Sheldon's "viscerotonic" (endomorphic) person loved sleep, hated exercise, had slow reactions, a slight sexual appetite but a grievously large appetite for food and society, gave a fine belch from a magnificent gut, and was passive and peace-loving. The viscerotonic person gave the impression of "soft metal, which has no temper in it and will not take an edge . . . a certain flabbiness or lack of intensity in the mental and moral outlook." Published during World War II, that description could hardly be neutral, given especially the profile of the "somatotonic" mesomorph, who loved physical adventure and exercise, took bold risks, was energetic, assertive, competitive, courageous and at times callous and ruthless in the climb to power—in brief, the heroic soldier. Even the "cerebrotonic" ectomorph, introspective, emotionally restrained, hypersensitive to pain, a quick eater and restless sleeper—even this type had more virtues in wartime than the endomorph, for Christ himself had been traditionally portrayed as an ectomorph, and the cerebrotonia inherent in Christian America could give the Yanks that extra spiritual pull they would need to overcome the "unsublimated somatotonia" of the Nazis.[80]

I am not making this up. Sheldon was. Few later researchers could find reliable correlations between the somatotypes and any of Sheldon's "viscerotonic," "somatotonic" or "cerebrotonic" traits. But body typing did not have to carry with it so flagrant a set of moral judgments in order to isolate the fat person. Clinical psychologists and sociologists of the 1950s and 1960s, using only a series of silhouettes, showed that most people, even most fat people, considered endomorphs distant and unlovely figures. It might as easily have been concluded that most people, even most fat people, considered endomorphs from a distance and therefore found them strange and unlovely.[81]

Discouraged by the distant prospect of themselves, fat people had the most distorted images of their own bodies. They were, according to psychiatrist Hilde Bruch in 1957, akin to schizophrenics. They came from similarly debilitating family situations with domineering mothers and weak fathers. They had similarly extreme fantasies of consuming and being consumed. They experienced the world as a similar series of unpredictable distortions; dimensions kept changing around them, their personal space was always being violated.[82]

That fat distorts was a fundamental principle of the new moral architecture of the body. Yet fat, not weight or bone size or specific gravity, was the visually determining factor for the recognizing of body types. In the common silhouettes of endomorph, mesomorph and ectomorph, the quantity and distribution of fat set one profile off from another. People did not think of the short rounded figure as being the most muscled or the tall thin figure as being the most thin-blooded. Those were older, preindustrial associations. The visual continuum by the 1940s was from least fat to most fat, from least distorted to most distorted.

So, ironically, fat people would appear to have the most unreal of bodies even as they were found to be the most unrealistic about their bodies. Fat distorted elemental structure even as it defined elemental type. This flamboyant contradiction was made worse by the cultural suspicion that sight itself might be fattening. It was a dictum of the portrait photographer, the television producer and the fashion designer that the camera put 10 lbs on a body. This was nonsense. The focus, depth, lighting and angle of the shot, the proportions of the frame around the photograph or picture tube or movie screen, and the angle from which one looked toward the captured image made the figures appear fatter or thinner. But the camera seemed to distort consistently toward the endomorphic. And mirrors too, especially those full-length mirrors set into long, thin rectangular frames so that one's body seemed to fill up the entire visual field, mirrors too were fattening. This cultural fantasy about the distortions of camera and mirror would make it less likely than ever that fat people would want to look at images of themselves. Fat women least of all, for they had to contend with narrower tolerances for physical beauty. When Weight Watchers posted old photos of themselves on refrigerator doors, the photos became Evil Eyes, wardens of desire. The very act of looking warned one of fat.[83]

Images of the fat body were thus doubly distorted, first by the fat itself, slippery and deceptive, and next by the act of looking, conditioned as it was by the triumvirate of body types. The distortions were worse for women than for men, not because Paris designers change the "look" from season to season, but because women's bodies naturally have twice as great a percentage of adipose tissue. Women's bodies would therefore be more visually ambiguous. Ernst Kretschmer had found "more indefinite and atypical forms" when he tried to type female physiques; Sheldon thought women more "viscerotonic" than men. Psychologist Sidney Jourard in the 1950s should have been well prepared for his discovery that women themselves were never as satisfied as men with the way they looked. Women wanted to lose weight, change breast shape, reduce waists and hips. They wanted to maintain a clear perimeter to their bodies. Flabbiness, looseness, heaviness would make them seem visually hazy, ill-defined and (it would follow) endomorphic.[84]

As one's image was primarily determined by fat, so one could master that image only by mastering fat. With the underlying "build" one could not do much of anything. Build was built-in. It was hereditary. Insurance examiners had early been advised to consider build, and by the 1930s physicians were grumbling that standard height-weight charts made no allowances for build. The Metropolitan Life tables of the 1940s finally did incorporate columns for small, medium and large frames, but those tables came without good instructions on how to determine build.[85]

Fat people could claim that they were big-boned, large-framed people. Build, however, was far more arthritic an apology for overweight or obesity than metabolism had been. With a faulty metabolism you could bury the blame in the past while letting the future puff out as it might. Metabolism was at once an inheritance, a current investment and a future trust. But build? Build gave you 10 to 15 lbs leeway at most. It granted you no new purchase on fat, nothing to bank on in the days ahead. Build meant only that whatever you did, you had a certain skeletal structure. That structure could be filled in or out as you chose. An ectomorph *could* be fat; an ath-

letic mesomorph *could* go to pot in middle age. Conversely, an endomorph *could* by dint of diet and deft costume appear slender.
Build was far less comforting than metabolism, especially when fat
was so active a presence, eager to transform a real mesomorph into
an apparent endomorph.

Builds were merely the ramparts from which one watched for
fat. Fat could come at any time, and it favored the night. ("Night-
eating" was a syndrome first associated with the obese during the
1950s.)[86] Fat could lay siege from any direction; it knew instinc-
tively where the heart was and how to reach it, by hook or by crook.

Most sieges are won from inside, by betrayal. Call such bodily
treason "constitutional." The more resolute fat was, the more it
seemed that there must be inside help, some internal disposition to
fat. Such dispositions had been remarked since the 18th century,
and estimates of the relative importance of heredity had risen considerably over the years in tandem with Darwinism and then Men-
delian genetics. In the mid-19th century, some 30–40% of cases of
obesity were attributed to hereditary factors; by the mid-20th, the
estimate was up to 60–70%. Those percentages were computed
from medical histories: 60–70% of fat people had at least one fat
parent. In 1923, Charles B. Davenport, America's leading eugeni-
cist, proposed that fatness was a dominant genetic trait, slenderness
recessive. A slender woman mating with a fat man would produce
offspring who were medium-to-fat. A child of two fat parents would
be encumbered with all the flesh that heirs are ill to. When C. H.
Danforth in 1927 located hereditary obesity in a strain of yellow
mice, it seemed entirely possible that humans might also carry a
gene for fat.[87]

If such a gene there be, we have not found it. Nor would things
change were we to find it tomorrow. People must eat, and how they
eat will always be a function of the society in which they live—its
food taboos, its childrearing practices, its food processing techniques, its economic system, its compromises with climate and terrain. Chromosomes would only assure a *tendency* toward the accumulation of fat.[88]

The idea of a genetic obesity was therefore less important than
the appearance of a cultural belief that fat itself had an historical,
even a prehistorical, momentum which continued on inside certain
bodies. Those who could store fat easily had held an evolutionary
advantage in primitive hunting-and-gathering societies, or so the
belief went. Unlike pastoralists and agriculturists, who could accu-

mulate surpluses, hunter-gatherers were subject to the immediate vicissitudes of nature. Body fat was their only stockpile. In modern society, fat-storing endomorphs were atavisms, neolithic remnants, more cautious, more retentive than they had any reason to be. Like the squat, fat, fleshy statuette of the Venus of Willendorf, unearthed in 1908 and described in 1929 by medical historian Fielding H. Garrison as a fine example of endocrine obesity, the endomorph was the figure of a Stone-Age culture.[89]

Active *and* historical, fat would be doubly hard to root out. As obesity came to seem more dangerous, striking at the heart and the arteries, it came also to seem more intractable. The prospects for successful permanent weight loss grew dimmer. Dr. Robert H. Rose, who had written his own diet book in 1916, was estimating a 75% failure rate in 1928. Dr. William M. Ballinger wrote in 1930 that with cooperation and perseverance, the obese patient might be assured of an excellent prognosis, "but in actual practice, if you are able to reduce fifty per cent of your patients to ideal weight and keep them there for at least one year, you may consider yourself eminently successful in the treatment of obesity." Ballinger was an optimist. Dr. Hugo R. Rony in 1940, following up his most promising weight-loss cases three to five years later, found all of them overweight and some of them heavier than before. In 1944, Yale researchers reported an 80 percent failure rate over the long term, this in the midst of wartime food-rationing. By 1959, in an article so widely quoted that it has become a citation classic, psychiatrist A. J. Stunkard and Mavis McLaren-Hume reviewed all the follow-up studies in the medical and psychological literature, noting that "a majority of persons regain a majority of the pounds lost." Seven years later, the Public Health Service would declare, "The treatment of obesity is one of the most exasperating experiences in clinical and preventive medicine." By 1981 the reported failure rate was up to 95 percent for those seeking the permanent loss of 40 lbs or more. Wrote one physician in 1982, "a person is more likely to recover from most forms of cancer than from obesity."[90]

Haunted by heredity and history, the dieter's life had to be "one long unending struggle, with one eye constantly on the scales," a life of "unceasing vigilance." Readers of the *Ladies Home Journal* were advised in 1941, "Don't say you are dieting for a week or a month or three months. Say you are adjusting your food to your circumstances, forever." The Harvard physiologist Jean Mayer, one of the nation's most academically respected experts on nutrition and obesity, testified before the Senate in 1972 that "the cost of thinness may be eternal vigilance, and where you may have to impose on yourself ten years, twenty years, thirty years, a lifetime of a certain discipline."[91]

Wholeheartedness: The Romance of Exercise

Vigilance and discipline were not enough. "Old Debbil Fat" was sly, active and quarrelsome.[92] The dieter had to be thoroughgoing, assertive, and energetic. Counting calories, keeping weight charts, measuring out food on kitchen scales—these were defensive maneuvers, ritual acts of penitence, gestures of restraint. Now was the time for heroism and romance, acts of transformation, gestures of power. Where ritual dieting might stave off heart attacks and possibly renew life, the dieting romance *began* with a change of heart. If the fat person was a sad person, empty and insatiable, wasn't it foolish to insist at the start on restraint? If the fat person was beset by history, what grounds were there to expect cheerful perseverance? Rather, begin with the transformation of the inner person and so engage fat from a position of strength. Anxious for autonomy, restless with the chains of time, the romantic dieter was an adventurer. Someone with style. Courage. Vitality. Vitamins.

Vitamins were the charms that drew dieting out of ritual into romance. "Minute, elusive, mysterious" and strangely powerful when first named by the Russian scientist Casimir Funk in 1912, vitamins were popularly conceived of as "the life of the food." Somehow vitamins gave food an enormous inner strength. They appeared to substitute for protein, as in the 1922 cookbook, *Eating Vitamines.* They might stand in for fat, to offset depression and hunger. They could take the place of calories in low-calorie diets or diet foods such as Min-amin (1935) or Kyron (1948) or Unicap-M Diet Formula (1984). They revitalized the neurasthenic, restored sanity to the victim of pellagra. They could bring beauty in times of peace and "fortify" staple foods in times of war. By 1943, when eleven vitamins had been identified, nearly a third of American families were using vitamin concentrates such as Vita-Kaps, which was advertised explicitly as a supplement for those on home-made reducing diets. A trim model of 114 lbs stands on a sleek penny scale reading her fortune; she has an "inherent power for organization, great determination—and a vitamin deficiency!" Those not on diets were drinking vitamin D–enriched milk or eating vitamin A–enriched margarine on vitamin B–enriched breads. But even as vitamin manufacturers sold $200 million worth of vitamins in 1944, eight out of ten housewives could not explain the difference between a vitamin and a calorie.[93]

The confusion was crucial. Vitamins were both a source of energy and a source of health. Vitamin deficiency was known as "hidden hunger." The Kellogg Company in 1942 would show "How You Can Help Others Combat HIDDEN HUNGER" by serving its vitamin-enriched wheat cereal, Pep. Hidden hunger is exactly what this chapter has been about; vitamin theory was perfectly coincident with the ballad of the fat café. People got fat, explained Hollywood's National Institute of Nutrition in 1935, because they overate, and they overate because something invisible was always missing from their food. The National Institute's Min-amin reducing food (primarily wheat germ) would satisfy the appetite because it had the missing ingredient. In the first part of this chapter, that missing ingredient would have been love; now it was vitamins.[94]

The idea that sickness could be due to something *missing* had been hard to swallow during the 19th century. With the positivism of modern science, physiologists and medical investigators were looking for active agents of disease. Despite evidence for dietary deficiencies in the cases of scurvy, anemia and goiter, scientists warmed to the presence of bacteria, and scoffed at the apparently medieval supposition that something could arise from nothing. Deficiency diseases were most thoughtfully considered by agricultural chemists familiar with the problems of soil depletion and trace minerals. It was through academic departments of agriculture and agricultural experiment stations that vitamins gained professional and then popular ground. Vitamins, even when synthesized and produced in laboratories, would therefore seem earthy and natural. They also would seem filling, because they ended hidden hunger.[95]

Once accepted, vitamins were to exogenous obesity what thyroid preparations had been to endogenous obesity. Like the thyroid drugs, vitamins stimulated the body and kept it growing. They were synonymous with freshness, sunlight, bright eyes and smooth skin. They solved the problem of appetite without adding a single calorie. They were nonfattening and, it seemed, always on the side of good. It was avitaminosis—the lack of vitamins—that could produce "a puffy appearance of the skin simulating obesity."[96]

Of themselves, vitamins could not remove weight or fat. They

were the waybread romantic dieters would take to sustain themselves in the midst of their transformation. The transformation itself
had to be more athletic.

The Depression shift of emphasis from metabolism to appetite,
from glands to calories, had done little for the physical approach to
dieting. As beauty columnist and nutritionist Ida Jean Kain explained in her R_x *for Slimming* (1940), "Exercise is no match for calories." One might bend and stretch for spot reducing, but for general weight-loss, exercise was "a practical joker." With 3,600
calories to the pound of flesh, a dieter clambering up 2,240 steps to
the top of the Empire State Building would lose ½ lb. To work off
an entire pound, a dieter must lay 14,731 bricks or scrape dirty
laundry across a washboard 2,100 times an hour for 28 hours
straight. Such equations were common in diet books. Dr. William
Engel, responsible for the lamb-chop-and-pineapple diet of the
1920s, choreographed calories according to dance steps in 1939. The
rumba, at 8.85 cals/lb body-weight/hr, was outclassed by the Big
Apple (10.75), the polka (16.75), and the mazurka (24.03). Yet a
150-lb person dancing the mazurka full out for an hour would lose
no more than a pound. And after all that exercise, a few innocent
pieces of bread and butter would put the weight back on again. A
pat of butter was equivalent to climbing all the steps inside the
Washington Monument, a single doughnut meant conducting an or-
chestra for 2½ hours. Hazel M. Hauck's *How to Control Your
Weight* (1942) put everything most prosaically (and therefore most
pessimistically) in terms of distances to be walked off. A Graham
cracker took .7 mile, an ice cream sundae 5 to 7 miles. Would a person unlikely to walk a mile for a Camel walk seven for a sundae?[97]

Put this way, exercise ran dieting aground in the middle of Zeno's
paradox: No matter how many steps one took, there would be yet
another step to take or stair to climb. One could never reach the
end. But if one thought of reducing in terms of fat rather than of calories, exercise had virtue. Exercise could turn flab into muscle,
change shape, improve endurance, strengthen the heart. Exercise
could transform. It set the dieting romance in motion.

Popular advice in 1908 was that "standing erect half an hour after eating helps in an even distribution of fat."[98] The practice depended for its success upon the inertness of fat, drawn down the
body by gravity as one stood in postprandial suspense. When fat became aggressive and invasive, such moderate devotions would not
do. Though the World War I calisthenics of Susanna Cocroft were

neglected during the 1920s in favor of gland treatments and calorie-counting, exercise slowly returned to favor in the next decades. As radio listeners in 1932 heard on the Columbia network from the Voice of Experience, "Reducing from diet alone . . . does not build good, firm, shapely muscle tissue and vigorous vital organs; it takes exercise to accomplish that. Exercise oxygenates the body and oxidizes the fat; then if you eat a non-fattening diet, you will surely produce a more normal, shapely, vital physique."[99]

That shapely physique had—a new word—"streamline." Let Celia Cole explain, as she did for the popular middlebrow magazine, the *Delineator*, in 1934: "When a thing is streamline, it's so built—isn't it?—that nothing impedes its progress. It's stripped for speed . . . it goes where it means to go and with the least possible friction. That's streamline." Originally a term in hydrodynamics, by 1934 "streamline" meant "Intelligence. Health. The will-to-achieve. Strength of character. Courage. Faith." Where to find a better profile for the romantic adventurer? This was, to be sure, the profile of the modern romantic, "revealing up-to-date lines—the new 'streamline' body—not too heavy, not too thin—a body that will fit our civilization." It was the body of the Franklin car advertised in 1930, "as smart and as modern as youth itself." It was the body the dieter wanted, "functional, firm and active."[100]

The streamline(d) body was a dynamic, athletic body, lithe rather than light. It was the body of such fashion models as Choo Choo Johnson, Stretch Smith, and the young Gerald Ford, all models for Harry Conover. His was the agency responsible for the Cover Girl of the 1940s—the Noxzema Cover Girl, the *Cover Girl* movie of 1944, the first cover girls for *Mademoiselle*. Unlike the "Slender, Tender and Tall" women of the 1942 popular song or the "long-stemmed American Beauty Roses" of the John Robert Powers agency (founded 1933), Conover's women (and men) looked more robust, more wholesome, more middle-class, more Midwestern—as he was himself. Conover had been a top male model for Powers, but in 1939 he broke away to form his own agency with the help of two other Powers models, Phyllis Brown and her friend (later President) Gerald Ford, then at Yale Law School and confident enough to invest $1,000 in the Conover enterprise. The new look, with Brown and Ford, reached *Look* in 1940 and *Cosmopolitan* in 1942. American Airlines stewardesses and WACS recruiters adopted it in 1944.[101]

During the war, while young men were run through basic training, women who had swapped skirts for greasy overalls were given

Joe Bonomo's *Health Manual for War Workers*. Published by the National Foremen's Institute, the manual promoted efficient work as exercise toward beauty. "There is no reason why physical toil should forever rob you of your glamour and fragile femininity," wrote Bonomo, a former movie stuntman and serials star. His emphasis, however, was on glamour, not fragility, as appropriate for the winner of the 1919 Modern Apollo Contest. It was healthy to sweat, good to get tough. An active war job firmed up the body and reduced weight. "There's no need to visualize yourself as a barrel-shaped, waddling peasant" just because you do physical labor, Bonomo added. The right shape and the right weight were extra benefits of war work.[102]

So too were pantie girdles. Industrial welfare directors promoted the pantie girdle as support against fatigue. Previously pantie girdles had been "soft little roll-ons for the junior trade," but now they were part of the war effort. A corset company in 1942 even hired physical fitness lecturer Olga Ley to create a course of exercises for women. That was a big change, as Ley noted, since corset companies had customarily considered themselves in competition with calisthenics. Now, shaping garments were advertised as flexible enough to accommodate the active physical life.[103]

After the war, Jantzen began to produce "Lastex-powered figure-control swim suits" whose elastic panels worked in a manner surprisingly parallel to the theory of containment broached at the start of the Cold War. As George F. Kennan wrote in *Foreign Affairs* in 1947, "Soviet pressure against the free institutions of the western world is something that can be contained by the adroit and vigilant applications of counter-force at a series of constantly shifting geographical and political points." Elasticity, exercise, pressure and power became national defense policy as they became instrumental in the battle against encroaching fat. President Harry Truman did pull-ups on the Charles M. Pierce slanting board and took morning constitutionals; Eisenhower was on a low-fat diet and playing golf while he established a President's Council on Physical Fitness (1955). When Bonnie Prudden reported on the poor physical condition of American youth, Eisenhower would establish a second Council on Youth Fitness. Gallup pollsters interviewed Americans in January 1957, asking, "Do you think young people in the United States get more or less exercise than young people in the U.S.S.R.?" More than half of those who had any opinion on the question believed that the Russians were getting more exercise. Exercise was becoming a part of the Cold War and an index to national character.[104]

Bonnie Prudden was herself a national character. She was head of the Institute for Physical Fitness, fitness editor for *Sports Illustrated*, and a regular attraction on NBC-TV's "Today Show." Her 1959 exercise record, "Keep Fit/Be Happy," was, according to TV host Dave Garroway, "Another step forward . . . in helping us to be an alive, alert nation in these difficult times." To the tunes of "The Most Beautiful Girl in the World" and "Wait Till You See Her," Prudden took her audiences through bends, stretches, twists, jumps and kicks. Her constant refrain was to keep the "abdominals" tight. "Tighten those abdominals. You never give them any peace." These were difficult times, and the center had to hold. The free body (the free world?) could relax to the strains of "Sophisticated Lady" only after it had mightily exerted itself.[105]

Prudden's counterpart, the "Norman Vincent Peale with muscles," was Jack LaLanne. LaLanne began leading calisthenics on television in San Francisco in 1951. By 1960 he had the biggest national daytime TV show, and forty thousand orders came in each month for his Glamour Stretcher, "a whole gym in a rubber cord." His first book, *Way to Vibrant Good Health*, sold more than 150,000 copies in hardback and 250,000 in paper. "I'm as dedicated about this as Billy Graham," LaLanne said. "He puts people in shape for the hereafter, and I get them fit for the here and now."[106]

LaLanne's here and now was a "great adventure," a "quest." "Not for the Holy Grail like crusaders of old, not even the Fountain of Youth like Ponce de Leon. Yet there is something of both in my adventure. It has been a crusade and a quest for foods to fulfill a dream.

"The dream? To put a fairer face on an ugly duckling. (Me.) To create health out of the chronic illness I knew as a child. A strong physique for one that was puny and embarrassing." He had been "a pathetic little world-hating, heart-aching boy" with "an ungovernable hunger for candy and soft drinks." He had not grown fat, like his father (a former dancing master), but thin and weak-eyed, weak-spined. His father died of a heart attack and chronic "pooped-out-itis" while still in his forties; Jack would start exercising and eating wisely late in his teens, influenced by the health lecturer Paul Bragg. Jack's mother had babied him; now he would strike out on his own and find glamour, become a "G-man" like Franklin D. Roosevelt or Winston Churchill. Glamour-men and Glamour-women were charming, fascinating, exciting, enchanting and adventurous. Norman Vincent Peale had glamour; so did Gandhi and General Douglas MacArthur. Glamour came from the inside of the person. It was the flash in the eyes and the spring in the step. It was faith and the sharing of faith. It was wholeheartedness.[107]

This was the transformation implied by the dieting romance: from the empty, sad heart to the full, joyous heart. It could hardly be incidental that the nutritionists Frederick J. Stare and Jean Mayer of the Harvard School of Public Health should press for more exercise for everyone—including the sluggish endomorph—even as Bonnie Prudden equated fitness with happiness. And it could hardly be incidental that such heart specialists as Dr. Paul Dudley White should advocate more exercise—to *strengthen* the heart—even as Jack LaLanne reinvented glamour before the TV camera. The dieting romance was the final way out of those hearts of darkness—the broken heart, the bursting heart—which made the lives of fat people at midcentury so hopeless and so threatened.[108]

"No," wrote diet author Vance Thompson as early as 1914; "the fat man may clown and slap himself and wag a droll forefinger, but he is not merry at all; and if one should sink a shaft down to his heart—or rather drive a tunnel through to it—one would discover that it is a sad heart, black with melancholy."[109] I have not meant here, or at any moment in this book, to play fast and loose with the heart, or with sadness, or with the lives of those who are fat. I have meant these pages on broken and bursting hearts to take us across the Depression, World War II, and the Cold War with some sense of the depth of emotions behind the monotrophic diets, amphetamine pills, group therapies and fitness records of the times. Only when the emotions run so deep, only when the symbols are so primitive, do rituals take such hold or romances gain such footing.

There was to the culture of slimming between 1930 and 1960 an elemental fear that the more one had, the emptier one would be. The overprotective mother made for hollow-hearted, insatiable children. The round fat man had constricted arteries and a weak heart. The endomorph was soft, passive, out of focus. Overweight and obesity were, ironically, symptoms of emptiness, not signs of fullness. The emptiness was disturbing because the desire that lay behind it was remorseless and unquenchable.

This was, at heart, the fantastic nightmare of the consumer who finds that the more one has, the less one is. Americans of the Depression and the Cold War projected onto fat men and women their own basic fears of abundance, their own confusions about how to handle themselves in a world that seemed to offer so much and yet guaranteed so little.

On such fears and such confusions an entire economy could be built.

CHAPTER EIGHT

Thin Bodies, Fat Profits

As dieting became a national way of life, Americans were caught up in a market system that profited by offering more of less. "Anyway you look at it," read an advertisement for Diet Delight foods in 1983, "you lose." But the lo-cal economy was not just a question of ironically effective advertising. It drew upon a fundamental change in basic patterns of living and attitudes toward food. The culture of slimming has gradually asserted the primacy of flavor over substance. It has put in question our very sense of what is and what is not a food, what is an imitation and what is real.

Don't Stay Fat
$1.00 Box
Free

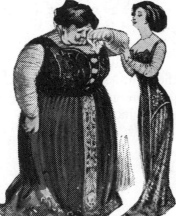

My treatment is prepared scientifically. It does not stop or hinder digestion: on the contrary, it promotes proper digestion and assimilation of food, which 99 fat people in a hundred haven't got, and that's why they are fat.

Don't Cry Because You Are Fat. Send To Prof. Kellogg and He Will Reduce You As He Did Me.

Free, posi:·· ly free, a $1.00 box of Kellogg's Safe Fat Reducer, to every sufferer from fat, just to prove that it actually reduces you to normal, does it safely, and builds up your health at the same time. I want to send you without a cent of expense on your part this $1.00 package of what I am free to call a really wonderful fat reducer.

From Woman Beautiful *(1910). Frank J. Kellogg's Rengo obesity cure and Safe Fat Reducer ads drew some 135,000 replies by 1914.* Courtesy of the Library of Congress

Past and Present

THOMAS WOOD, a miller of Billericay in the county of Essex, was fat, fair and forty in 1759. He had eaten well of fat meat, ale, butter, bread and cheese, and he felt fine. Four years later he was an insomniac with a sick stomach, bad bowels, vertigo, rheumatism and gout. A clergyman showed Wood the autobiography of Luigi Cornaro, who had cured himself of a similar run of ills at a similar age by choosing to drink little and eat less. Wood was convinced. Within months he was off all malt liquor, taking cold baths and exercising with dumbbells. Within a year he was out-abstaining the abstinent Cornaro, denying himself water, moist vegetables, butter, cheese and meat. He maintained his newly restored health on daily meals of seabiscuit pudding. At the age of fifty, to use his own expression, he was "metamorphosed from a monster to a person of moderate size." He died in 1783 at the age of sixty-four from an inflammation of the bowels.[1]

Thomas Wood was the old breed of dieter. He never once weighed himself. (Friends thought he might have lost as much as 150 lbs.) The story of Wood, often repeated in the 19th-century

239

English literature on dieting, bears repeating again as foil to the late-20th-century culture of slimming.

Though he could have been weighed on the steelyard scales of a butcher or wine merchant, Wood had no recourse to penny platform scales at local drugstores or city halls. For him there were no streamlined bathroom scales with "graceful, flowing beauty, free from all obstructions," no oval or hexagonal bathroom scales, no bathroom scales in mint green, hot dots, maize, Dubonnet, autumn wheat, French provincial, butcher block, leather, cane, fur, fashion sable, marble, wicker, wood-grain or nostalgia. No Stow-A-Way or Hide-A-Weigh scale, no personal scale to carry with him in a trim plaid case. No bathroom scale designed for a bride, "made like a fine watch—feather-light, slim as a wafer, handsome as her silver itself!" No semiconductor strain-gauge (load cell) pressure transducers to make electronic digital scales possible. No Datatrim, "The amazing scale that talks to you . . . and predicts your weight in the future!" No Sunbeam Motivator with a General Instrument voice synthesizer, 400K bits of ROM memory and a Hitachi microprocessor, saying "Congratulations, I am pleased. You are making progress. Today practice taking more time to chew each mouthful."[2]

Indeed, there were few voices, natural or synthetic, alive or dead, to advise Wood on losing weight. Aside from Cornaro, Wood could have read the works of George Cheyne, as he did, and treatises by two other contemporary Englishmen, Thomas Short and Malcolm Flemyng. If literate in Latin, he might have leafed through two dozen foreign dissertations produced between 1670 and 1778 on the subject of pinguitude. In spare moments he might have come across books and articles on beauty with passages about reducing "Bodies of an unwieldy Bulk." All this was a far cry from the 6,397 technical works on obesity published between 1964 and 1979; a far cry from the 300 diet books in print in the United States in 1984; a far cry from the average of 1.25 dieting articles per issue in the *Ladies Home Journal, Good Housekeeping* and *Harper's Bazaar* between 1980 and 1984, or the 66 articles on dieting that appeared in 22 contemporary magazines in January of 1980. Five million copies of Dr. Irwin Stillman's *Quick Weight Loss Diet* (1967) were not yet in circulation, nor were nearly four million people watching the "Richard Simmons Show" on television to learn to "be the best you can be" and "never-say-diet." There were no professional journals such as *Obesity and Bariatric Medicine* (1971), *International Journal of Obesity* (1977), *Appetite* (1980) or the *International Journal of Eating Disorders* (1981), nor could he find more popular periodicals such as *Slimmer* (circulation 250,000), *Slimming* (United Kingdom, circulation over 400,000) or *Weight Watchers Magazine* (circulation base 825,000).[3]

Wood had to design his diet by himself, as he had to create his own diet dish, that seabiscuit pudding. He could not benefit from the Graham cracker, let alone from the dieters' Basy Bread (1918), Cellu cellulose wafers (1921), diet zwieback, Slim Krisp, Ry-Krisp and Norwegian Ideal Flat Bread (late 1940s), or from Profile Bread (late 1960s) or Less (1976: "Soon you can eat more bread by eating Less. Less . . . at last"). Wood could not substitute soy protein mixes for his "fat" meat or buy new, leaner cuts of ham. He could not fill his ale cup with low-calorie carbonated beverages (1952), light beers (1953, first successes 1973) or light wines (1981). His butter might have been rancid or adulterated, but it was still fat and full of calories, unlike the emulsions called "spreads" in the 1970s. Skim milk was not considered fit for human consumption until the 1920s, nonfat dry milk appeared after World War II, instant nonfat dry milk in 1955, advertisements for the "Mooraculous Moo Juice" in 1978. If he had thought to, Wood might have gone on the cottage cheese diet first popularized in 1956, but Kraft Light-n'-Lively and Borden Lite Line cheeses escaped him. In 1973, Barbara Kraus could list a low-calorie version of practically every kind of food in her *Dictionary of Calories and Carbohydrates*—including Aunt Leah's frozen concentrate diet borscht. In 1983 alone, ninety-one new light foods were introduced.[4]

Wood's seabiscuit pudding was hardly an innovation. It belonged to a tradition of invalid and infant foods of the same consistency and same starchy base, recipes for which could be found in medical texts and cookbooks throughout the 18th and 19th centuries. Wood was not blessed with that shelf of diet cookbooks we have now. As a genre apart from recipes in diet manuals, the diet cookbook owed its origin to promotional booklets distributed by food manufacturers and their trade associations. In 1938 the American Institute of Baking rolled out white bread as "a proper part of modern *reducing* diets" in its *The Right Way to Right Weight*. Around 1940, the Ralston Purina Company produced two booklets on weight reduction with Ry-Krisp as the centerpiece. In 1942, the Knox Gelatine Company published its *Reducing Diets and Recipes*. By 1951, the National Dairy Council had published a full-scale diet cookbook, Margaret A. Ohlson's *Weight Reduction Through Diet with Everyday Foods Everyone Likes*, emphasizing, of course, the use of whole milk or of skim milk and butter.[5]

Commercial publishers entered the diet cookbook field in 1950 with Annie W. Williams-Heller's *Reducer's Cook Book*, then Bernard Koten's *The Low-calory Cookbook* and E. Virginia Dobbin's *The Low Fat, Low Cholesterol Diet* (both in 1951), then Dorothy M. Hildreth's *Low Fat Diet Cook Book*, Llewellyn Miller's *Reducing Cookbook and Diet Guide* and Marvin Small's *The Special Diet Cook Book* (all in 1952). These were plain titles for plain books with relatively plain recipes, remarkable only in their increasing devotion to vegetables. Almost immediately it became evident that dieters needed tastier foods and livelier titles. New diet cookbooks concentrated on spices and flavorings, elegant place settings, the pleasures of gastronomy. Their titles were upbeat and upscale: Elaine Ross's *Reduce and Enjoy It Cookbook* (1953), Martin Lederman's *The Slim Gourmet* (1955) and, later, Naura Hayden's *The Hip, High-Prote, Low-Calorie Easy Does It Cookbook* (1972).

If Wood went out to eat, he would not find Sweet 'N Low in the sugar bowl, a dieter's special on the menu or a salad bar across the aisle. (Indeed, he would not find in any tavern or inn a sugar bowl, a menu or a salad, period.) There would be no diet fast-food chain until D'lites opened in 1981. Even at the grocer's, Wood was out of luck looking for a low-calorie prepared meal; he would never taste Stouffer's cheese cannelloni (Lean Cuisine), Celentano's Lasagne Primavera, or Weight Watchers Frozen Pizza.[6]

Aside from his one diet food, seabiscuit pudding, Wood also used exercise: dumbbells. He could as well have walked long distances, wrestled, rowed, run, leaped, maneuvered across a wooden horse, or gone a-hunting. There were sports to play, gardens to hoe, bricks to lay, logs to chop, fields to sow. These were fine on good summer days, but what could Wood do indoors in winter without a Schwinn Air-Dyne exercycle with its true Ergometer, a wind-vane system providing programmable workload resistance, a pedal RPM indicator, trip odometer and electronic digital timer? Or the Vitamaster Pro*1000 totally electronic fitness system from Allegheny International, a hi-tech exercycle with read-outs for calories, pulse, speed and distance? How long could Wood persevere without a Relaxicizor (400,000 sold 1949–70) or a Jack Feather Sauna Belt (600,000 sold 1968–70)? And if Wood did not jog, was this because Nike had yet to advertise its designer sweatsuits or because Adidas had yet to attach a microcomputer to its running shoes to keep track of calories and miles?[7]

I am being facetious, but Wood was truly on his own, without much advice or equipment. He might go to spas at Bath or Bristol, but there were no environments primarily for weight-loss, such as those a century later in Marienbad or two centuries later in Waterville, Maine, and in Phoenix, founded by Elizabeth Arden in 1936 and 1946. The water and the phoenix were most appropriate totems for a woman who had begun life as Florence Nightingale Graham, just as the Golden Door was a fine totem for spas in Tecate, Mexico, and Escondido, California, which were meant to gild as they groomed. For the poorer sort there were illusions of *minceur* at Safety Harbor in Florida and out on the barren California desert in Lancaster, where the Bermuda Inn cast its triangular spell as "the best blubber bargain in the world."[8]

Wood might stay at home and consult his local doctor, but there were no specialists in obesity. Even now, the American Society of Bariatric Physicians has second-class professional standing. Established in 1950 as the National Obesity Society, it was renamed the National Glandular Society, then the American College of Endocrinology and Nutrition, then in 1961 the American Society of Bariatrics. "Bariatrics" was a new word marking the shift in the treatment of obesity away from glands toward appetite and exercise. In the shift, bariatricians (400 in 1972, 600 in 1982) gained a Latin title only to lose professional ground. If a psychologist could deal with appetite and a dancer with exercise, the bariatrician was left to prescribe drugs—appetite suppressants, diuretics, glandular substances—that were themselves in growing disrepute within the medical community.[9]

Among the lay specialists in obesity were Monty MacLevy, B. H. Stauffer, and Lawrence L. Mack. Their reducing salons might well have appealed to Thomas Wood. Each featured vibrating tables and machines whose motions Wood the miller would have found curiously similar to the rotary grindstones of his own occupation. (Had he lived into the 19th century, the new roller milling process would have presented an even more striking parallel.) Monty MacLevy, former assistant general manager of the Madison Square Garden Swimming Pool and Gym, opened his salons in the 1930s with Roaler Massagers, Back Ring Rollers and the Slendro Massager Table. Lying on his Slendro Massager was "like a silent movie where you see yourself being spanked and await with dread the stinging pain which never arrives." This was neat therapy for the Depression, and MacLevy had two hundred salons by its end. In 1938, B. H. Stauffer invented a mechanized table called "the magic couch," which could double as a davenport and had an attachment for rocking the baby's cradle. The Stauffer chain had 225 salons by 1959. Lawrence L. Mack had been a door-to-door salesman in Missouri during the Depression. Coming out of the Navy after World War II, he was on the lookout for a market opening, an enterprise. In 1950 he established Slenderella (initially, Silooette) to "civilize" reducing salons. He enlisted a professor at Ohio State University to design a table to slenderize a woman with her clothes on, got Dr. William Fishbein (brother of the roly-poly AMA potentate, Dr. Morris Fishbein) to test and approve the new table, and drafted size 12 Eloise English, former WAVES lieutenant commander, to supervise national operations. He installed Muzak in his anterooms, purchased a *Good Housekeeping* Seal of Approval, and talked about "figure-proportioning" rather than weight reducing. In 1956 he had 145 salons and was handling 300,000 people from the age of nine to eighty-six.[10]

Then there was Vic Tanny, the Rochester, New York, newsboy whose first gym failed in 1935. He moved to Santa Monica, California, and began again. By 1961 he had eighty health clubs or gyms, forerunners of the fitness centers of the next decades. Tanny's program did not rely upon the subtle vibrations of passive ergotherapy but upon the hard-sell and Tanny's wonderfully ambiguous philosophy that "health can be banked like money."[11]

Thomas Wood had neither Vic Tanny nor vibrating tables. He was literally without support. There were no heart associations or cancer societies to assure Wood that he was on the right track, no insurance company weight charts to give Wood a sense of mortal purpose, no toll-free long-distance numbers to dial to ask about the caloric properties of seabiscuits. He could not join Weight Watchers or call his sponsor from Overeaters Anonymous at the start of a binge. Neither could he enroll in a Diet Workshop to learn "healthy eating habits for weight loss now and forever," nor walk to the nearest Diet Center to "Become Less Of A Person In Just Two Weeks." Nutritional Management, Inc., had not expanded from Boston to Billericay to bring him "A shared commitment. . . . Empathy and expertise." Thin Forever! Inc. of Manhattan had no franchise in Essex for individual counseling, survival techniques, group rap sessions and assertiveness training. There was no 18th-century salon run by Gloria Marshall, "The Best Friend Your Figure Ever Had." No Schick Easy Start Diet Place with "supportive, fun group meetings" could be pinpointed on a map of Georgian England. Wood had no local

YMCA offering a "free fitness-related calorie counter/slide rule, just for stopping by," no local clinic with weekly group sessions on such topics as the effects of stress and anxiety on eating, and how to stay *"Forever Thin."*[12]

Expanding Markets

I have sorely abused poor Thomas Wood. I have beset him with ana-chronism, transported him from Great Britain to the United States, forced upon him the company of dieting women. May he forgive me this exercise in unlikeness. The exercise, of course, has been meant for us, not for him. Enmeshed as we are in a slimming culture, we need to disentangle ourselves for a moment in order to appreciate the fineness of the web. With Thomas Wood we have stood just out-side that web and heard the distant spider call us to the parlor.

The parlor, with its Golden Door and magic couch, its talking scales and wheelless bicycles, its Less bread and no-alcohol wine (Seagram's St. Regis), has been as rich and well-appointed as it has been enticing. The sale of diet foods alone rose at a 10 percent an-nual rate between 1960 and 1980, amounting then to nearly 7 per-cent of all U.S. food sales. The diet soft drink market is growing at a 20 percent annual rate, stimulated by the approval of a new artifi-cial sweetener, aspartame (NutraSweet, Equal), from which G. D. Searle & Co. had $585 million in revenues in 1984. Diet food and diet beverage sales in 1984 were advancing at triple the pace of all other foods and drinks, with a market of $41 billion projected for 1990.[13]

Over-the-counter drugs for weight control have been even more profitable, their sales climbing at a better than 20 percent annual rate. Stimulated by the 1979 FDA approval of phenylpropanol-amine (PPA) as a safe and mildly effective appetite suppressant, and then in 1982 by $150 million in sales of "starch blockers," the proprietary diet drug industry has benefited as well from comple-mentary sales of laxatives, diuretics, vitamin and mineral supple-ments and liquid diet formulas. Thompson Medical Company, the leading advertiser of over-the-counter diet drugs, had sales of $29 million in 1978; on the strength of its Appedrine, Prolamine, Con-trol and Dexatrim, Thompson expected sales of $1 billion in 1985.[14]

The Relaxicizor, promising to build "a living girdle from the muscles" with its electric dashboard, switches, cords, belts and soothing tingle, grossed $400 million in twenty years. Jack Feather's simpler plastic Sauna Belt grossed $6 million in three years or less. In 1947 gyms across the country were making a total of $50 million a year; in 1959, Vic Tanny alone was making $21 million from his health clubs, Stauffer System Salons and Home Plan were making $40 million, and Slenderella $25–35 million.[15]

When it first became a business, Weight Watchers had revenues of $160,000 (1964). In 1970, revenues were up to $8 million, in 1977 to $39 million, with nine million people registered in thirteen years. Even accounting for inflation, this was more than a hundredfold increase in business. Harold Katz, creator of the Nutri/System Weight Loss Centers, had 1981 revenues of $48 million from 352 franchises, enough money to allow him to buy the Philadelphia 76ers basketball team. With such horizons, the Carnation Company in 1983 launched its own weight-loss business to promote its line of Diet Chef foods and take advantage of the expanding diet market.[16]

The market was expanding because the percentage of people considered overweight kept growing. In 1933, one-fifth of Americans were thought to be at least 10 percent overweight; in 1949, one-quarter; in 1973, one-third. (This meant, in absolute numbers, 79,000,000 people—a composite figure of those who thought themselves overweight and those who were overweight but denied it.) If the data were confined to adults over thirty, proportions were even more impressive: one-half to two-thirds. If one imposed a stricter 5 percent margin on acceptable weight, nine out of every ten adults could be overweight.[17]

The market was expanding because more people believed that they were overweight. In a 1950 survey, 21 percent of men and 44 percent of women believed that they were overweight; in a 1973 survey, it was 38 percent of men and 55 percent of women. Indeed, many more people believed that they were overweight than actually were. A 1980 survey of college women found that 70 percent saw themselves as overweight while only 39 percent were overweight according to insurance charts. During a small poll in 1981 asking people what they feared most in this world, nearly 40 percent said "getting fat."[18]

The market was expanding because more people who believed that they were overweight or feared being overweight were doing something about it. In 1950, 7 percent of men and 14 percent of women surveyed were on a diet at the time; in 1973, 34 percent of the men and 49 percent of the women were dieting and/or exercising to control their weight. Perhaps most telling, at least one person in almost half of American households had been on a weight-control diet during 1977.[19]

The market was expanding because the people who were doing something about weight and fat were not only more numerous but more various. More men were dieting, especially businessmen. The muckraker Vance Packard in 1962 reported that "even plump men are hard to find in the larger executive suites." Prudential Insurance, C. I. T. Financial and Chase Manhattan Bank offered calorie-count menus in their dining rooms. Business lunches were becoming lighter, smaller. While dairymen in the 1960s were trying to adjust feeds for a low-fat milk and hog-growers were scouring the Alleghenies for the lean-pork razorback, a packinghouse executive could claim, "We're all Jack Sprats now." Men's double-breasted suits, apt for disguising stout figures, were going out of style; the tapered look was in. Weight Watchers advertised in 1969 with a picture of a middle-aged executive stuck in his swivel chair as he attempts to rise: "An executive should carry extra weight on his shoulders. But not on his hips." Personnel agencies noted that overweight junior executives earned less money and moved more slowly up the corporate ladder than their leaner competition. While the Matrix Corporation advertised in *Computer World* in 1971, "Get rid of that UGLY FAT in your data processing budget," corporations were hiring Executive Health Examiners to check on the health and weight of their leadership. By 1984 even the corset was back, tightly laced around a steel cylinder, in an *Iron Age* ad about squeezing the fat out of steel inventory. This was a neat and significant reversal of images. Where before, in the early part of the century, men's industrial techniques—efficiency, economy, streamlining, flowcharting—were applied to women's bodies, now women's devices for figure control were being applied in the most masculine of industries.[20]

Not just the male executive was serious about dieting. Roly P. Oly, chemical engineer, also had to watch his weight. And blue-color laborers too, though perhaps they worried less about executive privileges than about manhood. The more invasive fat was, the more the burly working man in his forties had to struggle against it. A good sign that such men might be thinking about dieting came as early as 1942 with the war effort and an ad for Ten High Straight Bourbon Whiskey, a man's drink if ever there was meant to be one. Glen Fleischman drew the ad as a comic strip called "The Ribbers." Four men were playing handball, but Toby there in the center, like the 18th-century Toby jug, is pudgy. "'Smatter, Toby—weight slow-ing you down?" asks one of his friends, with a loud aside to the oth-ers: "He must add a balloon tire every birthday, boys!" The image of the man gone to pot, fat and feminine, was increasingly common as appetite and exercise became more important in the 1950s and 1960s. If fatness was not caused by a deficient thyroid, fat nonethe-less seemed to diminish another set of glands. The association be-tween fatness and sexual impotence was as old as capons and eu-nuchs, and it had been frequently invoked to explain the growth of fat in women past menopause and in old libertines. But there was a newer, less folkloric association. Peter Wyden, double-chinned exec-utive editor of the *Ladies Home Journal*, wrote about *The Over-weight Society* in 1965; three years later he co-authored *Growing Up Straight*. With his wife Barbara, woman's editor for the *New York Times Magazine*, Peter Wyden found that the same constella-tion of overprotective mother and weak father that lay behind obesity was also responsible for homosexuality. To be fat not only threatened an immediate sexual neutering but an imminent sexual inversion. Jack LaLanne had been quoted in Peter Wyden's earlier book: "With men you gotta use the scare thing. You gotta get down to the masculinity!" Thus the peculiar constitution of light beer ad-vertisements of the 1980s, which promised the working man as well as the rising executive a taste to match the power and drive of "man's" work.[21]

More black men—and women—were dieting. This is much harder to prove because of the strong stereotyping of black mothers as fat and of black men as admirers of heft in both sexes. But as early as 1950 the *Crisis*, an organ of the NAACP, had received so many re-quests for more information on weight-reducing that the editors de-voted a rather thorough article to the subject, complete with daily caloric needs for housekeepers, clerks, laundresses, workmen and day laborers. Cecile Hoover Edwards in 1952 was writing diet columns for Tuskegee Institute's *Service* magazine and citing a sur-vey showing that 31 percent of women (black women?) were at least 10 percent overweight. Not until the 1970s, however, did major black magazines regularly feature black personalities fighting off fat. While a Gallup poll found that 41 percent of "non-whites" be-lieved themselves to be overweight, *Ebony* was describing the exer-cises and diets of Grace Bumbrey, Fats Domino, Eartha Kitt, col-umnist Carl Rowan and the TV actresses Gail Fisher and Jayne Kennedy. *Essence* spotlighted model Diane Johnson. *Sepia* profiled

Harmony McCoy, a chef who learned his diet cooking at the Golden Door spa, though he himself was a meat-and-potatoes man. *Jet* ran a story on how Maynard Jackson, mayor of Atlanta, lost 110 lbs. If he preached discipline in the body politic, Jackson had reasoned, then he must practice what he preached on his own body.[22]

Diets in black magazines were meant to be permanent and practical, suited to normal people, not just to the "rich spinster computer" with the money to buy salmon and the time and skill to tote up vitamins, minerals and calories. *Ebony* in 1978 warned that black women, a third of whom were overweight between the ages of twenty and forty-four, were most susceptible to the appeals of faddish, dangerous drugs and devices—like those advertised in *Sepia's* December 1979 issue: the Doctor's Diet Reducing Tabs, the Sauna Slim Suit, the Vib-a-Way Tummy Toner, the Body Taper-Trim Shirt, the Trim-a-Bod slimmer, and the 3-Way Diet Program that would turn your body furnace up so high "IT LITERALLY MELTS THE FAT OFF YOUR BODY—LIKE A BLOW TORCH WOULD MELT BUTTER." It was better to go on a sensible diet that was *not* laden with fattening soul foods or starchy down-home dinners. After the singer Barry White, 360 lbs, stood naked in front of his mirror and shouted at his image, "You big . . . fat . . . awkward-looking m----- f-----!" he began eating Chinese food. Other blacks moving up the economic ladder would also leave behind the lard and sweet potatoes of black poverty. According to an *Ebony* article, "Did Your Mother Make You Fat?" successful blacks would also have to leave behind that ancestral African equation of fat with wealth and health. Weight control as "a lifestyle . . . a *permanent* lifestyle" had come to seem both a cause and a consequence of social mobility and black achievement within the wider (but thinner) American middle class.[23]

Among Puerto Ricans, weight control was an extremely sensitive index to acculturation. Emily Massara's study of the Puerto Rican community in Philadelphia in the 1970s revealed that, although husbands expected their wives to become plump (*gordita*), this was not because they thought of the plump figure as a beautiful figure. Rather, plumpness was the mark of a married woman's proper devotion to children, health and home. First-generation immigrants shared from the start the mainland ideal of the youthful figure as a slim figure and the slim figure as an attractive figure. Young men and women, unmarried, were very conscious of their weight, and some parents were aware of the medical weight standards for their children. Married men prided themselves on their youthful appearance, but a married woman too concerned with her weight or shape would be accused of selfishness and coquetry. When the second and third generations began to encourage their mothers to reduce, for reasons of health or fashion, they were implicitly redefining social roles and rearranging the cultural calendar. Where before slimness (and beauty) had been restricted to the young, now it was appropriate to the rest of life.[24]

As they aged, Puerto Rican men took to wigs and secret dieting to keep their youthful looks. In general, in all of American society, more of the elderly were dieting and exercising. For centuries physicians had been reluctant to reduce the diet or increase the physical activity of the old, especially of the old and fat, believing that such bodies could not take much strain. This attitude changed dramatically with the introduction of weight charts that stopped abruptly at age thirty and with the national inventory of diseases affecting the heart, the arteries and the gall bladder. The longer people lived now, the more they had to concern themselves with chronic diseases and encroaching fat. Twice as great a proportion of Americans were over the age of sixty in 1974 as in 1900; close to a third of the population was over the age of forty-five. The older the population was, the more important weight control would seem. Louis "Satchmo" Armstrong, the great black jazz trumpeter, went on a diet in 1956 and lost 98 lbs. Satchmo was fifty-five. He sent a copy of his orange-juice-antacid-laxative regime to the dieting Dwight D. Eisenhower, then sixty-six. "I told the President to do it the Satchmo way and he'd feel ten years old. He wrote back and said as President he isn't supposed to feel like he's ten years old." Most diet books did not promise such exorbitant rejuvenation, but they did increasingly encourage the middle-aged and elderly to eat less and exercise more. Bonnie Prudden at fifty-five rewrote her popular book, *How to Keep Slender and Fit After Thirty*, to show that "You can't turn back the clock—but you *can* wind it up again!" Irwin M. Stillman in his *Doctor's Quick Weight Loss Diet* (1967) held up the elderly as models for other dieters, since the elderly were most likely to stick to their diets. Dr. Barbara Edelstein in 1977 produced a chart on "The Best Times of Life for Dieting" which made it clear that women in their sixties had the fewest obstacles in their way. Of the case histories and testimonial letters in the *Pritikin Program for Diet & Exercise* (1979), the majority came from people in their fifties and sixties, like Nathan Pritikin himself; most of the others came from people in their seventies, eighties, nineties.[25]

The market was expanding, then, because more people and more kinds of people were working to control their weight throughout their (longer) lives. When Dr. Frederick J. Stare at Harvard's School of Public Health warned that growing fat was more dangerous than actually being fat, then slim people were under as much obligation to watch their weight as fat people. When psychiatrist Hilde Bruch insisted on talking about "thin fat people" and Dr. Gulielma Alsop cautioned, "Let no person who has been fat think he is now a thin person in nature, tastes and temperament," even the unusual successful dieter had to be on guard, for "he is only thin in silhouette, in weight, in flesh." When the most popular television cook, Julia Child, was on a 1,200-calorie diet "practically all the time," gourmets had no excuse for unwary indulgence. Weight-watching was fitting for every stage of life and every condition, from the chubby preteen to the pregnant mother (as we shall see in detail in the next chapter); from the army recruit at boot camp to the executive in the business suite; from the former athlete to the retired stewardess. Kathy Keeton, editor of *Viva*, looked up the noun "diet" in a dictionary in 1978: "Daily food allowance, from the Greek *diaita*, way of life."[26]

Dieting as a Way of Life

It used to be, in the 1930s and 1940s, that dieters had to learn elaborate forms of etiquette so as not to offend at dinner parties. Gradually, the burden of *politesse* was shifted onto their hosts, who were instructed not to force food upon dieting guests, either by obvious ploy or by subtle blackmail. Dieters in 1937 were advised to fast beforehand, then at the dinner party to look as if they were eating. By 1985, a guide to fitness etiquette in *Woman's Day* had more rules for nondieters than for dieters. (Nondieters invited to dinner at a dieter's home should not bring their walnut fudge brownies; they should bring flowers.) The shifting of the burden of *politesse* from the dieter to the nondieter was strong evidence that dieting had become a "way of life."[27]

As a way of life, dieting could be even bigger business. Diet food companies before 1960 had been small affairs. Rose Straka Fowler, a hospital dietician, founded Chicago Dietetic Supply (CDS) in 1919 to provide foods low in carbohydrates for diabetics on medically supervised diets. The CDS market was primarily institutional, as it would be for Jules Bernard of Chicago after he began Bernard Foods

in 1947 with soup mixes for schools, then no-salt soup mixes and sug-
arless gelatin products for hospital kitchens. The first low-calorie
food line to be marketed nationally on a retail basis came from
Flotill Products in central California. Myrtle Ehrlich, daughter of a
Brooklyn music store proprietor and herself a rags-to-riches Wall
Street stockbroker, ventured into the tomato canning business in
1935. By 1951, as Tillie Lewis, she owned the world's largest tomato
cannery under one roof and headed a multimillion-dollar enterprise, which was the largest packager of C-rations during the Korean War. For ten years she had been on a strict sugar-free diet and
for ten years she had been searching for a way to produce saccharin-
sweetened canned foods that would not turn bitter during the canning process. In 1951 she introduced Tasti-Diet Foods. A year later
the women's page editors of the Associated Press voted her Business
Woman of the Year.[28]

Still, the diet food business was a small business, a *dietetic* business, with Tasti-Diet and other more local brands segregated in dietetic sections of groceries and supermarkets, neither widely advertised nor widely sold. The change came in 1959 with the decision by
Mead Johnson and Company to "go public" with a national advertising campaign for a product first advertised in medical journals.
Accustomed to selling its infant foods Dextri-Maltose and Pablum
through physician recommendations and hospitals, Mead Johnson
took its diet formula Metrecal, "not exactly a drug product, not exactly a food product," to the upper-income urban/suburban audience watching a 1960 television series on Winston Churchill. As
Churchill stumped through "The Valiant Years," Mead Johnson was
by his side, stylish and soft-spoken, agreeing that "we must be ever
alert to preserve our freedom" and "it can happen again." So, it
might seem, Metrecal was devoted to protecting our way of life.
"We hold our freedom by extending it," said one commercial, "and
by deserving it every day." And fat—was it not as much a threat to
liberty as any other foreign power? In another commercial, the
camera followed the broad back of an overweight man as he
climbed a lonely path in snowy Central Park, plodded through a
playground, tried to pick up a basketball, could not, kicked it instead. "Through the years, overweight has been pictured in terms of
pity, and, at times, scorn." Now, the narration continued, it was a
question of mortality: one way or another, fat led to the loss of life.[29]

Metrecal made the transition from the medical office to the
kitchen table with such success that by 1961 it had $100 million in

sales and competition from other large companies: Sears Roebuck's Bal-Cal, Quaker Oats' Quota, Korvette's Kor-Val, Jewel Tea Company's Diet-Cal, Ovaltine's Minvitine and, in 1962, Pet Milk's Sego, which stuffed more protein and more ounces into the same 900 calories featured by Metrecal. Pet Milk focused on the women's market, with Sego ads using the actress Tippi Hedrin and Catalina swimwear. Mead Johnson pushed further into the men's market with the "Metrecal for lunch bunch" and a 1965 print ad, "Not one of the top 50 U.S. corporations has a fat president." Astronaut Scott Carpenter was using Metrecal as he prepared for his mission; Senator William Proxmire used it during a filibuster. Combined sales of Sego and Metrecal were more than $450 million in 1965.[30]

Such big business enticed Duffy Mott to market a line of fifty-eight Figure Control Foods (1962), based on its purchase of the Pratt-Low Preserving Corporation, which had been selling low-cal products through the medical network. The diet food business was big enough by 1972 to force General Mills on the defensive with a Counterweight educational program to convince consumers that healthy dieting did not mean abandoning foods with flour in them. CDS in 1975 initiated its first national advertising campaign for its line of Featherweight Foods, and in 1976 even Bernard Foods went retail with lo-cal cake, custard and lemonade mixes. As advertising budgets expanded to match the growing variety of diet items, grocers and supermarket managers were persuaded to desegregate diet foods. Food companies with products that were naturally low in calories began to highlight their weight-control virtues; Star-Kist spent $12 million in 1980 advertising "great taste, great for the waist" water-packed tuna. A CDS research study in the late 1970s found that diet food buyers "do not think of themselves as being in any way unusual. They prefer to think of special diet foods as only slightly different from the regular products purchased by the average person." Dieting was a way of life. A perfectly normal way of life. A national way of life.[31]

"During the past twenty-five years," wrote psychiatrist Albert J. Stunkard in 1973, "interest in weight reduction in our country has grown from a mild concern to an overriding preoccupation. At present, interest in obesity almost assumes the dimensions of a national neurosis." A few years before, a survey had shown that more people had heard about the danger of fatty foods than the danger of strontium-90 fallout in milk or of insecticides in the food chain, and that more people saw cholesterol as a danger to their health than fallout or food sprays. In 1969, the National Academy of Sciences advised a national reduction of daily caloric requirements by 100–300 calories, and in 1977 the Senate's Select Committee on Nutrition and Human Needs urged a reduction of at least 10 percent in daily fat consumption. In 1978, Dr. Edwin Bayrd wrote in *The Thin Game* that overeating caused the "vast preponderance of modern health problems" and that "the time has come for a concerted, coordinated assault on the nation's leading health hazard, one conducted with missionary spirit and zeal." Blue Cross/Blue Shield had placed a thirty-second spot on television just the year before to emphasize that "there is no free lunch. Sooner or later we all pay for it." Entitled "Family Dinner," the coaxing mother hugs her chunky grown son and says, "Son, when you eat like this, I just love you to death." Blue Shield's national print ads went after fat with true missionary zeal. One featured the bulging midriff of an obese male, his shirtbuttons about to pop, his trousers grotesquely wrinkled, with the caption, "When God created man, is this what He had in mind?"[32]

Light Foods

Blue Shield would seem to have overplayed its hand here, as I have overplayed mine. Not everyone in the United States was buying diet foods, diet drinks, exercise equipment or appetite suppressants. The market research profile of the typical dieter remained that of the white urban/suburban married man or woman, employed, well-educated and well-off, in the age range 25–44 (women) or 35–54 (men). A 1978 Lou Harris poll suggested that half of all Americans had never been on any diet. Not every Bostonian rushed out to get a copy of the Special Diet Shoppers Guide distributed by Stop & Shop Supermarkets, and not every diet product was a success—Nestlé's New Cookery line, introduced in 1980, was a major flop.[33]

But the promotion and sales of diet-related products and services do not take us to the heart of the lo-cal economy. Nor do those cigarette advertisements which confuse sensations of taste with sensations of weight and visions of svelte loveliness: "This little cigar brings out the Tall N' Slim in you"; "It's More you. It's long. It's slim. It's elegant"; "Long, lean and low with lots of style. Silva Thins"; "Wear a Max Today. Long, lean, all-white, tasteful. Max 120s."[34]

Rather, at the heart of the lo-cal economy was a long-term shift in fundamental eating patterns, habits of exercise, and manners of speech. To become a national way of life, weight control had to be built into the culture as if it had always been there. Diet foods had to seem to be basic foods. The Pepsi Generation that drank Pepsi-Cola in 1954 because it was "the LIGHT refreshment for today's active people" would be ready for Pepsi Light in the 1980s. The 40 percent of families using lo-cal products in 1962 and the 70 percent of families using them in 1970 would be ready in 1984 for the slogan of Weight Watchers Frozen Foods: "This is not dieting. It is living." The 20 percent of Americans regularly exercising in 1961, the 47 percent in 1977, the nearly 60 percent in 1982 would be ready for jogging shoes and sweatsuits as everyday wear. Americans who in 1961 used the adjective "thin" twice as often as the adjectives "thick" or "fat" would be ready in 1978 for the fifty-eight products registered under the name Trim (Trim Beer, Trim-Thi, Trimcycle, Trimfit hosiery . . .) and the seventy-three products registered as Slim (Slim Away girdles, Slim Jills stationery, Slim Jim contact-lens cases, Virginia Slims cigarettes), not to mention the thousands of products in the 1980s called Light or Lite.[35]

Between 1916 and 1958, the very definition of basic foods groups changed in a manner most accommodating to the Trims, the Slims and the Lites (see Table 3). Americans were redefining their categories of essential foods so as to identify fats with sweets and then to wash both of them clear of the conceptual slate.[36] This is not to say that the national taste for fat or sugar had changed dramatically, but fats and sugars could no longer be commonly acknowledged as

TABLE THREE
BASIC FOOD GROUPS

1916–23 *Basic Five*	1941–42 *Basic Seven*	1950 *Basic Five*	1954–58 *Basic Four*
bread/cereals	bread/cereals	bread/cereals	grains
veg's & fruits	veg's & fruits	veg's & fruits	veg's & fruits
meat, eggs, milk	meat	meat & eggs	meat & eggs
	eggs		
	milk	milk	milk
butter & fats	butter & fats	fats & sweets	
simple sweets	sweets or citrus fruits		

independent essentials under the terms of a weight-watching culture. Within the final Basic Four, fats and sugars could be—and
would be—plentiful. But they would be less visible, less apparent,
more open to compromise and masquerade.

   To make sense of the compromises and masquerades, we must
first take stock of a set of far more fundamental changes that lay behind the restructuring of food groups. Throughout this century,
Americans have qualified foods as either light or heavy, strengthening (invigorating) or weakening (calming).[37] The more powerful the
cultural presence of weight-watching and weight control, the more
commonly were foods realigned across these two axes. We can see
this process most clearly by mapping it on a series of simple graphs.

1.   THE RED SHIFT

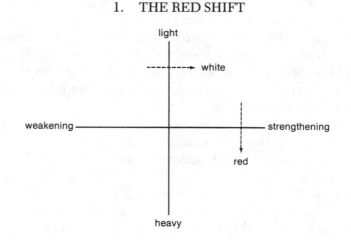

Americans since 1910 have been edging away from red meats
toward poultry, canned tuna, cheeses and, most recently, fresh and
frozen fish. Total protein consumption per capita has grown during
this century by only 1 percent, and the proportion of daily calories
from protein has remained at about 12–13 percent, so it is not that
people have changed their attitudes toward protein foods *per se* but
that they have increasingly associated *good* protein foods with lightness and whiteness. The same association operates with other foods,
in particular flour, onions, grapes and wine. (Red wine is not necessarily higher in calories than white wine.) The belief that there is especially light protein which is especially good has been responsible
for the popularity of the liquid protein diets of the 1970s, the overnight amino acid reducing tablets of the 1980s, as well as Lifetech's
1984 "Slimtech" food with its "cytogenic nutrients to maximize uti-

lization of the amino acids arginine, ornithine, tryptophan and phenylalanine." The increasingly common association of lightness with glamour, strength and protein had been made explicit in 1960 with Knox Gelatine's proclamation in *Cosmopolitan*, "Beauty is protein."[38]

2. THE FAT EXCHANGE

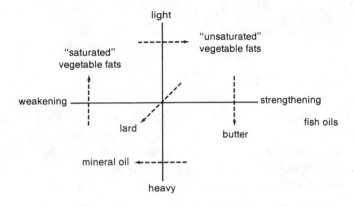

In 1899, the nation consumed 20 lbs of butter per capita. Since then, the use of animal fats has declined—lard precipitously and butter slowly—so that by 1957 more margarine than butter and more vegetable fats than animal fats would regularly be consumed by Americans. Between 1910 and 1976, however, total per capita fat consumption rose by an estimated 28 percent. The preference for vegetable fats over animal fats was not therefore a simple result of competition for a fixed percentage of the consumer's dollar or diet, but an active choice, especially since consumers could well afford lard and need not fear rancid butter once they had their own refrigerators. Butter and lard were increasingly associated with fatness (butterballs, piggishness) and with heart attacks (cholesterol, arteriosclerosis) while Nucoa Margarine could be advertised in 1942 as the "Cinderella of Table Fats," a thin-waisted girl in a large ball gown. By midcentury most margarines were entirely free of animal fats— and consequently had a "lighter" odor to them than lard or medium-priced butters and left a less visible residue of grease. Consumers could believe that they were eating less fat than ever before, though much of the fat in their diet was hidden as shortening in prepared foods and baked goods, as salad oil in dressings and as the natural oils of nuts and grains.[39]

3. THE SUGAR FIT

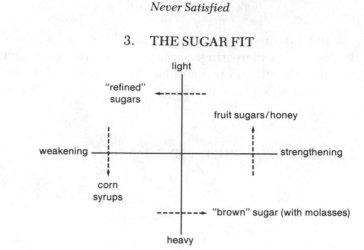

In 1884, Mary J. Lincoln in her *Boston Cookbook* added a table-spoon of sugar to her bread recipes to compensate for the sweetness lost in the steel-milling of the new fine flours, and she noted, "All children have a fondness for sugar, which should be gratified in moderation rather than repressed," since it was a natural fondness. In 1917 Americans were consuming 85 lbs of sugar per capita, up tenfold from a century before; sugar rations of soldiers had nearly tripled from 1.6 oz a day in 1838 to 4 oz during World War I. People were beginning to worry about all that sweetness as they noticed more diabetics and overweight women indulging in those small packages of candy and the delightful Eskimo Pies which appeared in the 1920s, as did the first 5-lb retail packages of granulated sugar. By 1941, per capita consumption of refined sugars and corn sweeteners was up to more than 110 lbs, or a third of a pound a day. Then, gradually, consumption of visible refined sugars began to level off as they were associated first with tooth decay, then with obesity and by the 1970s with hyperactivity, hypoglycemia, aggression and the "sugar blues." Between 1962 and 1982, refined sugar consumption fell by 23 percent and more than half of all consumers had altered their food purchases to avoid excess sugar. It was not the taste for sweetness that was in flux but the definition of the most desirable kind of sweetness. Good sweetness would be light and strengthening and (therefore) less fattening. The growing consumption of fruit juice and honey, as well as of the high fructose corn sweeteners and syrups hidden in canned, convenience and ready-baked goods, was in fact enough to make up for any drop in the use of the more obvious table and baking sugars. If "the greatest culprit

4.   THE SPICE TRADE

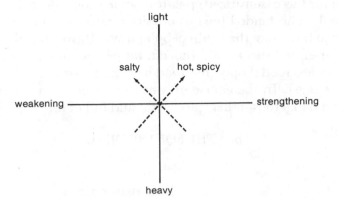

in modern civilized diet is refined sugar," this did not mean that Americans would move toward a sour palate. Indeed, they could still be seen using candy as a reducing aid to "spoil" the appetite.[40]

Grahamites had despised pepper and other seductive spices, although they did take a bit of salt. Salt in fact has been nearly inescapable in the American menu, since it has been used as the primary food preservative as well as one of the primary seasonings and food tenderizers. Athletes were the first to be hostile to salt, since it causes water retention and may add pounds to body weight. From this came the association with obesity, Bright's disease and diabetes in the early part of this century and the first suggestions that dieters should watch salt intake. Then came stronger associations with heart disease and high blood pressure, until in 1973 Cosmopolitan's *Super Diets & Exercise Guide* would claim that most Americans consumed ten to twenty times as much salt as they should. In 1984, over half the shopping public avoided buying certain food products because of the salt in them. Concomitant with the cultural suspicion of salt arose a cultural demand for a menu that was more highly but more innocently flavored. Diet cookbooks began to introduce ethnic dishes with foreign spices, believing that "taste is the key to joy and slimness." Ernest Dichter, premier market research psychologist, told manufacturers in the 1960s that their diet foods should emphasize strength and flavor. In 1985 Dr. Susan S. Schiffman of Duke University argued that the relatively bland taste of much processed food was itself responsible for the epidemic of obesity in the industrialized world. Fat people were actually people who craved more flavor and who had therefore to eat more food—more of this salty but otherwise unflavorful food—in order to satisfy their unusually sensitive (or less desensitized) palates. Some experiments had shown that people who tended toward obesity tended also to be more responsive to taste cues than thin people; it was flavor that the fat person was after, not sheer bulk. Indeed, fat people might be easily satisfied with less food if only that food had "zest" (from the French for citrus peelings). In the course of a century, salt had come to seem heavy and dangerous, other spices light and full of life.[41]

5.   THE SQUARE DEAL

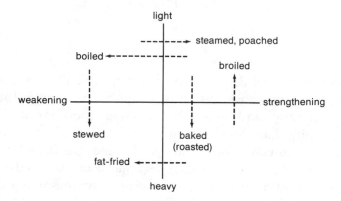

American cooking has been moving toward the principle of least transformation: the less done to a food the better. The obvious reason may seem to be that we use many prepared foods—canned, instant, frozen, concentrated, dehydrated—which need only be mixed with a liquid or reheated. These foods, however, have already been mightily transformed, out of our sight, by the food industry, so they hardly prove the point, except that they do encourage an illusion of least transformation. At home we have miniature factories—blenders, pressure cookers, food processors—that make the modes of transformation less time-consuming and less physically strenuous, consequently less demanding and less sensuous: less real. The technological masking of the stages between the raw and the cooked has progressed from the wood-burning fireplace and brick oven to the coal stove to gas and electric ranges to the microwave oven, whose operations are entirely invisible and to most people entirely mysterious. (How *does* a microwave cook anything?) In company with a host of peripheral technologies such as nonstick frying surfaces and sprays, the microwave oven reduces the audible and visible signs of transformation. It speeds up the cooking process and accommodates "grazing," our increasingly common habit of small frequent meals and snacks. We are abandoning stewing and slow roasting not just because they are lengthy processes but also because they are internally complex, while we associate flavor with what is closest to the "natural" or raw state. The recent popularity of salad bars and the recent return to dietary fiber and bran are perfect expressions of the movement toward the principle of least transformation. The more intense the belief that transforming a food makes it at once heavy and feeble, the more intent the search for foods that are, to begin with, light and invigorating. Foods subjected to heat and steam for hours cannot possibly be strong (they lose their vitamins, minerals, or fiber); foods encumbered with salt, fat, grease and additives cannot possibly be light (they are, after all, carrying death with them). The principle of least transformation is ideally suited to dieters who must ever desire foods that are light and strong. Advertisers saw the connection early on. In 1956 National Presto Industries claimed for its Diet-Master pressure cooker, "Now It's Easy to Stay on Your Diet!" Their cooker gave high satiety value to foods by retaining their flavors without added salt or fats. The producers of the Osterizer claimed in 1968 that "Spin Cookery Is Slim Cookery." Meanwhile, diet experts, traditionally opposed to snacking, had begun to advise small, frequent meals for weight control. Don Gerrard's "simple concept for controlling body weight" was the *One Bowl* (1974), an elegantly meditative practice of eating always out of the same bowl, one course at a time, one food at a time, in accordance with such philosophies as Søren Kierkegaard's *Purity of Heart Is to Will One Thing*.[42]

The ironic outcome of the Square Deal—as of the Red Shift, the Fat Exchange, the Sugar Fit and the Spice Trade—has been to exalt flavor over substance. Though it would seem that the move toward simpler meals should yield a more "honest" cuisine, a one-bowl "Purity of Heart," it has instead opened the way to imposture. Americans now tend to welcome "lighter" foods which solely by their flavor and texture can masquerade as something they are not. The 1984 slogan for Banquet Light and Elegant frozen food entrees— "What You See Is What You Get"—was certainly the credo of the Square Deal, but it was also an illusion fostered by the new food technology. The Square Deal assuaged the dieter's fear of hidden calories while in practice encouraging food technologists to come up with more synthetic flavorings, stabilizers, surfactants, flavor enhancers and acidulants.[43]

Asked near the end of World War II what one commodity then rationed was hardest to cut down on or get along without, more people named sugar or butter than anything else, including gasoline and shoes. (Beef was tied with butter.)[44] Since, as we have seen, the taste for fats and sugars remained despite their elimination from the Basic Food Groups, it was most likely that the masquerade would begin with them. As indeed it did, with margarine in 1869 and saccharine in 1879.

Imitations: 1. Margarine

A century before, in 1766, students at Harvard had led a Butter Rebellion against unwholesome butter. Butter was an often and easily adulterated commodity, since it had no standard color (that changed with the season and the grazing crop) and was usually highly salted. Some fifty years later, the French chemist Michel Chevreul isolated a fatty acid whose pearly drops tasted something like butter. He named it margaric acid, from the Greek for "pearl," *margarites*. In 1866 Napoleon III, at the behest of the French Navy, offered a prize for the best butter substitute, one that would be proper as a table spread but less likely to spoil. Three years later the prize was won by Hippolyte Mège-Mouriès, whose previous inventions included a sugar-refining process and a machine for removing the husks of wheat so that whole grain could be ground into a flour almost devoid of bran. His first "margarine" or "oleomargarine" (*oleum*, Latin for beef fat) was prepared by reducing beef suet to an oil; churning it with the finely chopped udders of cows, hogs or ewes; then adding carbonate of soda, salt and skim milk. Production in the United States began in 1874; by 1886 there were thirty-seven American manufacturers, all using beef by-products from a meat-packing industry whose stockyards were now filling with corn-fed cattle fatter than the traditional range cattle. [45]

That same year, 1886, a national law put stiff licensing fees and taxes on oleomargarine to protect the dairy industry. At first, however, oleomargarine was in direct competition not with butter but with cooking fats such as leaf lard. Oleomargarine still had a strong beef odor and an awkward consistency; it did not seem meant for the table. With the 1895 use of superheated steam and vacuum processing to deodorize animal fats, and with the 1902 development of hydrogenation to harden edible oils, oleomargarine took on more of the characteristics of butter. Attacked then as a fraud and impostor, it came under as much suspicion as those wholesalers and retailers who had been using the cheaper product to redeem rancid butter or to mix into new butter to cut costs. In 1902 a national tax was imposed on all colored margarines—that is, on all margarines that pretended to the "standard" yellow color of good butter.

With the gradual replacement of animal fats by vegetable oils between 1890 and 1940, margarine could shed its *oleo* prefix and also its reputation as a fraud. Made with skim milk and peanut oil, coconut oil, cottonseed oil and/or soybean oil, margarine took on a life of its own. When vitamin A was added in during the 1930s, margarine was no longer butter's poor city cousin but a full-fledged competitor which gained popular acceptance as a table spread during World War II. (Packages came with packets of food coloring so that homemakers could give a butter-like hue to the margarine.) National taxes on margarine were finally repealed in 1950. Margarine consumption per capita first exceeded butter consumption in 1957, and was double that of butter in 1970.

By law, margarine had to be 80 percent fat. Butter and margarine had, pat for pat, the same number of calories. They also had much the same texture. Thanks to lipid research using gas-liquid chromatography to determine the chemical components of butter flavor, margarine by the late 1950s could also have much the same taste and aroma as butter. There were no remaining restrictions on color, so margarine could also look like butter and be packaged like butter. That nobody could tell margarine from butter was the constant pride of margarine manufacturers.

Margarines cost half as much as butter, especially after taxes were lifted, so claims for identity were claims for superiority: the same product at half the price. But the real virtue of margarines was that they seemed lighter, not because they had any fewer calories but because they had fewer associations with animal fats, saturated fats, cholesterol. The more expensive corn oil and safflower oil margarines of the 1960s appealed to higher-income consumers on the basis of lightness, not cost. Lower-calorie margarines (called by law "spreads") were slow-growth products since margarine itself was considered light to begin with.

Margarine was light because it had one sort of fat rather than another; diet margarine was lighter simply because it reduced the proportion of fat to 60 or 40 percent. There was no "lower-calorie" variety of any given fat.[46] This short history of margarine has been the history of the acceptance of a "real" imitation—that is, of an imitation that was itself a legitimate food.

Imitations: 2. Sweeteners

The history of the masquerade of sweeteners is quite different, for it begins with an artificial or "non-nutritive" sweetener. In 1879 Constantin Fahlberg of Johns Hopkins discovered a thiazol derivative which he called saccharin. It was entirely without calories and 200–300 times as sweet as beta-D-fructofuranosyl alpha-D-glucopyranoside or sucrose, what we popularly call sugar. First employed as an antiseptic and food preservative, saccharin was soon sold for table and cooking use for diabetics and dieters. President Theodore Roosevelt was using it every day by doctor's orders. Told by his pure-food-and-drug investigator, Dr. Harvey W. Wiley, that saccharin might be dangerous, he responded, "Anybody who says saccharin is injurious to health is an idiot," In 1910 a national committee of scientists agreed that in moderate doses saccharin was acceptable, although it did have a disagreeable aftertaste. By 1981 more than 8,000,000 lbs of saccharin were being produced in the United States for a $2 billion domestic market. At least a third of all Americans were regular consumers of saccharin, either indirectly in diet soft drinks and lo-cal foods, or "straight" in the tabletop sweeteners Sucaryl and Sweet 'N Low.[47]

As of 1985, Sweet 'N Low was being used by more than twenty-nine million people more than thirty million times a day. It was, according to the advertisements, the one diet product "poured more often than any other." It was the registered trademark of Cumberland Packing Corporation, which had begun with real sugar.

Benjamin Eisenstadt ran the Cumberland Cafeteria near the Brooklyn Navy Yard during World War II. After the war, business fell off and he looked for something else to do. His brother manufactured tea bags, so he tried the tea business, then had the profitable idea of using a teabag machine to put sugar into small packets. This was a fast, cheap method of preparing individual servings for restaurants. As a contract packager for major sugar companies, the Cumberland Packing Company was asked by a drug company in 1956 if it might develop a packaged sugar substitute. Saccharin until that time had been available only as a pill and a liquid (Abbott Laboratories' Sucaryl), while Eisenstadt's company was prepared only to handle granular products. In order to make saccharin for single-serving packets, Eisenstadt had to find a filler to combine with the saccharin. He read a baking magazine and tried lactose, which gave the proper texture to the compound and leeched out some of the bitter aftertaste. (He also added some cyclamates, approved as sweeteners for commercial food uses since 1951 and present in a 10:1 concentration in Sucaryl to cut the saccharin aftertaste.) Meanwhile, the drug company had lost interest, so Eisenstadt in 1958 decided to market the product by himself as Sweet 'N Low, the title of a popular tune from his youth and derived ultimately from Tennyson's romantic lullaby. Soon there were posters in buses, "I call my sugar Sweet 'N Low," and in 1966 the Cumberland Packing Company dropped its traditional sucrose products to devote its affections exclusively to the new romance.[48]

It was a tricky romance. On a Friday night in the fall of 1969, Marvin Eisenstadt, son of Benjamin and now president of the company, was watching television with his mother. On the news he learned that cyclamates were likely to be banned as cancer-causing agents. That would mean a terrible blow to low-calorie soft drink manufacturers but a much worse blow to Cumberland Packing, all of whose Sweet 'N Low contained cyclamates. Fortunately, Marvin Eisenstadt had been at work on a new compound for the kosher food trade. Since regular Sweet 'N Low contained a milk product (lactose), it could not be used by Orthodox Jews at or just after meat meals. As a man with a degree in chemistry, Marvin Eisenstedt had figured out a different recipe which would contain no milk product whatsoever and would therefore be neutral, or *pareve*, and legal at all kosher meals. Incidentally, it had no cyclamates either; rather potassium bitartrate and a small amount of the nutritive sweetener dextrose were present to cut the saccharin aftertaste. When the cyclamate ban went into effect on February 1, 1970, Cumberland Packing had dumped all the old Sweet 'N Low and begun manufacturing the new, *pareve*, noncyclamate product.[49]

As if this were not enough, saccharin itself was under attack. The first reports of saccharin as a possible carcinogen had been published in 1951, but in 1971 evidence of bladder tumors in experimental animals was serious enough for the FDA to remove saccharin from the list of food additives "generally recognized as safe" (GRAS). After six years of controversy, the FDA proposed a ban on saccharin in the spring of 1977. Marvin Eisenstadt, more than a little upset, spoke out during a television interview, saying that saccharin was the only artificial sweetener left and that it was "up to you, America," to keep it on the market. The Calorie Control Council, a consortium of industrial users of artificial sweeteners and weight-watching groups, lobbied in Washington against the ban. Some 100,000 irate letters reached Congress—more, it was claimed, than ever arrived in any comparable period during the Vietnam War. In November 1977, Congress enacted an eighteen-month moratorium on the FDA ban. The moratorium has since been extended four times. It was enough to give a person ulcers.[50]

Working on a treatment for ulcers, Robert H. Mazur of the G. D. Searle & Company laboratories synthesized L-aspartyl-L-phenylalanine methyl ester and gave some to his colleague James M. Schlatter for recrystallization. When Schlatter was heating the substance in a flask with methanol, some of the mixture spilled over the lip onto his fingers. Later, licking a finger to pick up a piece of paper, Schlatter noticed "a very strong, sweet taste." He had come upon, most accidentally, in December 1965, the unusual sweetness of the substance which a lawyer for General Foods would some years later name aspartame.[51]

Aspartame is a nutritive sweetener, meaning that it has some calories and can be at least partly metabolized by the body. It is 180–200 times as sweet as common sugar (sucrose) and has no aftertaste, so it may be used as sparingly as saccharin and without any masking agents. Given final FDA approval in June 1981 (and again, for soft drinks, in July 1983), aspartame was sold to the public as an ingredient (NutraSweet) and as a table sweetener (Equal) in one of the most extensive advertising and educational campaigns ever mounted for an entirely synthesized product. A 1984 NutraSweet television commercial explained, "It's a sweetening ingredient that isn't fattening. A sweetening ingredient that isn't artificial like saccharin. Isn't bad for your teeth. Tastes just like sugar. And sounds just too good to be true."[52]

For G. D. Searle & Company, manufacturers of the motion-sickness drug Dramamine and the fiber product Metamucil, aspartame was true enough to be good for an estimated half of its total gross sales and 70 percent of its net profits in 1984. Medical disputes over whether it is too good to be true will continue for some time. Consider especially the intriguing hypothesis of Dr. Richard Wurtman of MIT that aspartame may block the body's synthesis of serotonin, a chemical that signals satiety. If this is so, then the more one uses aspartame, the less satisfied one will be. Is aspartame the ideal consumer-driven product?[53]

Aspartame *is* too good to be true—for quite another reason. It is a sweetener based on two amino acids, the building blocks of protein. As such it is exactly—too exactly?—what the shift in American food habits would demand just now: an edible substance associated at once with unusual lightness, unusual sweetness, and surprising strength. It tastes like common sugar but is not sugar. It is nutritive but practically noncaloric (four calories per packet of Equal). It is synthetic but is (almost) protein. Its masquerade is close to perfect.

A Food by Any Other Name

The lo-cal economy conduces to such carnival. The effect of the many masquerades is ultimately to call into question the very nature of food. When there can be such things as "empty" calories, noncaloric bulking agents,[54] low-fat fats, then we know that the cultural definitions of food are at great risk. In 1980 the FDA felt compelled by the many "light" foods on the market to issue new and complex regulations on food labeling. A "low calorie" food has no more than 0.4 calories per gram and no more than forty calories per serving. A "reduced calorie" food must have at least one-third less calories than a similar unmodified food. Mushrooms, naturally low in calories, cannot be labeled "low calorie mushrooms" but may be labeled "mushrooms, a low calorie food." What about newly synthesized foods that are (naturally?) lower in calories? Must we look around to see what (natural?) food they most closely resemble, as if all inventions were imitations? Some foods are labeled imitations, some "quiescently frozen confections," some "dietetic." Sometimes the euphemisms are synonyms, sometimes not. At what point does the reduction in calories so change a food that it is no longer the same food at all? (This is what, for decades, people thought of skim milk; it is what people now think of ice milk, which is neither ice cream *nor* an imitation.) Are vitamins foods or drugs? What about fiber sprinkled on our foods?[55]

When a society becomes confused about what is a food and what is not a food, what is real and what is an imitation, then we know that very strong forces are at work.[56] This chapter has been devoted to making clear the direction of those forces and the cultural momentum they carry. There cannot be a full resolution here, because the lo-cal economy is still abuilding.

At the start of this chapter, I lifted Thomas Wood out of a provincial 18th-century English village and set him down in the midst of a tumultuous fairground of diets, diet foods, diet drinks, diet books, diet doctors, drugs and devices. I have apologized to him, but we are without apology in the midst of that same carnival. Like all carnivals, this too has drawn crowds. Businessmen and laborers, businesswomen and housewives, black and white, urban and rural, the old and the not-so-old. And the children. Of course the children.

CHAPTER NINE

Baby Fat

American anxieties about overweight and obesity have settled fiercely upon children. First, during the 1940s and 1950s, on adolescents. Then in the 1960s on grade schoolers. In the 1970s, on the toddler, the infant, the newborn. These last years, on the fetus itself. Parents have projected onto the bodies of children their own fears of a lethal, permanent fat. With the advent of reducing drugs and diets for young children, we can see the full force of the culture of slimming at work.

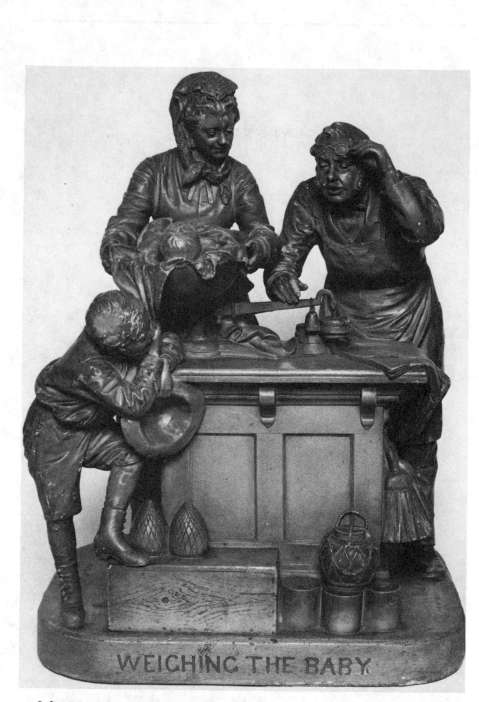

WEICHING THE BABY

John Rogers' popular sculpture, "Weighing the Baby," first produced in 1876. It cost $15 and weighed 120 lbs. Perhaps ten thousand copies were sold during the next twenty years. Courtesy of the Margaret Woodbury Strong Museum, Rochester, NY

Fine Fat Babies

D URING THE 1760s the Connecticut minister Ezra Stiles, later president of Yale, weighed each of his children at birth. As they grew, he recorded their heights and weights "fairly regularly," and on March 11, 1766, he weighed them before breakfast and after dinner, presumably to determine the weight they may have gained on a single day. Why he wanted to know this is not clear, except that in the rest of his affairs he took the same fancy for numbers, precise measurements, odd statistics. His counterpart, the Reverend Edward Holyoke, mathematician and president of Harvard, was doing the same thing: registering exact weights of his family to the ounce, the heights of his relatives, the number of feet of fencing. Stiles and Holyoke shared that growing American faith in numbers which would occasion a visitor's remark, some years later in 1833: "Arithmetic I presume comes by instinct among this guessing, reckoning, expecting and calculating people." As children at school were given prizes for reciting the multiplication tables, so their own multiplication—their growth in height, their gain in weight—was subject to a parental arithmetic. A vegetarian couple kept a journal of their infant in 1839; four weeks old, the infant was

271

9 lbs 9 oz, having gained 25 oz in the preceding two weeks. Health reformer William A. Alcott, who published the journal in his *Library of Health*, was alarmed. Though the parents were proud of the weight gain, Alcott "should by no means be disposed to boast of such rapid accumulation of fat. The child was undoubtedly overfed, and the growth morbid or diseased."[1]

Alcott's was a voice in the wilderness. The "fine fat baby" was the ideal, and parents did boast of gains in weight as proof of health. Indeed, there was a centuries-strong folk belief that weighing a baby was not only an act of measurement but an act of therapy. Weak, thin or sickly infants placed often on scales could be healed and fattened by the simple act of weighing. The Reverend David Macrae noted in 1860: "One of the first things to be done with a baby when it is born, seems to be to hurry it into a pair of scales. . . . It continues to be weighed at short intervals all through its childhood, and on to the time when the question becomes one of personal interest and it is old enough to weigh itself."[2]

Baby-weighing took place traditionally on grocers' counter scales. A portrait of such a weighing became one of the most widely diffused sculptures in Victorian America. Entitled "Weighing the Baby," it was one of the most popular works by John Rogers, the Norman Rockwell of his era. Patented in 1876, the sculpture had Rogers's wife posing as the mother, his newborn son David as the baby, and another son as the small boy pulling on the baby's blanket and so adding unusual weight to the healthy infant. This Rogers group, of which perhaps ten thousand copies were sold at $15 apiece, was so popular that an anecdote of the times had a tramp confiding to his benefactress, "You can realize how poor we were, ma'am, when I tell you that my parents could never afford to buy Rogers' Weighing the Baby." The *Medical Record* in 1884 recommended the sculpture for doctors' offices, and by 1890 there were stereopticon views and lantern slides of the sculpture for those who could not afford the 21-inch plaster casting.[3]

With all this weighing, people had a general sense of what a good weight was:

> How many pounds does the baby weigh—
> Baby, who came but a month ago;
> How many pounds from the crowning curl
> To the rosy point of the restless toe?

> Grandfather ties the handkerchief's knot,
>   Tenderly guides the swinging weight,
> And carefully over his glasses peers
>   To read the record, "Only eight!"

If 8 lbs was too little, then a birthweight of 11 or 12 lbs was safely on the large side. The wife of the actor Harry Watkins had an 11-lb baby in 1855; those who delivered the baby called it a "buster." Elizabeth Cady Stanton in 1852 was the happy mother of a 12-lb baby, "the largest and most vigorous baby I have ever had." More than this was overmuch; Mrs. Nellie Eaton's aunt of Worcester, Massachusetts, gave birth to a 15-lb baby in 1862 and suffered from falling of the womb ever after.[4]

The popular impression of what a good weight was followed a similarly inflated medical tradition. When Jonathan Swift in his *Modest Proposal* "reckoned upon a medium that a child just born will weigh twelve pounds," his reckoning was in agreement with the best medical authorities of his time. That imaginary number was subscribed to by most writers in English throughout the 18th century and well into the 19th. In 1825 Dr. William P. Dewees of Philadelphia reprinted the tables from the first report on the systematic weighing of thousands of infants at the Hospice de la Maternité in Paris. The Maternité's infants averaged, across the sexes, 6 lbs 4 oz at birth. This was a low figure, not just in comparison with today's standards (7 lbs 6 oz) but also in comparison with slightly later studies in France, Belgium, Scotland and Germany. The Maternité, a refuge for the distressed and malnourished, was hardly the place to issue norms for healthy babies, but Dewees had no others, and Americans would supply no official ones of their own until the end of the century.[5]

Accurate statistics on birth weight and early childhood weights would come with a sharp drop in infant mortality in the United States after 1880, due more to public health measures than to any improvement in daily medical practice.[6] The official weighing of infants ran under the steam of three related campaigns: the first, for a thorough registration of births and deaths to determine mortality rates—especially infant mortality rates; the second, for the establishment of babies' hospitals and pediatric wards to deal with infant diseases; the third, for changes in infant feeding practices to prevent those diseases.

Founded in 1912, the U.S. Children's Bureau shortly published a pamphlet on *Baby-Saving Campaigns*, announcing that "the infant death rate is the truest index of the welfare of any community." In 1911, the Census Bureau had regarded the registration of deaths to be "fairly complete" in twenty-three states, but the registration of births met its standards only in the Northeast, Pennsylvania and Michigan. Twenty years later, the Census Bureau would be satisfied with all but South Dakota and Texas.[7]

As babies were made official, so they were more often drawn away from lay midwives toward hospitals, scientific nursing and the medical profession. Dr. Abraham Jacobi, the first American professor of the diseases of children, had started lecturing in New York in the 1860s. The first American medical journal devoted entirely to children's health, the *Archives of Pediatrics*, appeared in 1884. In 1887, while the New York Nursery and Child's Hospital was being converted into the New York City Babies' Hospital (the first of its kind in America), Dr. Stanford E. Chaillé would already be writing that "parents should, throughout the first year, weigh their babies and record the result *every week*, as is now habitually done in the best hospitals and asylums for infants." Scales were an easy and accessible demonstration of that scientific enterprise to which the newborn field of pediatrics aspired, though the fifty or so pediatricians by 1900 had no special tools or diagnostic procedures.[8]

Pediatricians associated the majority of deaths and serious infant illnesses with gastric and digestive disorders. They therefore developed or laid claim to an expertise in feeding and nutrition, which could also be a professional badge distinguishing them from general practitioners. From regulating the feeding of sick infants they turned gradually to the regulation of all infant feeding, by breast or by hand.[9]

The course of breastfeeding is an intricate historical problem. A woman's choices—nursing the child herself, bringing in a wet nurse or sending the child out to be nursed, handfeeding (or "dryfeeding," unfortunately synonymous with the use of cow's milk and, later, bottlefeeding)—have been determined by her wealth, her social station, her husband's interest in heirs, her own worries about her physical appearance or her professional obligations, and by the concourse of medical opinion. Sometime around the mid-18th century in France and England, aristocratic ladies and the bourgeoisie resumed the breastfeeding which they had for centuries let out to women from humbler environs. There were several good reasons for the change, not the least of which was the terrible mortality rate of babies sent out to be nursed, a rate as high as 80 percent. If, with Rousseau's *Émile*, maternal affection had the stamp of literary fashion in the 1760s, the reclaiming of the infant was also a strong signal of class break at the start of industrialization. The nursing infant who had been a token of the sustained bond between women of separate classes was symbolically withdrawn, first to the mother's breast and then, within a century, to the bottle.[10]

For three millennia, physicians have spoken in favor of breast-feeding. In the event of a mother's illness or death, or in the rare case that a mother found herself constitutionally unable to produce milk, physicians would write out recipes for pap (a liquid concoction of starch, sugar and water) or panada (small beer and clarified honey) or cow's milk diluted with water and slightly sweetened. But foremost was mother's milk.[11]

Nonetheless, beginning slowly in the 1870s, working women and housewives turned their babies away from the breast, weaning them in tandem with a Second Industrial Revolution, which produced evaporated milk (Borden, 1856), dessicated or dry milk (Grimsdale, 1855), canned milk (Nestlé, 1866), unsweetened condensed milk (Myenberg, 1883), and a host of artificial foods—malt extracts, syrups, chaff from the food processing industries that was turned into feed for infants. Job Lewis Smith, whose *Treatise on the Diseases of Infancy and Childhood* became the new bible, warned women against artificial feeding and premature weaning, but he too had a recommendation for an artificial feed if one there had to be. He preferred the Swiss chemist Henri Nestlé's Lacteous Farina to Professor Justus von Liebig's Soup, and he printed in an appendix, by way of proving his case, the tedious procedure for preparing Liebig's formula of ½ oz wheaten flour, ½ oz malt flour, 7½ grains bicarbonate of potash, 1 oz water and 5 oz cow's milk, simmered, stirred, boiled, separated, sieved and thermometer-controlled.[12]

Formulas for infant food since the Egyptian medical papyri had resembled in syntax and possibly in flavor those prescriptions for the cure of colic, diarrhea and constipation which cluttered the small manuals on child care.[13] During the early 19th century, infant formulas advanced in precision as to the measurement of ingredients and the amount and timing of the feed. In 1792, Dr. Hugh Smith printed the quantities of undiluted cow's milk necessary to infants of different ages. In 1850, the Philadelphia physician J. F. Meigs published a widely imitated formula based upon an (inaccurate) chemical analysis of cow's milk. The formula itself (and not just the amount) was to be varied with the age of the infant.[14]

But how did these men know how much of what kind of food a baby required at each stage in its growth? They did not. Their formulas were guesswork, inspired by a common fear of that overfeeding which seemed to lead to the high mortality of infants with gastroenteritis. (Overfeeding implied then not obesity but vomiting, loose stools, indigestion—in brief, too much liquid in the system.) Disturbed by such awkwardly impressionistic medicine, researchers at foundling and baby hospitals in France began to weigh infants before and after they had been nursed. The babies would tell them, by what they demanded at the breast, how much they needed each day and month for normal growth. From the weight gains, the doctors would calculate the proper progressive amounts of artificial feed.

By the turn of the century, French statistics on infant weighing and feeding had become implacable. They were used as a rigid standard not only for handfeeding but for breastfeeding as well. Still distressed by infant digestive problems—even more worrisome now that mortality from infectious diseases was on the wane—French doctors inveighed against overfeeding regardless of method. Overfeeding was determined numerically, by the scale. A Scottish physician, recently returned from a visit to French infant clinics, described in 1913 how the weighing machine had become "an instrument of torture" for the young mother: "The fear of overfeeding has induced them to use the weighing machine in all cases, whether the mother have abundant lactation or not, and whether the child be normal or weakly. The attendant in labour advises the mother to weigh her child each time before and after giving it the breast, in order that the prescribed quantity of milk to be given be not exceeded. Many a young mother worries if her child has taken ten or fifteen grams more than she was told to give it."[15]

Americans would be no less emphatic about scales, and their formulas would be overwhelming. Though women in the kitchen had traditionally handled the confusing "Rule of Three" (a cumbersome method of figuring proportions), most were unprepared in the nursery for the pages of algebraic equations from the pencil of Thomas Morgan Rotch, professor of pediatrics at Harvard. His system, which took advantage of sophisticated analyses of milk protein and data on infant metabolism as well as infant weight, was called the laboratory method or percentage feeding or, simply, the American method. More forbidding than the most numerate of home economics texts, Rotch's American method was somehow in common use from 1890 to 1915, though it involved the long and fine computation of food mixtures for each month of the baby's life.[16]

Given such a demanding system, further elaborated in the widely read works of the pediatrician Luther Emmett Holt, there were several long-term consequences. For women who handfed their babies, weighing the baby before and after meals provided the best evidence that they had gotten the complicated formulas right. They also began to appreciate the time-saving virtues of prepared, premeasured baby foods. For breastfeeding women, only the scale could assure them that the baby had not taken in too much of a good thing. They also began to wean the child at an earlier age, encouraged by the commercial food companies who stressed the importance of accurate nutrition. For both the handfeeding and the breastfeeding mothers, the notion of feeding a child on demand became suspect. Too many children suffered summer diarrhea and digestive failures; only the scale and the pediatrician knew how much food a baby should have.

Everyone knew that the food should be pure. In the 1890s a rather lordly class war was fought between advocates of certified raw milk and advocates of pasteurized milk, that new French procedure. The AMA stood behind certified raw milk, more expensive than regular fresh milk, privately produced and sold but medically supervised. Nathan Strauss, millionaire partner at Macy's Department Store, stood behind pasteurized milk, which was sold at cost through Strauss's milk depots in New York City and through municipal depots across the country. In 1908 Chicago required pasteurization of all milk sold, and in 1914 the discovery of tuberculosis among certified (raw milk) cows effectively silenced mainstream opposition to pasteurized milk.[17]

The milk stations were also and eminently weigh stations. Pediatricians and public health nurses used the depots as occasions to examine babies and to educate mothers on patterns of physical growth in infants. By 1911 the Chicago Milk Commission had become the Infant Welfare Society, with public health nurses taking weekly weight records on infants and giving lectures on feeding schedules. In 1915, there were more than five hundred baby clinics in the United States as well as numerous day nurseries where weighing was also a commonplace. In 1921 the Sheppard–Towner Act created a federally funded health care program to reduce infant and maternal mortality rates through prenatal and child health centers, most of them (three thousand by 1929) in rural areas and small towns.[18]

Everywhere there was a clinic or a public health nurse, there was a scale. Perhaps an elegant infant's scale with a wicker basket, measuring up to 50 lbs by the half-ounce, or a Portable Combination Child and Baby Scale for Rural Schools and Welfare Stations, which could be "easily carried about by a nurse in a Ford car." "Frequent weighing," read a 1920 Howe Scale Company catalog, "indicates the effect of proper nutrition and points out the need of changes in diet. The Nurse and Physician regard a consistent record of your baby's weight as a sure guide to diet regulation." The 1924 catalog was more insistent: "A scale tells whether or not a child is thriving. You want a scale that would tell you the truth to such an extent that you will know a gain or loss, if even only ¼ of an ounce."[19]

The scale, one critic claimed as early as 1907, was usurping the mother herself: "Mother-love as a guiding star gives place to a pair of scales on which the New Baby is weighed each week, and if its weight comes up to standard for that week of life, that does just as well." An underweight baby would mean an unloving mother, or at least a very worried mother. Dorothy Reed Mendenhall, after a long and painful delivery under ether in the hospital, gave birth to a 9-lb baby. She wrote to her friend Margaret Long from the hospital about the baby, "He is not gaining well, like all my babies he is a poor nurser—as I a scant provider. He weighs now 8-11—and refuses to change either way. As soon as I am home and both of us outdoors, I hope to do more with his weight."[20]

The fortunate mothers, those with weightier babies, entered them in baby shows. The great promoter Phineas T. Barnum had sponsored his first Grand National Baby Show in 1855, with prizes for the finest baby and the fattest. The show was hardly grand or national, but it was good publicity, especially when the irate mothers of losing children stormed the Barnum Museum in New York City. They had cause to be upset, for the judging had been entirely arbitrary. Some fifty years later, the baby shows would be "scientific," with pediatricians, nurses, and age-weight charts. The first such baby show was at the National Western Stock Show in January 1913; while the American Breeders Association had mastered eugenics for livestock, now the Child Welfare Bureau would keep track of human offspring. In March 1913, the *Woman's Home Companion* established a Better Babies Bureau and provided cash prizes, medals, certificates, wall charts, and instructions for Better Babies contests across the nation. Within a year there had been contests at twenty-five State Fairs, as well as 117 county and local competitions in thirty-seven states; 5,000 doctors had examined 150,000 babies. Nearly every month for the rest of the decade, the magazine published dozens of photos of Better Babies, often a page or two away from advertisements for baby foods, which featured identically round and healthy infants. As the contests spread and more babies were measured uniformly, Frederick S. Crum was able to compile a new standard height-weight table based on 2,945 selected baby contest babies. Because Better Babies were truly larger and heavier than average babies, the presence of this new standard aggravated parental concerns about the weight of the normal infant. The anthropometric distance between the sick baby and the well baby had widened, and the distance was computed in pounds.[21]

The weighing of the baby redounded upon the pregnant mother. If infant mortality was falling, maternal mortality was not. In 1930, the United States had the worst record in maternal mortality of twenty-five industrialized nations. That resulted in part from the professional medical attack on midwives, whose gradual disappearance correlated with a rise in puerperal complications, and in part from the increasingly radical surgical interventions of obstetricians who conceived of labor as something "decidedly pathological." The death rate for hospital deliveries was twice that for home deliveries in the 1920s, and this would not improve until late in the Depression.[22]

In 1923, Dr. C. H. Davis cited German data which suggested that weight during pregnancy was diagnostic for eclampsia and edema, problems that complicated childbirth and could endanger the mother's life. He advised that the average woman should gain no more than 20 lbs during pregnancy. By 1925, Dr. Calvin R. Hannah had some data from Dallas which he interpreted to mean that average weight gain during pregnancy should be from 12 to 15 lbs, so as to avoid such complications as eclampsia, apoplexy, epilepsy and psychosis. By 1926, Dr. William Kerwin of St. Louis was arguing: "Observing the weight gain in the pregnant woman should no longer be a question for discussion among obstetricians."[23]

From then on, it was not. What remained for discussion was the exact number of pounds to be set as the average, and that depended upon two things: statistics on the average weight of newborns; estimates of the combined weight of the placenta, amniotic fluid, extra breast tissue and the enlarged area of the uterus. Hannah gave the total as less than 15 lbs. Davis, following the Germans, allowed for 15 to 20 lbs. For at least two decades, and occasionally into the 1970s, Hannah's number stuck.[24]

His number even then was low. Too low. Most women today, when they ask, are told to aim for 24 lbs, with a generous range of acceptable weight gains according to build, height, original weight, age and number of earlier pregnancies carried to term.[25] But from the 1920s to the end of World War II, the range was severely limited. The Hannah number was authoritative enough for obstetricians to insist on prescribing reducing diets for pregnant women who were initially overweight and also for those who became "overweight" in the course of pregnancy.[26]

If we realize that the average woman *would* gain more than 14 lbs during her pregnancy unless she were undernourished or particularly light-framed, and if we realize that she was being cornered into weighing herself not for the sake of fashion but for the sake of her own life and that of her unborn child, we can appreciate the sobering symbolic power of the scale and the height-weight tables of the 1920s and 1930s. For obstetricians and pediatricians, the control of feeding practices led back from the child to the mother, so that the physician entrusted with the health of the baby would soon command the obedience of the mother as well. To shape the body of the infant was eventually to shape the body of the woman who bore the infant.[27]

Women also tended to attribute the onset of their own obesity to weight gained during pregnancy and never lost. Their amplified concern with weight would extend beyond parturition to the years of early childhood. While they anxiously weighed their infants, mothers would with trepidation weigh themselves, hoping that by some sympathetic magic their babies would take on the extra fat they as women no longer needed. This curiously conflicted attitude toward weight would underlie their fearful but ferocious attachment to height-weight tables as their babies crawled beyond infancy toward childhood and adolescence.[28]

Childhood Incorporated

Infant weighing was a private, familial or clinical ritual of investiture, the newborn taking on the flesh of its ancestors. The weighing of older children was a public ritual of incorporation, the child being placed on an American grid to become part of an American curve. In the early 19th century, such incorporation had been worked primarily through religious revivalists and Sunday School leaders, who counted the children they converted and measured their piety by verses memorized. In the late 19th century, incorporation had less to do with civic millennialism, more to do with the charting of a mean. Those who counted and measured the children considered them less as an index to the spiritual health of the nation than as a national physical fund.

Was that fund being bankrupted by the waves of spindly immigrants to the American shores after 1880? Was it bankrupted by the increasing number of older girls receiving a public education, suffering from mental strain and the consequent womanly troubles, for "ovaries will always be arrested if the brain is forced"?[29]

Between 1870 and 1920, answers came from the avid anthropometry of such as the Harvard physiologist Henry P. Bowditch, scion of one of the oldest Boston families, who was worried that his people had a low birthrate and were destined to be swamped by the reproductive powers of immigrants. And from W. Townsend Porter in St. Louis, who saw a connection between physical condition and intellectual strain, especially in the tender prepubertal years of girls. And from Franz Boas, physical anthropologist at Columbia, interested to reveal the positive influences of the American environment on the supposedly fixed racial types arriving from Europe. And from Arthur MacDonald, he who had put advertisements in personals columns to study "Abnormal Women" and was now wondering whether unruly (immigrant) boys weighed more or less than well-behaved (native) boys. And from a phalanx of physical education instructors determining how best to measure the possibly inferior American physique in an age of increasingly competitive international athletics, which culminated with the reestablishment of the Olympic Games in 1896. All of these men weighed children. Not once but often.[30]

They found that Americans were taller and heavier than Europeans, that the second-generation immigrant was larger than the first generation, that better physical condition promoted better school work, that a healthy body made for a healthy mind. But their results were of less significance than the very fact of the weighing as a primary means of integrating children into a specifically American (and patriotic) statistical web.

These were at first white urban children and elite private college students, but the scales reached far beyond them as people came to believe that "frequent weighing is the most practical and, in the whole, the most certain method of detecting the presence of the influences that are working injury to the development of the child." With the legislation of mandatory school medical inspections during the first decades of this century, there would be a campaign for "A Pair of Scales in Every School." The Bureau of Education in 1918 created a Division of School Hygiene, which printed up classroom weight record forms and weight cards. "The children themselves mark their own weights upon the classroom record. They are weighed thereafter once a month, and the keeping of these records stimulates friendly rivalry and gives the children a real motive for forming health habits." In Wisconsin in 1919, there were Modern Health Crusader tournaments to get boys and girls to measure up to weight standards. During the 1920s, anthropometrists began to accumulate data for representative height-weight standards for black children, rural children, and the large communities of Asians on the West Coast. Massive longitudinal studies of children's growth, careful to account for race and ethnic origin, were inaugurated in Boston, Cleveland, Yellow Springs, Iowa City, Denver and Berkeley. The scale companies produced schoolroom scales, while the *Delineator* advised mothers that if their children were more than 7 percent underweight (at the age of ten, this could be as little as 4 lbs), they should "drop all other interests in life and set to work to remedy this condition."[31]

By the Depression, the national ritual of incorporation by weighing would encompass rural and urban children, the poor and the well-to-do, black and white, those of European and of Asian ancestry. As usual, conscientious statisticians would warn parents against a blind faith in height-weight charts even as they produced new ones whose weights were steadily higher. As usual, the complexity of standard deviations and acceptable variations was popularly ignored. Weight in relation to age and to height was too potent a number to be clouded over by dithering probabilities and percentiles.[32]

The Overweight Child

So many pages about the weighing of children, and nary a paragraph about slimming. Everywhere, in all the baby contests and school crusades, the overriding concern was with an ominous thinness, not with obesity. Proof might best be drawn from the inordinate controversy stirred by a 1922 article in the semipopular press. Charles K. Taylor of the Carteret Academy, Orange, New Jersey, wrote an article for *Outlook* on "The Great 'Under-weight' Delusion." He was writing against the tyranny of the weighing machine: "How often have you seen this common sight? A slender, wiry mother places slender, wiry little Willy on the station scales, drops in a penny and gasps in horror. Tables printed on the scales say he should be *x* for his age and height," but he is under. The mother tells the father, who is shocked. "He can't see how an aggressively noisy and obstreperous boy like his Bill can be 12½% below 'normal.' . . . The boy certainly doesn't look anemic. But there it was—right on the scales! One has to pay attention to such things." No, one does not, Taylor wrote. Consider build and hereditary physical types, and consider the well-muscled athlete. Malnutrition was the issue, not a pair of scales. Taylor was right, and the statisticians were soon to speak out against the "Worship of the Average." But in jumped pediatrician Luther Holt and Mrs. Ernest K. Grant, director of the Children's Health Crusade, to protest that at least 20 percent of the nation's children were malnourished and that child weighing was not a fad. Wrote Holt, "The weight of a child is the best simple method we have of estimating the state of his nutrition." In hindsight, Grant and Holt were being overly defensive; Taylor had all the debater's points on his side. But the overreaction was a clear demonstration of the preciousness of weighing in 1922 and shows us with equal clarity how much the scales tilted against underweight.[33]

Before 1940, only a baker's dozen articles on obese children had appeared in the American medical press and just a handful in popular magazines. In 1924 Dr. Borden S. Veeder of St. Louis could find but a single previous discussion of height-weight tables in reference to overweight children. That same year, Dr. Bird T. Baldwin of the Iowa Child Welfare Research Station, co-designer of the height-weight tables for children most consulted through midcentury, suggested that the "decidedly overweight child should be as much a subject of pathologic study as the underweight child" and that children who rose more than 8 percent over the proper weight for height (and age) should receive special attention. Still, ten years later, addressing the staff of the Los Angeles Children's Hospital, Dr. Norman K. Nixon would observe that the "undernourished child has so usurped the attention and worries of the modern mother that his counterpart, the overweight child, usually is ignored." In 1927,

Adelaide R. Ross, director of health education in Malden, Massachusetts, could call the overweight child the "forgotten child."[34]

One person who had not forgotten the overweight child was the popular diet author Dr. Lulu Hunt Peters. Through her syndicated health column she received many letters from unhappy fat children, and in 1924 she published the first calorie-counting book explicitly for them: *Diet for Children (and Adults) and the Kalorie Kids*. "I was an obese child myself," she explained, "and I know that there is genuine mental suffering in being an obese child." Kathryn McHale, in the first American monograph on the *Comparative Psychology and Hygiene of the Overweight Child* (1926), found overweight girls the most fearful and unhappy of her large sample of New York City schoolchildren of all weights. In a study of junior high schools in the West at the same time, it was discovered that nearly 10 percent of the children (most of them girls) were going without breakfast because they were afraid they would get fat. Sixth-grade pupils at Garfield School in Lakewood, Ohio, put on a play called "Dieting" in 1931. The doctor tells Mr. James Williams to reduce his weight, but James proceeds to eat a $1.95 dinner of soup, pork chops, potatoes, date and nut salad, hot muffins, marmalade, olives, celery, four pats of butter and two pieces of pie. He says at the end, feeling a bit sick, "I wonder—I wonder—if something I ate went to my stomach."[35]

After years of being put on scales from infancy through high school, fat children were becoming as sensitive to their overweight as others to underweight, and *any* deviation from the norm was reported by schools and clinics to their parents. We know from the experiments of Jean Piaget conducted just about this time that children appreciate number long before they appreciate mass. The school and clinic charts and scales confirmed for children from the very start that there was an immediate and preternatural relationship between numbers, bodies and weight. But this was an unrooted, floating weight, a burden without purchase. A quarter of the students of Adelaide Ross's fourth, fifth and sixth graders were not sure whether their teacher wanted them to gain, lose or keep their weight where it was. Teachers and nurses spoke about fatness as a sign of malnutrition, which must have been even more confusing: how could eating too much mean eating too little? Since teachers were trained to praise those who gained weight, the position of the fat child was especially perplexing. The numbers on the scale would seem to be arbitrarily punitive, the numbers on the weight chart impossible to fathom. Subject to a stiff regimen of weighing from birth through adolescence, children of the first decades of the century would become the first adult generation of constant weight-watchers, and the fat children would become the first generation of full-scale if inconstant dieters.[36]

Parents of the 1920s and 1930s, however, did not yet take seriously the problem of childhood overweight. It was just baby fat. Children would grow out of it. They themselves had grown up surrounded by images of the healthy child as a round child, pink and fleshy. This wide-cheeked, round-faced, round-armed, round-legged child had come to the fore in American art around 1850 with the many cheap portraits produced in Boston by William Prior, his wife and his brothers-in-law. The Currier & Ives prints of "Pretty Dolly" (1873) and "Home Treasures" (1887–1907) perpetuated the round child, as did the Sunbonnet children drawn for postcards at the turn of the century and the Clapsaddle and Brundage postcard children of the same era. Most of the kids in the comic strips were round too: the Katzenjammer Kids, Hans and Fritz (1897), the Roly Polys (1898), Freckles and His Friends (1915), Dolly Dimples (1915), Little Lulu with Tubby Tompkins (1935) and Nancy (1940). Grace Wiederseim Drayton, who drew Dolly Dimples, also designed the famous Campbell Kids advertising dolls. Like them, the most popular dolls early in the 20th century were plump and round, not the thin-waisted, long-legged fashion dolls whose basic body form had changed little since the 17th century. For children, doll contours did not follow the lines of tailor's dummies or women's clothing. They followed rather the fattish outlines of printed fabric dolls sold as promotion for Diamond Dyes, Clark's Spool Cotton and Kellogg's Corn Flakes, or the new full-bellied Kewpie Dolls of Rose O'Neill, whose designs in 1913 would lead to sales of more than five million kewpies in the next decade. The hoopla in the 1920s was over Grace S. Putnam's "Bye-Lo Baby," round, short-armed and modeled on a real infant, as had been at least one of Maud Humphrey's round postcard babies in 1899. While the Humphrey baby grew up to be actor Humphrey Bogart, the favorite doll of the Depression was modeled on another star, Shirley Temple, pink-kneed, dimpled and spheroid.[37]

"The question may properly be asked," Dr. Veeder had written in 1924, "whether it is necessary to bother with or consider the overweight child at all."[38] But a trap was being set. The tension and the torque had been built in by 1940: a high cultural sensitivity to numerical child weight and an exaggerated alertness to subtle changes in that weight. What had gotten in the way of the jaws of the trap had been the belief that overnutrition was the child's prerogative—that abundance was meant for children—and that children would naturally grow out of their fat.

By 1940 the trap was sprung. Why 1940 as opposed to 1939 or 1941, I do not know. Why 1940 instead of 1930 I can explain.

It had surprisingly little to do with the Depression. True, in 1932, the American Friends Service, which organized relief for children in mining communities, was basing its distribution of free meals on the weights of the children, but across the length of the Depression the average weights of children remained about the same; they were neither thinner nor fatter, whether they were black or white, rich or poor, than they had been in the 1920s. The nutritional quality of the diet may even have improved during the Depression and World War II, despite poverty and rationing. (There were less fats and sugars in the ordinary diet during hard times, though the sales of candy bars did go up tremendously.) The economic effects of the Depression were not such as immediately or directly to provoke a special concern with overweight children.[39]

The question is, why in 1940 did it seem that childhood fat might be permanent? Dr. Veeder had written in 1924, "So far as we know, the degenerative changes that go with obesity in the adult world do not occur in childhood; but whether carrying around excessive weight early in life predisposes to a similar condition in adult life is another question on which I can find no data." Bird T. Baldwin had claimed in 1921 that "The heavy boy or girl at six or at nine or ten will be a heavy boy or girl six years later," and Kathryn McHale in 1926 had shown that overweight tended to be transmitted across generations, but there were no statistics on whether overweight children did or did not lose their baby fat. And no data had been published by 1934, when an anonymous mother looked at her son David, a plump baby become an overweight six-year-old, and "began to fear that he might grow up to be one of those fat boys who are so severely handicapped by their weight." Where did that fear come from? How did Mildred Hatton Bryan in 1937 get the wherewithal to urge parents "to start fighting fat when you first see it coming on," and not to delude themselves with the vain hope that their fat daughters would thin down in a few years? Why did she think that fat would stick?[40]

What we are looking for, then, are not statistics but adult convictions that what happens in childhood is somehow permanent and, more particularly, that what a child does with its body somehow determines its later physical life. Although we might wade into the literature of any century and skim from the surface passages with just those assumptions, only in the 1920s and 1930s can we find a national movement fervently applying such convictions to the rearing of young children. This was the mental hygiene movement, with its child guidance centers for older children, its behavior clinics for kindergartners, and its habit clinics for preschoolers.

The mental hygiene movement took official root in the United States in the 1920s and had by 1931 more than two hundred clinics and centers across the country. While Dr. Arnold Gesell at Yale and other experimental psychologists studied the stages of sensorimotor activity, their contemporary mental hygienists supposed that the habits developed in young children would open up neural pathways of intimidating resilience. Those habits were not habits of thought *per se*; they were habits of behavior, actual physical activity that could be recorded and controlled. Behind the propaganda of health and growth lay the principle of good rhythm, which implied smooth private and interpersonal relations—from the "normal nursing rhythms" of the infant to the athletic flow of the playground to the give-and-take of social intercourse. Bad rhythm meant bad habits (bedwetting, stealing, fighting, refusing to eat). "Although no claim is made at this time that there is any relation between these undesirable habits in childhood and the mental breakdowns of later life, it is not difficult to see that these infantile reactions closely resemble the psychoneurotic manifestations in adult life." So wrote the psychiatrist Douglas A. Thom, whose Habit Clinic for Child Guidance (established 1921) was the leading model.[41]

Thom wrote in the same article, "I have not lost sight of the fact that many of the foregoing conditions described as 'undesirable habits' might well be considered self-eliminating, yet this in no way justifies us in ignoring them." The problem of childhood obesity was slowly caught up in such logic. The mental hygienists were very alarmed by child feeding problems—tongue-sucking, thumb-sucking, clothes-sucking, holding food in one's mouth, refusing foods, vomiting, gagging—as signs of the failure of socialization and of later psychological disturbance. They were much concerned, too, with physical fluency and the development of the neuromuscular structure, so they collaborated with playground directors and modern dancers who were bringing movement classes to young children. From table to teeter-totter, the fat child would not have been left alone.[42]

But while the mental hygienists meddled everywhere with all ages, they also promoted childhood independence. Their ideal of the healthy adult was the figure of the adventurous American entrepreneur, canny, resourceful, smooth, in touch with the rhythms of the commercial world and quick to move to meet the demands of the market. So the child should learn dexterity, ingenuity, regular bowel movements, manners and promptness.

The children's clothing industry in the 1920s moved quickly to meet the demands of *this* market, the self-help market, by advertising shirts, blouses, jackets, dresses and pants which children could work themselves. Manufacturers produced better fitting clothes, resizing for children according to height and age, and (something very new) asking in mail order catalogs for weight as well. They allowed for build and for movement. They introduced more stretch material. Around 1928, they put Talon slide fasteners where before there had been tedious rows of buttons or snaps. In all this, the advertising emphasis was upon preparing the child for a healthy life, free of the constipation caused by burdensome fastenings, free of the overheating and cramping caused by layers of clothes. Swaddling had disappeared from the American nursery early in the 19th century, but babies had been so bundled for the rest of the century that the lighter buntings and baby bags of the 1930s could appear highly progressive, and children's zippered snowsuits positively revolutionary.[43]

Would it follow that the fat child might seem now to be a backward child, or a slow child, or at least a child whose adulthood would be haunted by the visible failures of early life: constipation, or clumsiness, or fatigue, or the chubby-fingered ineptness at shoelaces (and, eventually, at the knotty problems of maturity)?

This was a subtle path toward an assertion of permanence. People around 1940 had far more dramatic proof of unchanging bodies. The first (small) American epidemic of polio was reported in 1841 in West Feliciana, Louisiana. In 1894 there were 132 cases in Vermont, in 1907 some 2,000 cases in New York. The Northeast was struck by a massive epidemic in 1916, with 29,000 cases and 6,000 deaths. Franklin Delano Roosevelt, stricken in 1921, held a President's Birthday Ball for Polio in 1934. In 1938, behind the singing of Eddie

Cantor, the American March of Dimes began: posters everywhere of a smiling child on crutches, long metal braces up his legs. The incidence of polio, relatively stable in the 1920s and 1930s, quadrupled between 1940 and 1955. Children were put in plaster casts, splints, steel corsets, Bradford frames. "Crucifixion frames," Sister Elizabeth Kenny called them when she came from therapeutic triumphs in Australia to set up her polio clinic in Minneapolis; "plaster prisons." She was fifty-three, a self-taught physical therapist putting hot cloths on children's legs, teaching children "joint consciousness." She could work miracles. It's spasm, not paralysis, Kenny told America; muscle tone. Six years later, Rosalind Russell played her in the movies. In 1952, fond of capes, pearls, and enormous hats, Sister Kenny was voted highest in American esteem, ahead of Eleanor Roosevelt and Emily Post. There were 58,000 cases of polio that year. The Salk vaccine was sixteen months away.[44]

Throughout the 1940s, it was the image of childhood paralysis that gave force to the image of abiding childhood fat. In the 19th century, paralyzed infants had often been mistaken for obese infants, and in their immobilized state, many young victims of polio would grow fat or would be further handicapped by the baby fat they already had. In 1941, Albert B. Sabin and Robert Ward pointed at the mass of evidence "which established with certainty that the stomach and gastro-intestinal tract are the usual portal of entry of infantile paralysis into the body." Polio, then, had something to do with eating. Asked in 1949 what they would do if there were an outbreak of polio in their neighborhood, some 15 percent of respondents said they would rest and eat well; 12 percent thought that polio could be prevented by a change of diet. Between 1948 and 1951, Dr. Benjamin P. Sandler received national publicity and some national cooperation with his theory that polio was caused by low blood sugar; the way to defend against polio, therefore, was to reduce the starches and sugars in the diet. "Several observers have remarked on the fact that polio frequently attacks children and adolescents who are larger and heavier than the average for their age," Sandler wrote. "Some of them are actually obese."[45]

So polio could make a child fat, and a fat child could invite polio. There was a cultural conjunction between images of permanent immobility and images of fatness. With adults, obesity led to heart attacks and crippling strokes, partial paralysis which might leave a person half dead. Parents would then hear Sister Kenny say, "Infantile paralysis is a damnable thing. It leaves a child neither alive nor

dead."[46] That, despite the dancing elephants of Walt Disney's un-
popular *Fantasia*, was the issue of 1940: the fat child becoming the
immobilized adult, the isolated adult, the adult who could die early.

When the trap was sprung, it was sprung with a vengeance. Like
the invisible polio virus, fat was an invasive consubstantial villain. It
entered through the stomach (through eating) like the virus, and
eventually it could paralyze. Fat was polio in slow motion. Children
writing to health education director Adelaide Ross in 1937 talked
about their obesity as if all were already lost. "Do you think I am too
fat to be healthy?" asked David, age twelve. "I weigh 141 lbs. If I
reduce do you think I will be healthy?" "I am only nine," wrote
Phyllis, "and I weigh 112 pounds. Please help me if you can."[47]

The Hungering Child

"Give the fat child a chance," Beatrice Black was pleading in *Parents' Magazine* in 1941.[48] She was anchoring her plea on the articles
of Hilde Bruch, a physician who had come to the United States in
1934. Startled by the number of really fat boys and girls here, Bruch
tried to establish objective criteria for the diagnosis of endocrine disorder among obese children. In 1900 the French neurologist Joseph
Babinski had found a pituitary tumor in an adolescent fat girl. In
1901 Alfred Froehlich published a report of a fourteen-year-old boy
grown rapidly fat; he explained the fatness as a result of a pituitary
tumor. Dr. Froehlich did not mean thereby to explain all childhood
obesity as pituitary in origin, but when the syndrome was given an
official name ("dystrophia adiposo-genitalis") and linked to pituitary insufficiency, it became as popular as the diagnosis of thyroid
insufficiency among obese adults. Seemingly confirmed by research
on pituitary gland disorders and Cushing's Syndrome, the diagnosis
of hypopituitarism was soon extended to any child—especially any
boy—with a girdle of fat around the abdomen, an infantile appearance, and retarded genital development. Since fat children almost
by definition looked infantile (with the round faces and bodies of
healthy babies) and usually did carry their fat at the hips, and since
folds of fat could obscure the apparent size of a boy's genitals, the
majority of fat boys could be lumped under the blowsy umbrella of
Froehlich's Syndrome. Froehlich himself was very unhappy about
this; over some forty years he had found no more than half a dozen
authentic cases confirming his initial report, "though every little fat

boy has been named after me." In 1936 Dr. Gavin Fulton of Louisville would claim that 99 percent of fat children had endocrine
problems.[49]

But true to the Depression shift of emphasis from metabolism to
appetite, Hilde Bruch could make no sense of this endocrine theory.
Hypothyroid children were thin, not fat, and obese children were
generally advanced in skeletal and genital development. As Bruch
wrote after several years of psychiatric training, the problem was
not physiological so much as it was psychological. Bruch maintained that the hunger of fat children was deeply rooted in the family. Since food was a substitute for something lacking or a defense
against an overprotective mother, the child's hunger would not necessarily disappear with time or glandular injections. Baby fat might
be physiologically temporary, but childhood fatness was an expression of an insatiable, enduring hunger.[50]

In the switch from "Is your child too thin?" (1926) to "Don't let
your child get fat" (1945), the specter of permanent fat stood in the
shadows of permanent hunger. This was the mother's hunger for her
child's approval; it was also, as with Walt Disney's *Dumbo* in 1941,
the child's hunger for the mother, Mrs. Jumbo. The fat child was
discovered to be a problem at the very moment when mothers were
moving away from rigid feeding schedules and when the first real
spate of American studies of anorexia nervosa was appearing in the
medical literature. It was in fact "that clean-plate bogey" that had
created the eating problems, wrote Gladys D. Shultz for *Better
Homes and Gardens*. In the 1920s, when mothers first became
nutrition-conscious, "We were armed then . . . with diet lists calling
for nice large servings of lots of wholesome foods, but we had too little knowledge of how to get them into small human beings. We created the biggest problem we've had to meet with children these past
twenty years, that of the child who 'wouldn't eat.' "[51]

The child who would not eat and the child who never had
enough were both products of the same era in which, as anthropologist Margaret Mead saw in 1943, there had been a sharpened distinction between the foods that people thought were good for them
and the foods that people thought were tasty. "In the average
home," Mead explained, "the right food and the wrong food are
both placed on the table; the child is rewarded for eating the 'right'
food and so taught that the right food is undesirable—for parents do
not reward children for doing pleasant things." With the fixing of a
moral line between what is good and what is delicious, every meal

would become a moral battle. The finicky eater fought back by eating less of anything, the fat child by eating everything.[52]

Appetite then was a psychological and social issue, not a question of glands. There were injections for thyroid and pituitary deficiencies, but what could one do with a deeply bound sense of hollowness and frustration? While psychologists explored family therapies, physicians began prescribing amphetamines for children as young as two. The drugs worked in the short run: children in 1940 lost .831 lb per week. . . . We need not follow the history any further; amphetamines would remain in diet pills for children until the 1970s, and psychotherapies are still in progress. The point is that now the same methods of reducing used on adults were being used on children because something quite powerful seemed necessary to break the child's habit of hunger—which would, otherwise, make for frighteningly permanent fat.[53]

Children Reduced

Closest to adulthood, teenagers were least likely to grow out of fat newly taken on or long maintained. Girls over the age of sixteen—college girls—had essentially stopped growing, so they were the first to attract national attention for their dieting practices. Barnard students in 1937 adopted a high-vitamin, low-carbohydrate, low-calorie diet and went for mile walks in order to reduce. But most of them also smoked, and like their smoking, their dieting and their long city walks may have been an assertion of maturity.[54]

It was more important to catch fat at its advent in early adolescence. A Chicago pediatrician made it clear in 1941 that "obesity is seldom a problem in early or late childhood. It usually becomes one at or near puberty." The appearance of awkward, disturbing fat ran parallel to the appearance of awkward, disturbing sexual desires. And the doctor paraphrased Hilde Bruch: The sudden taking on of fat could be a mask to avoid the tensions of sexuality, adolescent sex play, or the fears of sexual maldevelopment. Weight-control diets, cautioned nutritionist Lulu G. Graves, could be successful only if they prevented "an empty feeling." Those were her quotation marks, and she was using them to indicate more than a scientific mistrust of appetite or a psychological mistrust of the overprotective mother. That "empty feeling" was in contrast to the sexual fulfillment tacitly and ungrammatically promised teenage girls who did reduce: "Properly done, figures slim down, fleshy rubber tires turn into wiry muscles, piano legs grow slender and symmetrical, acne clears up, skin becomes smooth and glowing, elimination improves, and she begins to look like a model."[55]

Teenagers did seem in need of weight loss early on, around puberty and high school. At least 10 percent were overweight in some Boston high schools in 1952–53, 25 percent in Berkeley in 1962–65. And teenagers—especially teenage girls—often felt that they should be dieting. Of fifteen thousand surveyed across the country in the 1940s, nearly half the girls wanted to lose weight. Another survey in 1963 showed that 38 percent felt they had an overweight problem (boys 28 percent, girls 48 percent). During the 1960s, nearly two-thirds of high school girls had been on reducing diets by the time they were seniors; they had usually begun dieting at fourteen.[56]

From the mid-1950s, physicians and public health spokespeople began to cast their eyes even lower down the age column of the height-weight charts. Despite Dr. Benjamin Spock's kindly note that "mild overweight is common between seven and twelve" and likely to vanish by fifteen "without great effort," fewer people were taking seriously the old-fashioned idea that baby fat would disappear by itself. Adult obesity had to be caught by puberty, then at prepuberty, then by the age of six. Dr. Stanley Garn of the Fels Research Institute, one of the most prolific researchers on obesity, would be quoted by *Newsweek* in 1960 in an article on "Teen-age Gluttons": "Keep the six-year-old from eating his way into a premature grave at sixty, even if it means making life less joyous in the childhood period."[57]

The significant pressure downward to younger and younger children was in good measure due—at last—to some statistics on the intractability of childhood weight. In 1960, Abraham and Nordsieck reported on a two-decade follow-up of the physical examinations of schoolchildren in Hagerstown, Maryland. Of the overweight boys from their original sample, 84 percent of those located twenty years later were still overweight; of the overweight girls, 82 percent were overweight as women. Rounded down to 80 percent or up to 85 percent, this is the single most frequently cited datum in the modern literature on childhood obesity: 80 percent (or 85 percent) of obese children would be obese as adults. Other long-term studies in 1961 and 1966 confirmed the statistical unlikelihood of shedding childhood weight. "Overweight children," the 1966 study said, "cannot be counted on to 'grow out of' their obesity." These scientific papers were fed quickly into the medical mainstream and onto supermarket stands, as in the title of an article for *Good Housekeeping* in 1963: "Fat adults from chubby children grow."[58]

There were also demographic reasons for the downward pressure. Since the late 19th century, especially for females of the working class, average age at menarche had been declining—from 14.2 years in the 1870s to 12.8 years in the 1960s. Since the percentage of body fat and the gross body weight may very well be key triggers for menstruation, an earlier age at menarche could be attributed in part to long-term trends in average weight and average fatness among women. The greater the weight and the more fat, Stanley Garn suggested in 1959, the earlier the age of physical maturity and menarche. Getting a jump on the problems of obesity meant getting at it before puberty, which now meant before the teens. And the number of prepubertal children was just peaking in 1960, a result of the baby boom after World War II.[59]

Since birth, these children had been subject to an increasingly heavy fallout from advertising directed at their dieting mothers and exercising fathers. Low-calorie foods for adults made their way onto the kitchen table. The postwar codification of sizes for large women made itself felt in new clothing sizes tailored for chubby girls—not just the specialty fashions of 1940 ("Clever designing and artful cutting make Chubbette the gay deceiver that it is"), but mass-produced clothing sized for those "awkward years" between eleven and sixteen. Such sizes for girls, and the new "husky" for boys, may have been goddess-sends for working mothers too busy to sew clothes or to let out ill-fitting store-bought clothes, but they also marked obese children for what they were. This act of designation was nearly as important as the public weighing that continued in American schoolrooms. It established a system of visual models and public comparisons, oriented once again to numbers, by which children would come to see their bodies and their weight.[60]

Cultural models of children had been moving toward thinness. The new comic strips like "Peanuts" (1950), "Dondi" (1955) and "Miss Peach" (1957) presented far slimmer (though strangely bigger-headed) children. New age-graded toys had implicit size and weight differentials which put a fat child at a disadvantage. Playground equipment had pole circumferences, lateral rung distances and seat sizes geared to more slender hands, longer arms and narrower bottoms.

Most important were the new plastic dolls, climaxing with Mattel's teenage Barbie Doll introduced in 1958. The new dolls were visually slim and palpably hard, neither cushioned nor floppy nor indentable. They wore clothes obviously intended for those on the lighter side of the weight charts, and they begged for dozens of athletic outfits for their mobile, well-articulated bodies.

It should not startle if, just as physicians had come up with strong proof of the stubbornness of childhood weight, young children would believe that they ought to diet. The children had not been convinced either by modernistic velocity charts for the measurement of growth or by histories of the adult obese.[61] Many children seemed to want to diet when the charts gave them every right to a double malted, and by kindergarten age they had aversions to images of chubby peers. We are not faced with the happy results of an effective health campaign; rather, this was a generation of children with body image disturbances. While Fleischmann advertisements for liquid corn oil margarine pictured a young boy amid such captions as "Should an 8-year-old worry about cholesterol?" and "Is there a heart attack in his future?" and while the final report of the White House Conference on Food, Nutrition and Health in 1970 was urging screening for obese *pre*schoolers, young children were quite clear about their dislike of endomorphs. Little girls were more favorably disposed to ectomorphs (thin bodies) than were little boys, but both sexes agreed that fat bodies were obnoxious, sloppy, ugly, lonely, lazy and even stupid. By 1983 the round, smiling Campbell Kids (designed in 1910) had also been slimmed down; soup might be "good food" but it could not be fattening, not even for children.[62]

I do not mean to claim here that fat children are purely the victims of a cultural fantasy about the growing body, or that all fat children belong to a healthy but persecuted minority. Childhood fatness *is* an affliction—sometimes physiological, sometimes sociological, sometimes psychological, often all of the above. I am however less concerned with the still disputed medical realities of juvenile obesity than with the historical acuteness of those pressures imposed by the culture of slimming upon children at earlier and earlier ages. The seeming conspiracy against childhood obesity begun by the medical, parental and childhood worlds during the 1960s was an illusion produced by the coincidence of three separate movements culminating at the same time: a medical world with sadly triumphant numbers on the permanence of weight; a parental world with three generations' experience of weighing their children and dieting themselves; a childhood world with visual and tactile evidence that weight, like sin or size tags, might be carried forever.

The Fat Fetus

The same argument can scarcely be made for the spiral down to the toddler, the infant and the newborn. For them, of course, dieting would be imposed from above. The spiral was building from 1940, when Lulu Graves wrote in regard to fat children, "Fortunate, indeed, are the young people whose mothers have taught them right habits of eating from infancy." In 1941 the *New York Times* reported that "Weight Problem Bothers Dionnes: Quintuplets Are Going on a Diet." A quarter-century later, Dr. Alice Lake told the readers of the *Ladies Home Journal*, "In a sense, according to some of the most up-to-date pediatricians, a child should start dieting with the first mouthful he swallows."[63]

"Obesity starts in childhood," *Science Digest* announced in May 1969, followed by a popular account of new biochemical work on adipocyte (fat) cell tissue. Drs. Jules Hirsch and Jerome L. Knittle had developed a technique for estimating the number of fat cells in rats and then in humans. Lean people had twenty-seven trillion fat cells; obese people had seventy-seven trillion. It seemed that the number of fat cells in one's body was pretty much set in early childhood, and the greater the number of fat cells, the more likely that one would be fat as an adult. By 1972, Knittle would propose that childhood obesity was basically a problem in adipose tissue cellular development. "It would appear then," Knittle concluded, "that a critical period of development, with major consequences for one's adult weight, occurs somewhere between birth and five years of age."[64]

The fat cell theory appeared to be conclusive proof that we were "eating our way into the cemetery beginning in the perambulator." Mothers soon were telling their doctors that they did not want their babies to have too many fat cells. "Obesity is said to be the major pediatric nutritional problem today," wrote a leading pediatrician in 1981. "Many families request advice in an effort to prevent the development of obesity in children at one and two years of age."[65]

Striking, but not striking enough. Reviewing the subject in 1975, Heald and Khan decided that the time to prevent childhood obesity began with the last trimester of intrauterine life. In 1979, one of the premier researchers, Dr. June K. Lloyd, was suggesting that pregnant mothers avoid excessive weight gain in order to prevent "fetal overnutrition." The relationship between weight gained in pregnancy and newborn weight was, after a century of weighing, still contested, but diets for pregnant women sold well throughout the 1970s. As before, women had cosmetic and personal health reasons for dieting. They also had additional evidence that pregnancy was the runway toward their own obesity. And now came the anxiety about a fetus which might have too many fat cells, as if in retribution for the demand feeding of children since the 1940s.[66]

Yet this fails to convince. Trillions of fat cells there may be, all of them ferociously faithful to our bodies, but the extension of the notion of dieting to an unborn child was extraordinary enough to demand more than the passwords of science. As in the 1940s the image of the child stricken with polio was the sustaining cultural correlate of the child condemned to lifelong overweight, so in the 1970s there had to be some equally powerful correlate to the image of a fetus already fat.

If polio epidemics were, as they were, the national issue most focused on children in the 1940s, then for the late 1960s and the 1970s that issue was without doubt abortion. I do not claim that the two, abortion and slimming, are the same thing, but they have the same nerve endings. They are part of a synaptic gospel concerning permanence and loss, shape-changing, intervention and irreversibility, self-control and self-will, surveillance and security. They have shared the same physical strategies—horseback riding, harsh exercise, jumping off chairs—and the same preparations—vinegar, alum, boracic acid, diuretics, water douches. They share, especially in reference to the trimesters of a fetus, a semantic world of similar topography, with much the same turbulent emotional weather. There is talk of unwanted children or unwanted fat, of lust or gluttony, of social burdens. Though at first glance it seems that abortion is slimming's negative number, the loss of weight turned inside out, the relationship during the 1970s became more complex with the rise to national attention of anorexia nervosa.[67]

Anorexia is a slow self-murder, but unlike obesity it moves toward death by moving backward toward birth. In an era of campaigns for natural childbirth and breastfeeding, of the politicization of midwifery and of the "right-to-life" philosophy of abortion as "against nature" and "a murder of innocents," the anorectic child confronts us with the regressive antinatural act of slimming back toward the womb. The anorectic girl is this era's Mollie Fancher, whose fasting is meant to be magical but whose magic turns in the end upon herself. If she can cut up her food with geomantic precision, if she can hold certain images in her mind as she eats with Fletcherite economy, then the food will sustain her without clinging to her bones. Since anorexia usually begins with a more casual dieting, it may be that the anorectic girl (or boy) is born statistically fatter than the average and that her (his) infantile overweight is so worrisome within the family that she (he) confuses love's body with an infinitely thin embrace.[68]

If the semantic bond between abortion and slimming is more apparent for females, the syntax holds for males in a surprisingly mythic manner. I lift the following joke from our national repository, *Reader's Digest*, for July 1983:

> Friends of ours, worried about their father's middle-age spread, had been urging him to diet and exercise. The father, however, insisted he was in great shape for his age—until the day his grandson, fresh from observing the various stages of an aunt's pregnancy, approached him as he was watching TV. Patting his grandfather's paunch, the boy asked, "Grandpa, do you have a baby in there?"
>
> "Of course not!" his grandfather hastily retorted.

Shades of Cronus devouring his children? Of Father Time giving birth? But the joke goes on:

> "Oh!" the child replied. "You mean it's going to *stay* like that?"
> There was a new member at the health spa the next day.

So the slimming man removes the imputation of pregnancy, of the parturitive part of his self. A joke about slimming may be a joke about abortion.

A Child's Garden of Slimming

The joke also tells us something about children, male and female, tucked to the Damascene bib of obesity. "Oh!" the child replied. "You mean it's going to *stay* like that?" From the mid-1960s, children have been learning from Head Start programs, primary school teachers, 4-H clubs, television and their own books on dieting that fat—their own fat—is ornery. "Think thin, teach thin," advised the school nurse in Imperial, Missouri, in the journal *School and Community* in 1983. And so the teachers do, helped by syllabi from the National Education Association. Younger children study numbers by studying measurement; they make body bundles, compare their weights on teeter-totters and bathroom scales, use metric tapes to create height–weight–age charts. Soon they are ready to make daily charts of food consumption, defining obesity by caloric intake. In grades seven through nine, they will be asked to "list factors which will influence your weight throughout life." In high school they will draw graphs showing the relationship of heart disease, diabetes, high blood pressure and overweight. Their nutrition texts will tell them that "There are two peaks for the onset of juvenile obesity— ages 0 to 4 and 7 to 11 years. There is considerable evidence that obese children do not grow out of this condition but tend to become obese adults." By 1980 the fat cell was ensconced in a high school physiology text: "Evidence is accumulating that the feeding of large amounts of fats early in life results in the development of excess numbers of adipose cells. These cells "like to be filled" and tend to accumulate fat, which may lead to fat babies who are not necessarily healthy babies. Adults who are obese tend to have been obese as children, possibly from having more adipose cells 'crying for fat.'"[69]

"Crying for fat." That empty feeling was no vague element of a psychological model; it was situated in the craws of trillions of practically invisible bodies, a hunger as impossible to discern as, perhaps, to satisfy. Worse yet, scientists found that once the number of fat cells was set, all the dieting in this round world, however radical, however unwise, would do nothing but change the size of fat cells. The trillions would remain. "With the exception of cancer," a physician wrote in 1978, "there is hardly another childhood disease with such an unfavorable prognosis as obesity."[70]

And it was not just the fat cell; it was fat itself that remained. Skinfold tests taken during the Ten-State Nutrition Study of 1968–70 showed that by age seventeen, children of obese parents were thrice as fat as children of lean parents. Jean Mayer, Harvard's prominent nutritionist, turned up even more discouraging statistics in 1975: if neither parent was obese, a child had a 7 percent chance of becoming obese; if one parent, 40 percent; if two parents, 80 percent. Set those probabilities side by side with fat cells, and any parent the least bit overweight—overweight now, overweight in the past, overweight as a child—would be nervous about the prospects of the new generation.[71]

"Dear Girls and Boys," wrote Barbara K. Feig in the children's section of her *Parents' Guide to Weight Control for Children, Ages 5 to 13 Years* (1980), "You probably wonder why a fuss is being made about your weight. After all, you know plenty of kids who are heavier than you, they're really *fat!* Well, a couple of years ago, those kids were probably just like you are now." During the 1970s, in the company of books for parents, the first popular dieting books for young children appeared. Peggy Bolian's *Growing Up Slim* (1971) for teenagers was followed by Barbara Benziger's *Controlling Your Weight* (1973) for those at puberty; Sara D. Gilbert's *Fat Free: Common Sense for Young Weight Worriers* (1975) and Audrey Ellis's *The Kid-slimming Book* (1976) for grade six up; Bill Bluestein and Enid Bluestein's *Mom, How Come I'm Not Thin?* (1981) for grades two through five. James Marshall's *Yummers!* (1972) was for even younger children: Eugene Turtle advises Emily Pig to walk off her extra weight, but on her walk she has corn-on-the-cob, Eskimo pies, Girl Scout cookies and a free pizza sample in a supermarket. Will she ever learn her lesson?

The first preschoolers' picture-book on slimming was published by Lothrop, Lee & Shepard in 1972: Mary Lynn Solot's *100 Hamburgers: The Getting Thin Book*. The book begins:

> Sometimes I feel so HUNGRY that I could eat A HUNDRED HAMBURGERS but I'm not allowed to because I'm getting too fat. Not really, really fat like some people I see at the beach or the supermarket or on a bus, just fat enough so my mother is ALWAYS WATCHING ME WHEN I EAT.

The boy's parents are also and always on a diet.

> So are most of their friends,
>   even
>   the
>   skinny
>   ones.
> Maybe I will have to diet
> for the rest of my life,
> but I sure hope not.

Would he?

The answer, in fiction for older children, was no, not necessarily. Fiction about the problems of fat children flourished as never before during the 1970s and early 1980s. In these books, fat children start toward thinness only when they take control of their lives. Thinness means freedom—from overprotective or obsessively thin mothers in *Heads You Win Tails I Lose*, *Last Was Lloyd*, and *The Pig-Out Blues*; from an overprotective grandmother in *Jelly Belly*; from the harassment of peers in *One Bite at a Time*, *Blubber*, *Dumb Old Casey Is a Fat Tree*, and *Oh, Rick*; from the trauma of divorce in *Nothing's Fair in Fifth Grade*; from sadness and self-hatred in *Dinky Hocker Shoots Smack* and *Fat Jack*; from socially inhibiting or restrictive fantasies in *Next Door to Xanadu*, *One Fat Summer*, and *Dinah and the Green Fat Kingdom*. The children are often assisted by alter-egos: a scale and a gorilla in *Fat Elliot and the Gorilla*; horses in *White Pony* and *Panky and William*; puppies in *Mishmash and the Big Fat Problem*; athletic helpmeets in *Rinehart Lifts* and *Hey, Remember Fat Glenda?* In the very best book of this genre, Virginia Hamilton's *The Planet of Junior Brown*, the alter-ego is Big Buddy Clark or "Tomorrow Billy," a black boy so much the baroque angel that the novel ends with his rescue of the 300-lb Junior Brown floating down on a winch, almost weightless, toward the floor of an empty tenement, his new planet.[72]

Throughout this literature, written as much for boys as for girls, adult images of abortion are countered by childlike images of rebirth. The happy ending is not to accept one's weight but to accept oneself and so lose weight.[73] Where children are treated as convicts, as in Stephen Manes's tart *Slim-down Camp*, the protagonists rebel and will not lose weight. Where the children can escape being "It" at tag and "It" in life, where they can find themselves as people, then they become slim. Their new thinness is the curious badge of maturity.

In 1983, at the chronological end of the long spiral downward from the dieting co-ed to the fat fetus, some pediatricians began to pick up something they called "fear of obesity," which was not the same as the syndrome of anorexia nervosa.[74] Nine boys and five girls between the ages of nine and seventeen had imposed on themselves diets so calorically minimal that they were stunted in growth and sexual development. Otherwise they were healthy. They were good students and had few vitamin deficiencies, but as thin as they were, they behaved "like obese adolescents trying to lose weight." They were psychiatrically uninteresting, though somewhat shy and compulsive. They simply feared fat: it would make them less attractive and shorten their lives. Their families were usually preoccupied with achieving slim figures. The children had taken it upon themselves to begin the perpetual refrain of dieting.

Since the mid-1940s, our cultural problems with age, authority, abundance and love have taken on the iconography of the fat and the thin. What we say to each other every day about weight lost and weight gained is so fundamental to our notions of company, beauty, mortality and power that it should be no surprise if our children share the styles of our bodies which have become the measure of our lives. For children, however, fat and weight may be dangerously unrooted, like the "It" of tag, the It one never overcomes, only eludes. For children, the cultural burden of fat by 1983 had no purchase at all but a very heavy price.

CHAPTER TEN

The Weightless Body

The culture of slimming has reached its apogee when dieters imagine foods without calories and bodies without weight. In this context have appeared the most extreme of diets—the Christian evangelical romance, whose model for weight-reducing culminates in the glorious weightlessness of the Rapture, and the rituals of behavior modification, which treat the body as an unfortunate creature of time. Like the evangelicals and the behaviorists, who tend to make fatness a personal problem and slimming a private process, bioscientists have also drawn the dilemmas of obesity away from the social arena toward the inner world of neurophysiology. The weightless body (thin, energetic, private, impervious to time) is a body without any sense of gravity, detached from the body politic.

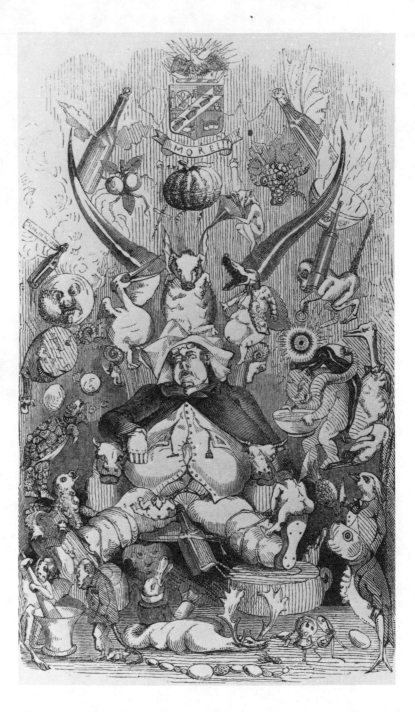

The ideal of the weightless body is an extreme reaction to this 19th-century English image of the fat body as heavy, bloated, torpid, and besieged by the demonic creatures of nightmare and medicine. From Sydney Whiting's Memoirs of a Stomach *(1853).* Courtesy of the National Library of Medicine

Essences

A MONG THE TALES of the *Arabian Nights* is the tale of the feast
to which a Persian lord of the great and generous Barmecide
family treats a beggar. As each course enters on its elegant
platter, the lord sings its praises in lavish detail. In fact, there is
nothing on any of the platters. The banquet is imaginary. The beggar, however, plays along, pretending to delight in each dish, and is
at last rewarded with a real dinner and a lucrative post.

The Barmecidal feast is the last word in dieting, the final exaltation of flavor over substance, the dream of the sumptuous meal
without a single calorie. It is, as Gail Borden would have understood, the ultimate condensed food. "I mean to put a potato into a
pill-box," Borden said as he experimented with his evaporated condensed milk in the 1850s, "a pumpkin into a tablespoon, the biggest
sort of a watermelon into a saucer. . . . The Turks made acres of
roses into attar of roses. . . . I intend to make attar of everything!"
When Henry Tanner was on his forty-day fast in 1880, his nemesis
William Hammond suggested that Tanner might be surviving on almost invisible foods: "There are all kinds of prepared food now,
some of it containing great nourishment in a very small space. A

quart of dried ox-blood can be compressed into a space the size of a walnut." Hammond was thinking in particular of Justus von Liebig's beef extract or Extractum Carnis, one pound of whose concentrated essence was supposed to be equivalent to 36 lbs of meat. Throughout the late 19th century, beef tea and beef extract were fed to invalids and children to strengthen them, though they were little more than attar of beef.[1]

In this century, the Barmecidal impulse has grown even stronger, sustained first by Fletcherism and then by the vitamin pill, liquid meals, starch blockers and the momentous announcement of minus-calorie foods. Sadly, no foods sport fewer calories than it takes in energy from the body to break them down and burn them, but there are low-calorie bulking agents that can give mass and texture to otherwise insubstantial flavorings, so that one may eat luxuriantly without fearing the consequences of indulgence, "in the same sense," wrote John J. Beereboom of the Pfizer Corporation, "that modern man can have the enjoyment of sex without the consequence of procreation." At the University of Illinois in 1977, contraception and Barmecidal feast were drawn together in the work—most appropriately—of Drs. Sarfaraz Niazi and M. Hussain, who suggested the use of perfluoroctyl bromide to coat the gastrointestinal tract and prevent the absorption of most food. We could have the taste, the aroma, the mouthfeel and the happiness of swallowing without the burden of the food itself.[2]

The Barmecidal impulse, most obvious among dieters, is integral to the "high intensity market setting" of our society, where what is imputed to a product is more important than what the product actually is. Not a cigarette but women's rights; not a drink but a fountain of youth; not a frozen dinner but a night on the town. The greater our bounty, the more fragmented our wants and the more tenuous the naming of things, the singing of praises. We think: If only we play along as the beggar did, we too must be rewarded with an honest meal. But instead there is an inevitable confusion of needs and wants, of hunger and appetite, and an equally inevitable disappointment. As the honey-coated words drift over each platter, each invisible offering, day after day, month after month, the language excites an indefinite longing, and we are not likely to be satisfied when the actual dinner is served.[3]

Dieting is a way of managing surplus. The less confident we are of our ability to manage surplus, the more we turn to dieting, that is, to trying to fool ourselves that we can have (and handle) everything by consuming nothing. Dieting in the midst of plenty may strike us as cruel or foolish or ironic, but it is not paradoxical. It comes with the territory. It is the other half of longing. The same forces that make us insatiable make us fat and make us frightened.[4]

In the 1930s, physiologists were fond of describing appetite as an outrider of nostalgia. Fat people were victims of nostalgia; they lived in a past where food was satisfying, comforting, good. Now, older, they ate not to consume but to be consumed. Hoping to return to the time of the primeval banquet, true and filling, they made themselves at once children and antiques.[5]

We would do better to apply the same terms to that culture of slimming which makes us so concerned about fat people. Dieting is an essentially nostalgic act, an attempt to return to a time when one *could* be satisfied, when one *was* thinner, when the range of choices in the world neither bewildered nor intimidated. To restrict one's range of choices, as all dieters must do, is not so much defiant as it is regressive. The dieter becomes an antiquarian, an annalist of calories, a collector of ancient recipes, a curator of before-and-after photographs. Imagining a miraculous future, the dieter is always looking back.

Dieting cannot subdue longing; it can only suppress it. The culture of slimming draws its enormous power from that longing and from two fears spawned by that longing: a fear of abundance and a fear of never being satisfied. The two fears feed on each other, as any dieter after a binge knows too well. The more extreme the longing, the more extreme the fears and the more extreme the strategies for slimming.

This chapter, the penultimate chapter, is about extremes. It is about the most extreme of romances and the most extreme of rituals. It is about a fascination not just with the thin body but with the weightless body. It is about being twice-born.

The Flesh and the Spirit

"The flesh that God hath given us is affliction enough," wrote poet and preacher John Donne in the 17th century, "but the flesh that the devil gives us, is affliction upon affliction and to that, there belongs a woe." Some three centuries later the fundamentalist minister Dr. C. S. Lovett found his calling to help God's people with this woe, and in 1978 he wrote a book, *Help Lord—The Devil Wants Me Fat!*

Consider: "If you were the devil, wouldn't you seek to penetrate lives at a point where you'd never be suspected? Sure. Well, what is more innocent than food? With Christians THANKING GOD for what they eat, what neater way to slip into their lives than with EXTRA spoonfuls of delicious food. . . . Subtle, right?" "Glutton," Deborah Pierce repeated to herself in the 1950s, "*Gluttony*. Suddenly I had a strange exultant feeling as I remembered something. It was as if I were on the verge of a miracle." If gluttony were a sin, then "perhaps God would help me overcome it." She began to pray, "Almighty God, when things seem too much for me, and my stomach begins to rebel, it is only through Thy presence and guidance that I may overcome my weakness." She went to Prayer-Diet Clubs and prayed, "The Lord is my Shepherd. He will lead me away from food and gluttony into higher paths of life." By 1960 she was a high-fashion model in Washington, D.C., and author of *I Prayed Myself Slim*. It occurred to the columnist Ellen Goodman in 1975 that "eating had become the last bona fide sin left in America"; in 1977 she reported on revivalist diet workshops led by Overeaters Victorious to the text of John 3:30, "He must increase, but I must decrease," or, as Joan Cavanaugh put it in 1976, *More of Jesus and Less of Me*.[6]

We have seen how, in the 19th century, Satan's boa constrictor of gluttony wrapped the dyspeptic in its coils. In this century Satan has reappeared as the mocking mouth of the dial on the bathroom scale, whose "red pointer flicks back and forth like a derisive tongue." And Satan has legions of Little Red Devils (or hidden calories) urging Mrs. Chubby to shoot the works at a soda fountain, as in the 1951 Metropolitan Life cartoon, "Cheers for Chubby." But the first overly Christian slimming book did not appear until 1957, with Charlie W. Shedd's *Pray Your Weight Away*. Pastor of the Memorial Drive Presbyterian Church of Houston, Shedd had lost 100 lbs and had found that "we fatties are the only people on earth who can weigh our sin." God could teach fatties to face their hidden selves while they followed diet recipes and did exercises to the psalms—leg lifts to Psalm 23, the side straddle hop to Psalm 118:24 ("This is the day which the Lord hath made; we will rejoice and be glad in it"). God, Shedd believed, had intended us all to be thin (the way He Dreamed You). Fifteen years later he wrote a second book, *The Fat Is in Your Head* (1972), after having sat on the board of a psychiatric hospital. The woeful truth was, "Scratcha fat man and you will find a neurotic. So that's how it stands. We can never get a lean body on a fat mind, permanently." If there was a cure, it lay with a soul turned toward God. The Christian watch against sin must also be a watch against fat, as well the apostle Paul knew, whose own "thorn in the flesh" was not epilepsy but, it seems, obesity. Like Paul, other fat people must be thankful for their affliction; their life of failed diets will eventually force them to put their faith in Christ, who was a good thin "photograph" of God. "We are out of shape because we are out of touch with the original."[7]

To get back in touch, the Reverend H. Victor Kane prepared *Devotions for Dieters* (1967), complete with such new graces as

> I promise not to sit and stuff
> But stop when I have had enough. Amen.

He spoke also of WILL, a Workshop in Lenten Living. In the 1970s, Christian dieting groups appeared, primary among them 3D, for Diet, Discipline and Discipleship. The wife of the senior minister of Parkminster Presbyterian Church in Rochester, New York, Carol Showalter founded 3D after a lumbering ten-year battle with her own 167½ lbs. At a Weight Watchers meeting held in a Sunday School room, she saw a school poster, "Smile, God has the answer," and soon she knew this to be true—if only she followed the advice of Luke 9:23, "If any man would come after me, let him deny himself and take up his cross daily and follow me."[8]

Such taking up of the cross, with its latent images of crusade and victory, was most romantic. It began with an inner transformation worked by the Holy Spirit, and it led to an inspirited battle against evil itself, as Evelyn Kliewer made absolutely clear in her *Freedom from Fat* when she cited Ephesians 6:12, "For we wrestle not against flesh and blood, but against principalities, against powers, against the rulers of the darkness of this world, against spiritual wickedness in high places." The Jesus System of Weight Control promised freedom and empowerment at the same time: what the romantic desires above all and what drives the evangelical Christian to testify as a witness for God. "With Jesus, you can't lose—or should I say, All you *can* do is lose!"[9]

Surrender and conquest at the same moment—this was the epiphany of both the romantic and the evangelical. "Jesus went to the cross so that His people no longer need be the victims of compulsive acts," Marie Chapian wrote in her book about Overeaters Victorious. "Jesus died on the cross for me to set me free from the addiction to wrong foods." Let Jesus therefore atone for your binges and weaknesses. "Loose the power of God in your life," wrote Frances Hunter, "and give Him your appetite. Loose it and lose it—for Jesus!" Her book, *God's Answer to Fat—Loøse It!*, sold more than 300,000 copies in the mid-1970s.

> Hurray! for the Holy Spirit
> Who has come to live within.
> Hurray! for my diet
> Hurray I'm getting thin!

Shirley Cook rhapsodized in her *Diary of a Fat Housewife*. The secret of slimming was enthusiasm, from the word *entheos*, to have God within. One could mount Melba toast on the dashboard in place of St. Christopher, as Totie Fields suggested, but it was far better to live with an inspirited self than to depend upon any saint or relic. The Christian diet programs were Protestant romances: faith above works. Though Evelyn Kliewer gave advice for Combat Cooking and though Charlie Shedd did leg lifts to psalms, thinness began with God's grace. Overeaters Victorious vowed, "I hereby refuse, in the holy name of Jesus Christ, to put my trust in fad diets, fasting, pills, surgery or any other false promise. I declare myself free from these 'natural appearances of wisdom.'" Frances Hunter paraphrased Romans 6:12–16: One could choose sin (food) with death (fat), or else obedience (and loss of weight). It was that simple. Those lifetime habits of eating (the Old Law) could be overcome only through faith in the risen Jesus, thin and triumphant.[10]

Feedback

Well, perhaps there was one other way: the Pharisaical path called behavior modification, which was as extreme a set of rituals as the Jesus System was an extreme romance. While evangelicals insisted on the priority of the soul and the inner life, behavior therapists insisted on the priority of the outward life. Instead of trying to deal with the invisible, inaccessible and therefore exasperating traumas and complexes of fat people, why not focus on what could be seen and manipulated? While some Christians like Charlie Shedd adopted behavior modification techniques as part of their programs, there remained a profound difference between the Jesus System of Weight Control and *Diet Cybernetics for Lean Lines*. With

Jesus and the Holy Spirit came an inner liberation and an inner peace; with the behaviorists, emancipation was never complete: "Obesity is a lifestyle disorder that can only be overcome through a lifetime of effort." While Evelyn Kliewer clearly meant the title of her book, *Freedom from Fat*, behaviorists talked about control, self-monitoring, maintenance. "So you say, 'What kind of emancipation is this? All my life I have to watch out.'" True, acknowledged Dr. Theodore Rubin, who incorporated behaviorist techniques with his psychiatry. "A fat man is never free. But then who is? Complete freedom doesn't exist."[11]

The evangelical worked with an open system, dependent upon moments of revelation, a New Testament of slimming. Behaviorists worked with a closed system of law and justice, history and prophecy, feedback and cybernetic loops: an Old Testament, datable at least to the spas and clinics of the 19th century whose rules and routines were formally designed to break conventional habits of eating. Christian authors anticipated an initial surrender to the Lord; behaviorists spoke of *How to Be a Winner at the Weight Loss Game*.[12]

Both systems required a personal stock-taking, but the behaviorists were not interested in the soul: "The fact is that you lose weight by controlling what you eat, not by knowing why you are overweight." So the behaviorists began with a Food Habit Inventory, an Eating Behavior Chart plotting meals against social and emotional rhythms. Then, while Christian dieters had prayer, the behaviorists prescribed slow eating, eating sitting down, eating quietly, eating and leaving food on the plate, eating in front of a mirror, treating food as you would treat a lover.[13]

The key to Christian weight loss, as Shirley Cook had explained, was enthusiasm; the key to behavior modification was acting *as if*. As if one were thin. As if one were full. As if one knew how to eat. "It's a strange world we live in, where there are whole books devoted to eating," wrote Dr. Edward M. Marshall in his behaviorist manual. "Not cooking, but eating. . . . Perhaps some day a librarian will unearth this little volume, shake the dust off, and say, 'How strange! You mean people had to *learn* how to eat?'"[14]

The Rapture of Weightlessness

Both the evangelical and the behaviorist programs were extreme responses to the problem of longing and the fears of surplus and of never being satisfied. Christian slimmers put their faith in the time-less source of all abundance; only in the embrace of God could one shed earthly flesh and still be satisfied. Behaviorists asserted the human mastery of time. When people are creatures of habit, they are creatures of history and of time; if they can break their habits, then they can assert their humanity. Once they realize their own powers over the daily rhythms of life, they can reconstrue their longings and so deal with abundance. Abundance overwhelms only when it is acute, when it *impends*. While the evangelicals hoped to escape time and to spiritualize all longing, the behaviorists hoped to use time as a tool to erode that same longing.

Evangelical and behaviorist programs for weight loss became popular in the mid-1970s, "at a point in time" (the stock phrase then) when the cyclical nature of things was most perplexing. There was a mystifying if momentary sugar shortage, a longer-term but highly controversial fuel shortage, a strange post–Vietnam War recession which had to be described by neologism as "stagflation." The birth control pill and the liberalization of abortion laws appeared almost in tandem with a movement for Zero Population Growth and an international concern with world hunger. It seemed that one could not trust to time. Time did not heal all wounds. "Our bodies are shot with mortality," wrote Annie Dillard in *Pilgrim at Tinker Creek*, which won a Pulitzer Prize in 1975. "Our legs are fear and our arms are time." She was awed and appalled by the fecundity of the natural world, by her rediscovery "that nature is as careless as it is bountiful, and that with extravagance goes a crushing waste that will one day include our own cheap lives." While the ecologist Garrett Hardin was raising a furor with his discussion of "lifeboat ethics" and the moral dilemmas of overpopulation, Annie Dillard found herself "a frayed and nibbled survivor in a fallen world, and I am getting along. I am aging and eaten and have done my share of eating too. I am not washed and beautiful, in control of a shining world in which everything fits, but instead am wandering awed about on a splintered wreck I've come to care for. . . ."[15]

Near the pivotal point of his magnum opus, *The Physiology of Taste* (1825), that "philosopher in the kitchen" Jean Anthelme Brillat-Savarin had paused to consider the End of the World. On the very next pages he would draw those distinctions between the gourmand and the glutton which we take for granted now, but first he had to speculate on the End. It could come, possibly, with the too-near approach of a comet whose burning tail would utterly scorch

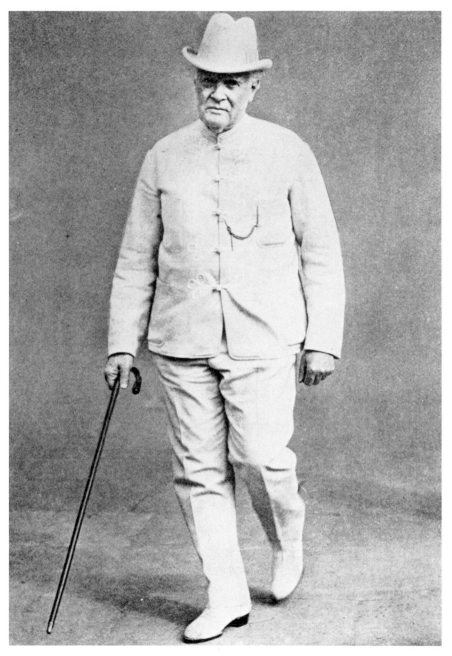

Horace Fletcher, the "Great Masticator," from his *Fletcherism: What It Is or How I Became Young at Sixty* (1913). Fletcher's devotion to slow chewing became a model for many who followed the ritual mode of dieting. His concern with proper mastication was accompanied by an equal concern for a spanking-clean colon. Like John Harvey Kellogg, also worried about intestinal asepsis, Fletcher dressed all in white. *Courtesy of the National Library of Medicine*

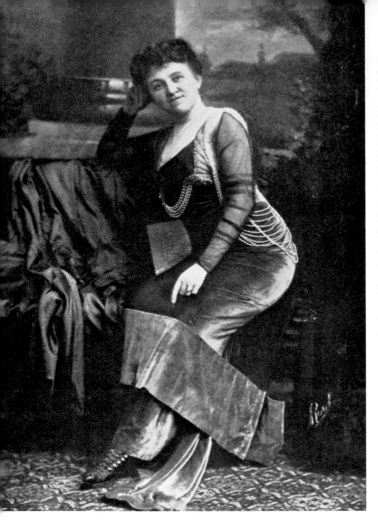

This "new and Improved Reducing-Corset" was at once a structural support and a steam bath. Henry Jacobs (a Brooklyn relative of the scale manufacturers?) attached pads of rubberized fabric to the inside skirting of the garment to promote sweating around the abdomen and buttocks. The invention brought together the old traditions of feminine tight-lacing and masculine sweat-boxes, so that such corsetry seemed fashionable *and* athletic. Patented in 1912, this corset was a progenitor of the many varieties of rubber and plastic reducing garments advertised today.

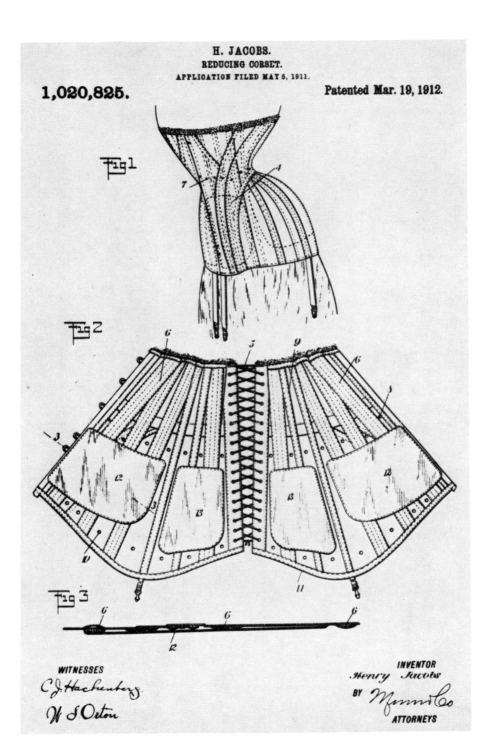

Fig1

Fig2

Fig3

From the *Corset and Underwear Review* (1922), copy written by Dorothy Dignam, one of the pioneering women in national advertising. The problem of fit became more traumatic for fat women during the 1920s, when the tolerances for the body were being progressively narrowed. If "It was the decade of the boyish form," as Dignam noted later at the top of the ad, it was also the decade of the measured body. For the first time, the copywriter had the statistics to claim with confidence that "One customer out of every three is 'stout.'" *Courtesy of the State Historical Society of Wisconsin*

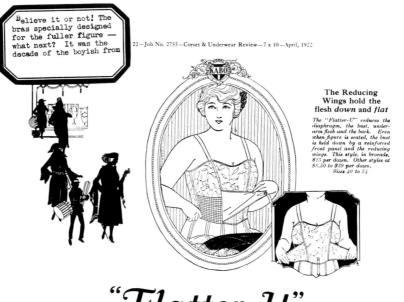

Believe it or not! The bras specially designed for the fuller figure — what next? It was the decade of the boyish from

22—Job No. 2755—Corset & Underwear Review—7 x 10—April, 1922

The Reducing Wings hold the flesh *down* and *flat*

The "Flatter-U" reduces the diaphragm, the bust, underarm flesh and the back. Even when figure is seated, the bust is held down by a reinforced front panel and the reducing wings. This style, in brocade, $15 per dozen. Other styles at $8.50 to $39 per dozen. Sizes 40 to 54

"Flatter-U"
The New Brassiere for Stout Figures
(Patent applied for)

Something new—something different for the Corset Department!

Here's the brassiere that's bringing new business to hundreds of corset departments. It's the only brassiere designed exclusively for stout women, and the reducing wings, which may be drawn as snug as desired, are an entirely new and unusually effective feature. One customer out of every three is "stout". You can sell her this stout size brassiere. The "Flatter-U" is being widely advertised in the newspapers. Write for immediate call from salesman now in your territory.

Two new KABO "Styles of the Times" Corsets also are being advertised — 9084 at $36 and 9090 at $36. Also the KABO "Comfort Top," 6039, at $24. Stock these numbers NOW You will need them.

The "Flatter-U" has so many good sales points and the effectiveness of the reducing wings is so apparent that these brassieres are unusually easy to sell.

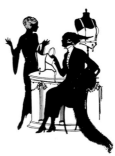

THE KABO COMPANY
Morgan, Milwaukee and Carpenter Sts.
CHICAGO

New York	Pittsburgh	San Francisco	St. Louis
23-25 E. 21st Street	609 Chamber of Commerce	278 Post Street	610 Victoria Bldg.

Start your diet
with a skinny waist.

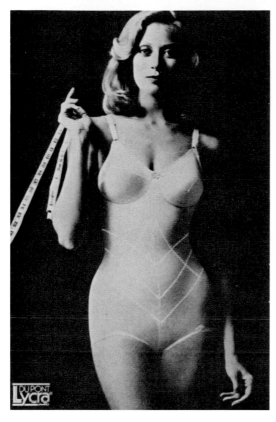

Now waist-watching is easier than ever.

Thanks to new Diet Skinny Waist by Young Smoothie.

Its unique criss-cross construction shapes you beautifully before you even start your diet. So you can show off a trimmer new waist without even shedding a pound.

Then, as you lose weight, the exclusive Diet Skinny Waist fabric follows your diet with you. So it always fits perfectly. And comfortably.

There's a complete diet wardrobe for you to choose from. Briefers, bodysuits, briefs, panties, pantsliners and bras.

Diet Skinny Waist. It makes waist-watching a real cinch.

Shown: #6650 Briefer. Beige. In Nylon/Lycra* Spandex B,C,D cup 34-46 $22.00 #6652 Matching Bodysuit. $27.00

Diet Skinny Waist°
with Lycra·
by Young Smoothie°

The Strouse, Adler Co., 90 Park Ave., N.Y.C.

A 1976 advertisement from the Strouse, Adler Company, in business since 1861. The corset now has become a "shaping" garment with a memory; as one loses weight, the elastic fabric will actually tighten up to accommodate a smaller size. The garment is not only an adjunct to weight-watching and dieting; it is a marker of success. Contrary to what might be expected, the corsetry (or "shaping" garment) industry has seen increased business over the last two decades. The desire for a "natural" look has simply led manufacturers to lighter-weight fabrics and more flesh tones. *Courtesy of the Strouse, Adler Company, with special thanks to Stephen D. Wayne and Trudie Berg*

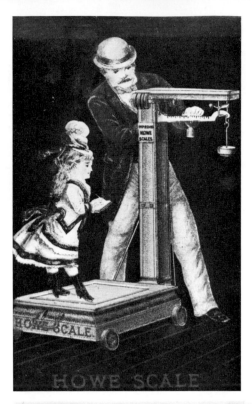

From a late 19th-century Howe Scale Company trade card. A somewhat exaggerated demonstration of the disproportion between the old commercial platform scale and the human body. *Courtesy of Special Collections, University of Vermont Library*

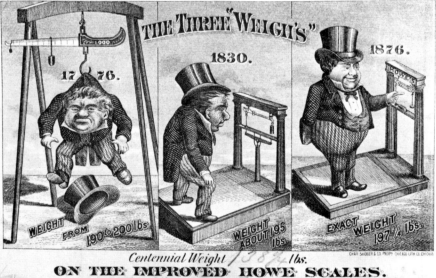

A weight-card given out by the Howe Scale Company at the Centennial Exhibition in Philadelphia in 1876. It is not only the precision of the weighing which improves as the man moves from old steelyard scale to new Howe platform scale; the body and the machine also become more compatible. By 1876, the weight markings are easily legible to the standing man, who need not squint to get the reading. The scale, however, is still primarily an industrial and commercial scale, inappropriate to the home. *Courtesy of the New York Historical Society*

Advertisement from *Woman's Home Companion* (1918). A very early illustration of a personal scale in a bathroom, this is clearly an idealized upper-class milieu. The scale itself is a streamlined version of the old penny platform scale with the large grandfather-clock face. The public world of weighing is slowly becoming private. *Courtesy of the General Research Division, New York Public Library, Astor, Lenox and Tilden Foundations.*

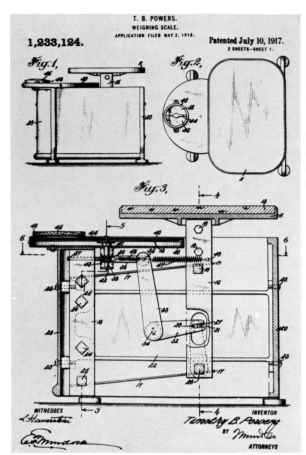

Similar to the Madaco scale patented by Mathias C. Weber, this Powers scale patent was used as the basis for the bathroom scales of the Jacobs Brothers. Its dial also resembled an automobile speedometer, and its inner mechanism also relied upon the Roberval or parallelogram principle. The person standing on the scale platform depressed one arm of the parallelogram in such a manner that a calibrated spring mechanism would pull the weight-indicator around to the proper number on the dial.

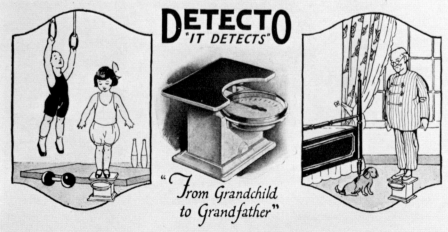

A Jacobs Brothers advertisement for the Detecto Scale, c. 1921. The bathroom scale crosses the generations and enters the bedroom and the playroom. Weighing is becoming part of life from birth to death, from the penny scale in the subway station to the Detecto at the foot of the bed. *Courtesy of Special Collections, University of Vermont Library*

the world of living things and leave the earth to revolve in silence for a time before the next round of life started up again. He wondered what would happen to the bonds of love and friendship as the heat grew, and what the heat would do to religious sentiment and faith just before the End. Then, on the next pages, he described the gourmand as an impassioned but reasonable lover of good food, the glutton as merely voracious. The gourmand's love of new tastes united the world in international commerce; the gourmand's good cheer at table strengthened the bonds of society; the gourmand's choice of a succulent and delicate diet could delay the appearance of old age. In short, the End might be forestalled by gourmandise, which could keep the nations at peace and time at bay.[16]

In the 1970s, there was a similarly tight conjunction between the act of dieting and the fear of an End. Could diet forestall not just a personal but a universal collapse? Would the critical mismanagement of surplus lead to famine, war and apocalypse? The bestselling nonfiction book of the decade—far ahead of its nearest competitors, Dr. Stillman's *Quick Weight Loss Diet* and *Dr. Atkins' Diet Revolution*—was Hal Lindsey's apocalyptic *The Late Great Planet Earth* (more than ten million copies sold by 1979). Strangely enough, Lindsey began his fundamentalist application of Christian prophecy not with the Book of Revelation but with the aroma of steaks sizzling on a patio grill. He and at least one other were at a party waiting for someone to give the signal to eat, but everybody else was inside waiting for a fortune-teller to read palms. So, wrote Lindsey on page one, "We were alone . . . with our appetites."

The longing to know the future surpassed any longing for food. On the cover of Lindsey's paperback edition was an empty eggshell with the continents painted on its two jaggedly cracked halves. The signs that the world was coming apart, wrote Lindsey, would include rampant drug abuse and the most widely spread famine in human history. Appetite and apocalypse.

The way out, for the committed Christian, was the Rapture. Before the Armageddon of global war, Jesus will come to meet all true believers in the air. As they rise, they will receive glorious new bodies and be transported to a glorious place safe from all the devastation below. In that glorious place, they will not have to eat, but they can if they want to. "For those who have a weight problem that sounds rather heavenly in itself."[17]

Lindsey put Commander Neil Armstrong's first words on the moon at the head of his chapter on the Rapture. If the moon landing was "one small step for a man—one giant leap for mankind," how much more extraordinary the Rapture would be, as millions disappear, lifted into the air "without benefit of science, space suits, or interplanetary rockets."[18]

As dieting and thinness were responses to the untrustworthiness of time, so this absolute weightlessness, this spiritual ascension, would mark the transcendence of time. Americans had become fascinated with weightlessness with the 1957 Sputnik and the push toward the moon inaugurated by jogger and swimmer President John F. Kennedy. Centrifuges had been used since 1814 to treat the insane and since 1898 for circulatory problems; in the 1950s they became attractions at amusement parks—I too enjoyed the sensation of being plastered against the green spinning wall as the floor fell away from me. At the same time, "zero-gravity" was being taken more seriously by the military, whose supersonic jets flying curves at high speed could produce forty seconds of weightlessness and feelings of euphoria. By 1968, scientists studying hypogravics could write with a marvelous lyricism, "Man still starts each new life with a simulated condition of weightlessness by suspension within the womb, and he now aspires to the weightlessness which awaits him in outer space." In the 1970s, while space physicians tested commercial liquid diets as possible concentrated foods for astronauts, down on the ground there was an Astronaut's Diet for fat people. Weightlessness was the finest counterpart to the Barmecidal feast. A banquet without food, a body without weight.[19]

If weightlessness was the ultimate escape and the ultimate return (to God, to new life), then fasting had to be "The Ultimate Diet." Evangelicals—and "moderately high-church cooks"—welcomed fasts in imitation of Jesus in the wilderness; behaviorists welcomed fasts as dramatic breaks in routine and as initial assurances of the possibility of real weight loss. Despite warnings against "acidosis" or ketosis, fasting regained a remarkable currency in the mid-1970s. As the protein-sparing modified fast or *The Last Chance Diet* or *The Ultimate Diet*, fasting attracted millions of dieters to *A Born-Again Body*.[20]

"Fasting can be a cheap 'high'—the cheapest 'high,'" wrote Dr. Allan Cott, who in 1970 had begun treating schizophrenics with fasts. Fasting was a way to "recycle" the human, according to one of Cott's advocates; according to another, it was the "Slowing down of time / Putting time into one act of now." It was a "trip," like the Ultimate Trip of Hal Lindsey's Rapture. And like the Rapture, it gave people a chance for a fresh start—this according to Joy Gross, direc-

tor of the Pawling Health Manor in New York, who wrote *The 30-
Day Way to a Born-Again Body.*[21]

There was more than hype to this coincidence of images. The es-
chatological language of the diet books fitted a much wider pattern
of desires to deal with abundance by reversing or transcending time.
When the minute hand was inches from midnight on the clock of the
Bulletin of Atomic Scientists, where industrial pollution had given a
signal irony to the name of the Love Canal in New York, fasting
could unite the transformative romance with rituals of purification.
Dieting itself was a means not just to health or to beauty but to new-
ness and perfection. A new skin: cellulite therapy. A new heart and
lungs: aerobics. A new intestinal arrangement: jejunoileal bypasses,
gastric stapling. A new belly: abdominoplasty. A new body—and a
new soul: hair stylist Michael Altamuro wrote of his fast, "It convinced me that I would have to keep trying for something I can only
call 'soul development,' the nearest thing to perfection on this
planet."[22]

"The attenuation, the slenderness, the deliverance of the body
from the encumbrance of much flesh, give us some assimilation,
some conformity to God and his Angels," spake Saint Jerome; "the
less flesh we carry, the liker we are to them who have none." If
Americans were not returning to an early Christian asceticism, it
was because the body, however slender, however weightless, remained crucial. The culture of slimming was relentlessly exhibition-
ist. No weight loss could be secure without being public; the body
had to stand as open surety for the miracle. Hal Lindsey himself was
at pains to assure believers that after the Rapture they would still be
recognizable despite their glorious new bodies. Even in a heavenly
setting, the person and the personality of the human form were inviolate.[23]

Energy and Light

Fasting would not be seen as an act of penitence, a mortification of
the flesh. Rather, it led in the same direction as the contemporary
fitness movement, toward something quite wonderful called energy.
Since the late 1960s, "energy" has had a quality to it that was not
there before. It bore all the past allusions to fuel, calories, vim, metabolism, libido, nuclear power and thermodynamics, but it meant
something more, something spiritual.

In 1978 a quotation from Friedrich Nietzsche appeared at the head of an otherwise straightforward book on dance/exercise. Judi Sheppard Missett chose as epigraph to her *Jazzercise* the philosopher's statement, "Energy is a source of sheer delight." What her half-million jazzercisers had in mind was a "new-found buoyancy," a love of life. What Nietzsche had in mind was the will to power: "Above all, a living thing wants to *discharge* its energy: life as such is will to power." The will to power was at once command and self-command, that strength of assertion which Nietzsche associated with Renaissance *virtù*. And when he wrote about *virtù* he was writing about eating and exercising. "The German spirit is an indigestion; it does not finish with anything," laden as it was with fat, flour and heavy pastries. The best food for the spirit was light (and Swiss-Italian); the best life was in perpetual motion: "Sit as little as possible; give no credence to any thought that was not born outdoors while one moved about freely—in which the muscles are not celebrating a feast, too. . . . The sedentary life—as I have said once before—is the real *sin* against the holy spirit." Energy led to command led to *virtù* led to the life beyond good and evil. George Sheehan, editor of *Runner's World*, would agree: "Once I discovered running, it became the key that unlocked all my energies. . . . [It opened] the world beyond health, fitness and wellness—the world of maximum human performance." This was, for Judi Missett—as, truly, for Nietzsche—the world of the four-in-one, human being as "animal, child, artist and hero," exultant and free. "I never in my life dreamed anything like JAZZERCISE would happen to me!" testified Louise Peterson, fifty-eight, of Sun City, Arizona. "It's like . . . going to heaven!"[24]

It was energy, then, in the midst of an "energy crisis," that could revive and transform, release and redeem. Youth was slim and vital; the twice-born would be slim and full of energy. Dance itself could seem to be therapy; movement (once again, as in the 1860s) could cure.[25]

How fluently the biosciences converged upon the same paradigm. Obesity in the late 1970s became a fascinating problem in energy conversion. Behaviorists had failed to demonstrate convincingly that particular eating styles were correlated with obesity or that obese people were regularly more responsive to food cues. There did seem to be a real metabolic difference between the thin and the fat. The old idea of *luxuskonsumption* was given new life. If some people who fast can reduce their metabolic rate to adapt to a lower energy intake, why might they not be able to increase their metabolic rate when overfed?[26]

The new password was thermogenesis, and the new secret agent was brown fat. Brown fat had been distinguished from white fat by the 1890s and identified with oxidation of fat tissues in the 1930s, but in the 1980s it was shown that brown fat was the primary site where fatty substances in the body could be transformed into heat. Put another way, brown fat, somewhat like an angelic mercenary, "can be recruited to regulate body weight by disposing thermogenically of excess energy." Bodies with more brown fat could burn off fat more easily.[27]

As the evangelicals espoused faith and the behaviorists acted *as if*, so the scientists too were moving away from any idea that obesity was a question of will power. In a society of increasingly fragmented wants and increasingly confused needs, the mere assertion of will could be of little avail. In order to escape the vicious circles of longing inherent in a high-intensity market setting, one had to put appetite out of the range of the market. The evangelicals did that by surrendering their appetites to the divine; behaviorists tried to do it by making appetite a creature of time; neurophysiologists hoped to do it by drawing appetite deep inside the brain.

Since 1912, when autopsies of obese patients had shown lesions in the hypothalamus, researchers had been looking for a specific center in the brain that might control appetite. The work of John Brobeck and of A. W. Hetherington in the 1940s further incriminated the hypothalamus—a part of the posterior section of the forebrain—as the appetite center. Adult animals with experimentally induced bilateral lesions of the ventromedial hypothalamic nucleus would stop eating. Named the Appestat in the 1950s, the exact connection between this part of the brain and the other hunger mechanisms of the body (gastric contractions, glucose regulators, lipid regulators, insulin regulators) remained unclear. With the 1982 location of specific receptor sites in the hypothalamus that mediate the actions of such appetite suppressants as amphetamines, interest in the "ventromedial hypothesis" was revived. At present, research seems focused on neurotransmitters and the neuroendocrine system.[28]

Like the evangelicals and the behaviorists, bioscientists have drawn obesity away from the perturbing social and economic issues of consumption. Whether fatness and hunger are factors of the concentrations of brown fat, serotonin, cholecystokinin (an intestinal peptide), or endorphins (opioid peptides), obesity becomes an issue of internal, possibly autonomic, regulation. The body's energy system is split off from the dinner table and the marketplace.

In 1985 the TV advertisements for a certain lower-calorie beer were drenched with the slogan, "O yes you can have it all." Like the brewers of Michelob Light, the evangelicals, the behaviorists, the jazzercisers and the bioscientists seem to be moving as far away as possible from any serious confrontation with the cultural origins of our (supposed) national overweight and overfatness. Adverting to the divine economy of the Spirit or to self-hypnosis[29] or to thermogenesis, we could very well have it all.

Weightlessly.

CHAPTER ELEVEN

Fat and Happy?

A coherent critique of slimming has been slow in coming. Satires of weight-watching date back at least as far as the 1711 hypochondriac's letter written by Joseph Addison and illustrated in the frontispiece to this chapter as a gouty mockery of Santorio Santorio. Recently there has been a growing protest against the despotism of slenderness, and a scientific debate over the dangers of a moderate fatness. Underlying the protest and the debate is a utopian vision of a Fat Society where neither overweight nor obesity stands in the way of social freedom or personal happiness.

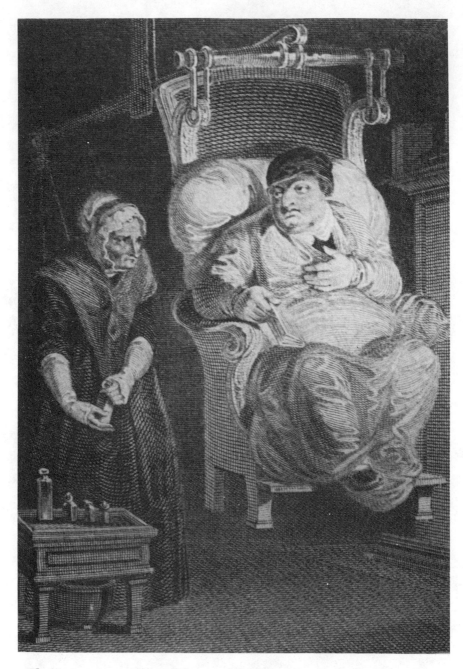

The first caricature of weight-watching, drawn as a parody of Santorio Santorio for an 1803 edition of The Spectator *—in which, in 1711, Joseph Addison had made fun of a hypochondriac who tried to keep himself always within one pound more or less of 200 lbs.*

The Vindication of Fat

FATNESS is fine.

If fat people are unhappy people, blame not their fat but their fellow citizens who bill them as clowns, clodhoppers, cannibals or criminals; who spread such commercial rumors as "To be fat is the end of life"; who sport bumper stickers on their vans, "No fat chicks"; who print posters which read, "It's in to be thin. It's out to be stout."[1] Blame the kindergarten teachers, the coaches, the friends and physicians who goad fat people into a maze of diets from which they may never return. Dieting makes everything worse, for the chances are high that fat people will fail. They will be saddened and frustrated by their failures, and they will come to agree with everyone else that they are failures in all of life. Because they have failed they are fat, and because they are fat they fail.

It is the taking off and the putting on of weight that endangers the body. Not the fat or the pounds but the dieting itself, the frustration, and the constant hunger. No one has been able to prove that fatness *per se* cuts life short. If left alone, 99 percent of human beings will reach a plateau weight, a set point at which their metabolisms will be satisfied and their bodies healthy. It is the dieting, the anxiety, and the perpetual scrimmaging with food that lead to illness. "What causes the most damage is not the actual weight itself, but the fear of weight." People who drive their weights down and up through a series of diets are those most likely to become fatter and unhappier than before, for they upset the natural equilibrium of their bodies. In self-defense, their bodies stockpile fat whenever and wherever possible, hedging as they may against the next (self-imposed) privation. Meanwhile hearts suffer through cycles of feast and famine, strained at each new feast, shocked at each new famine. "To fat, to starve— / Perchance to die of it! Ah, there's the rub." Pokeberry, dinitrophenol, rainbow pills, liquid protein—there is no end to death by dieting.[2]

And still the dieting goes on, as fat people are compromised and persecuted. Like other minorities, fat people are treated like children, given silly nicknames, considered socially and sexually immature. The "Diet Conscience," an electronic guardian, sneers when the refrigerator door is opened, "Are you eating again? Shame on you! No wonder you look the way you do! Ha! Ha! Ha! You'll be sorry, fatty. Do yourself a favor; *shut the door!*"[3]

Like other minorities, fat people are seen as throwbacks to a more primitive time. Neanderthals in museum dioramas are squat and fat; cannibals stirring pots are fat; Oriental despots are fat; harems are full of slothful fat women and supervised by fat eunuchs. The modern world is passing them by. Fat people are stuck in the past, so much so that modern businessmen and scientists prefer an employee who has been in jail or in a mental ward to one who is fat. Criminality and insanity seem less intransigent, less rooted, than obesity.[4]

If fat people are not such atavisms, why do they do so poorly in school and in business? The same vicious circle surrounding other minorities surrounds fat people, who have more difficulty getting into the best colleges and who are not promoted as quickly as their leaner rivals. How they look is more important than how well they do their jobs. The New York City Traffic Department in 1965 dismissed six meter maids for being overweight; National Airlines fired a stewardness for being 4 lbs overweight. As of 1982 only Michigan had a law specifically banning discrimination on account of weight. In 1980 a *New Yorker* cartoon depicted a judge sentencing a defendant: "It is the Court's opinion that, although innocent, you are dangerously overweight." This comedy had already been played out in Miami, where a woman being sentenced for a misdemeanor assault explained that at 315 lbs she was too heavy to work. The judge gave her three years' probation on the condition that she lose 65 lbs at 3 lbs per week; if she went off her diet, she would go to prison.[5]

Physicians are equally unsympathetic. They find fat patients distasteful. Fat people seem more difficult to examine, less likely to cooperate. Fat people are waddling reminders of the failure of medicine to come up with a safe, workable program for long-term weight reduction, just as poor people and homeless people are stark reminders of the failure of the economic system. Like politicians, physicians blame the victims. It is not the doctor's fault if fat people are weak, dishonest, lazy and childish. All one can do with such people is to threaten them with disease and death, play on their fears. "If, knowing these dangers—as you now do—you continue to overeat, it must be obvious that you are acting in a childish fashion. You are immature. This *alone* will prove to you that you are acting *like a child* if you continue to be fat. Now it is up to you. . . . Be childish and die, or grow up and live!"[6]

Yet nearly half of all dieters get their dieting information from such patronizing doctors, doctors who until recently have had no specific training in nutrition. In 1970, three-quarters of doctors surveyed found obesity and overweight to be very frequent among their patients, yet few have pursued the study of obesity (bariatrics) in order to improve their courses of treatment. Nor have they been in particularly good shape themselves; the Scarsdale diet doctor Herman Tarnower was 15 lbs overweight according to his own charts. Physicians are no better than gamblers playing "statistical roulette with the lives of fat people," prescribing diet pills that affect blood pressure and kidneys, dictating diets that are subtle forms of sadism, calling for a "grim, dour self-punishment. If we submit we become miserable, if not actually neurotic."[7]

And then? "Then you are told that your frustrations, your worries, your inhibitions, and your insecurities turn into fat." Tranquilizers will not work; they make you fatter. You need psychological help. A woman in the 1950s was given the name of a psychiatrist because she was fat. She wrote to Dear Abby, "Now Abby, I am not *crazy*, I am just a little overweight. Have you ever heard of anything so insulting?" Abby thought a psychiatrist might do her a world of good, but Abby had no statistics to support such a claim, and there are none now. Psychiatrists are as inept with fat people as they are, still, with the schizophrenics whom they often use as a model for the obese. Perhaps because they are so inept, they demand much more of their fat patients. "Goddammit!" cried one fat woman at her psychiatrist, "You call *me* insatiable; you're the one who's never satisfied."[8]

Society itself will not be satisfied until all fat people are gone. Aldebaran, a member of the Los Angeles Fat Underground, wrote an open letter to a doctor in 1977: "You see fat as suicide, I see weight-loss as murder—genocide, to be precise—the systematic murder of a biological minority by organized medicine." But not just by organized medicine. By society as a whole. In the United States, a fat person's prior identification is with fatness; as a status, fatness comes before religion, race, sexual preference, income, gender. Only in a society intent on doing away with fat people could fatness become so distinct and so negative a stigma. George Nathan Blomberg, fat hero of the 1978 novel by Mark Dintenfass, *The Case Against Org*, becomes defiant in the face of such genocide: "Listen, one must choose to be obese: it is an act of courage." Near the end he knows, "There is no skinny guy inside me struggling to get out. I am Org forever." And on the last page he imagines "I and the world and a chocolate cherry all melting together, becoming one and everything."[9]

The Fat Society: A Utopia

If the tables could be turned, if this were a fat society, a society that admired and rewarded fatness—a society that has never existed in this country for both sexes at the same time—things would be very much different and very much better. It would be like Servia, Indiana, in 1899, "A Town of Fat People," population 206, temperate, quiet and affluent. Or like Roseto, Pennsylvania, in the 1960s, population 1,700, nearly all of the residents obese and hardly a heart murmur among them.[10]

In a fat society, dinners would be scrumptious, sociable and warm. No Mixed Gelatinoids as hors d'oeuvres, no Strained Nitrogen Gumbo for the soup, no Grilled Proteids with Globulin Patties for the entrée, no Compôte of Assorted Vitamins for dessert. There would be 101 Things To Do With Cottage Cheese—use it as a facial, take it out on a leash for a walk, build a snowman—but no one would have to eat it.[11]

In a fat society, children would be fed and fed well when hungry. When they were fed, they would be satisfied, because there would be no snares laid around food. Feeding would be calm and loving, always sufficient, never forced. Children as they grew into adolescence would acquire no eating disorders, since fat people and thin people would be on equal terms and there would be none of that anxious dieting which so often starts off the career of an anorectic or bulimic. No one would be obsessed with food because all people would have the opportunity to be powerful and expressive beyond the dining table.[12]

In a fat society, fat people would dress expressively. Their fashions would no longer be called "oversize" or "halfsize," and they would have the same choice of fabrics and designs as everyone else. Not just pantyhose but all clothes would be "Just my Size." Full-size models would be featured in the salons of *haute couture*; full-size fiberglass mannequins would pose with others in the most elite shop-windows. Fat people would no longer need to buy their clothes at specialty shops like The Forgotten Woman and Catherine Stout, or discreetly through the mails from Lane Bryant, Roaman's and King-Size. A fat woman could wear dramatic colors and horizontal stripes when the fancy struck; a fat man could indulge a secret desire to wear a large-checked light gray suit.[13]

A fat society would be forthright about the body beneath the clothes. It would be relaxed about bodily functions, assured about sensuality, confident with sexuality. Compulsive weighing would disappear; no longer would the scale (always described as a male) lord it over anyone's body. The prudery of weight-watching, the overzealous guardianship of the body, would vanish. Beauty and sexuality would be independent of pounds and of calipers. The fat person would be a "strikingly *unavoidable* creature," and neither the fat man nor the fat woman would be typed as nonsexual or sexually corrupt. "I am touchable," fat people would say to themselves, and they would think of their pounds as "voluptuous planes." Like Sarah Fay Cohen Campbell in the novel *Fat People* (1982), they would accept their bodies as loving instruments and learn to play them in an open tuning.[14]

Women in particular would wear their weight with new conviction. They would affirm their physiological gifts, their genetic and cultural tendencies to put on flesh, their extra layering of body fat. Fat women would not live in the future conditional, suspended between what they are and who they will be when they are finally thin. Fat women would not have to invent fantasy selves a quarter their bulk and four times as lovely. "I've earned my wrinkles and padding," women would say with Ruthanne Olds. "They represent a lot of rewarding life experience." So everyone would at last welcome back the Earth Mother, the Venus of Willendorf, the female colossus, the grand diva, "La Stupenda," and divinity would once more be nurturant rather than vindictive.[15]

A fat society would be a comforting society, less harried, more caring. It would favor the gourmet over the glutton, slow food over fast food, matriarchy and communal affection over patriarchy and self-hate, eroticism over pornography, philanthropy and art over greed and blind technology. It would mean therefore an end to narcotics and narcissism. In a fat society, there would be no "flight from feelings," no need to resort to a form of privacy that kills as it protects. No one would have such stingy personal boundaries that the self would seem always under siege. Mirrors would neither frighten nor enchant. There would be more to the person than a mercurial reflection from shopwindows. "Sizing up" a person would be a wonderfully complex experience; tape measures and scales would have nothing to do with it.[16]

A fat society would be less harshly competitive, less devouring. People could be assertive without seeming aggressive or threatening. There would be no cannibalism, no fear of swallowing or being swallowed up. Accepting one's own bulk, one need not consume others or gnaw at one's self. Dieting is cannibalism. Dieters eat off their own bodies: "You start to get thin when you begin to *live on your own fat*." Dieters are encouraged to be cannibals: "If your body-republic doesn't get enough food to support all the citizens, some will die and be cannibalized to feed the others. . . . In this body-politic of cell-citizens, you can fool all of the people all of the time, and if you want to *get* thin and *stay* thin, that's what you must do." Dieters have no recourse but to be cannibals: "To reduce weight, an obese person must burn his own body fat. It's as simple as that. He must eat himself up! A bit cannibalistic? I'm afraid so. But it's the only way to lose weight." That legendary diet drug which was nothing but a live tapeworm was the folkloric representation of such cannibalism. In a fat society, no one would be eaten up from within and no one would be eaten alive. Fat people, weighted, solid, would not fear the desires of others or their own desires. If fat people now lie or steal or hide, that is because they are always trying to save face ("such a pretty face") and disguise their needs. They must act surreptitiously, with the night and the bathroom as their refuge. In a fat society, no one would be forced to such humiliating secrecy. All hunger would be honest hunger.[17]

Capitalism and the Culture of Slimming

A fat society would be a consumer's society, though not in the manner of the cannibal or the narcissist who "demands immediate gratification and lives in a state of restless, perpetually unsatisfied desire." In a fat society people would consume for the sake of the company they would keep. Consuming would become satisfying to the degree that it became social, generous and unburdening. People would consume not to hoard but to harbor. Abundance would not terrify them, for they would not fear that everything must be consumed lest it consume them. Abundance would be a quality of life rather than a test of appetite. There could be no food fetishism and no consumer fetishism, no worship of the consumed object or of the marketplace itself.[18]

The cult of slimness and the lo-cal economy are omens of Late Capitalism. Dieting strategies have followed the stages of capitalism so closely that one could be the model for the other. The primitive accumulation of capital comes through marginal efficiencies and personal saving; call this fasting or abstinence. During the next stage there is an expansion of markets and a mastery of the rhythms of distribution; call this thyroid treatment and the tuning of the metabolism. The third stage leads from the efficiencies of mass production to the control of the flow of market data; call this calorie-counting. The fourth stage is preoccupied with the discovery that in order to further stimulate demand to accommodate unceasing production, capitalists must arrange desires; call this psychotherapy or group therapy, whatever must be done to adjust the appetite to society. The fifth stage finds competition so narrowed and industrial networks so large that the most effective way to perpetuate desire is to promote fear; call this the low-fat diet to lose weight and forestall hypertension, or the low-fat low-cholesterol diet to lose weight and prevent heart attacks, or the low-fat low-cholesterol high-complex-carbohydrate high-fiber diet to deal with just about everything. In the sixth stage, capitalism runs aground on a shoal of *crises pléthoriques*, where neither the expansion of markets nor the manufacture of desire can keep pace with the extent of production. This is the last stage, the time of Too Much. The surplus must literally be run off in a fury of exercises, fast dancing and marathons. Call this fitness, capitalism's last best hope.[19]

This juxtaposition may seem surprising. Capitalists should be dead set against all dieters, whose professed object is to consume less. If dieters were permanently successful, such might be the case. But dieters ultimately consume more. The diet is a supreme form for the manipulation of desire precisely because it is so frustrating. Capitalists have as vital a stake in the failures of dieters as in the promotion of dieting. It is through the constant frustration of desire that Late Capitalism can prompt ever higher levels of consumption.

At each stage, capitalists have been beholden to dieters. From the first, industrial efficiency demands that all parts of raw products be used. Dieters, like infants, give the food industry the opportunity to profit from chaff, tailings and waste. Beef tallow and by-product vegetable oils go into margarines and then into lighter "spreads." Bran and wheat germ, stripped from grain during milling, become expensive food supplements for dieters who must assure their health as they eat less. Skim milk, whey and milk solids go into powders for liquid diets. The liquid protein of 1977 was compounded from animal hides and tendons. Drug companies find markets for glandular substances that would otherwise be discarded by slaughterhouses. With half a cent worth of vitamins—all it costs to provide 100 percent of the Recommended Daily Allowance of twelve basic vitamins—a manufacturer can make cellulose, soybeans, and spices into a vitamin-rich diet food.[20]

The culture of slimming collaborates with capitalism to adapt the body shapes of workers to machines that cannot abide loose flesh or imbalanced forms. The streamlining of the workplace demands a streamlining of the human body, whether by diet or by drug. Thus this advertisement for an amphetamine: "Swimsuit by Jantzen. Body by Dexaspan." Airplane seats, subway turnstiles, steering wheels in cars are designed to make fat people uncomfortable. People in motion in the modern world should be as streamlined as their vehicles.[21]

When capitalists in late stages face the prospect of glut, dieting works wonders. Dieters must constantly change wardrobes as their shapes and weights go in and out, up and down. Dieters must always seek out new diet foods, new diet books, new devices. Their cycles of famine and feast actually raise their physiological set points; after a time, those who have been dieting come to *need* more than ever before. People who go off a diet tend to gain back what they have lost and then some. Even the new "light" foods and the resurgence of exercise are compatible with Late Capitalism. The light foods, more synthetic, less substantial, give a greater return on the dollar; exercise puts workers to work outside the workplace, increasing the level of physical activity and so increasing the daily caloric expense, making possible greater food consumption. People buy more expensive scales in the technological pursuit of lightness. Food engineering is matched in sophistication by physical engineering or "fitness." On the one side there are flavorings and bulking agents, on the other side there are exercise machines and Family Fitness Centers.[22]

An expanding Late Capitalist world requires that no one ever be fully satisfied. In past times of shortages and new markets, most people knew what they wanted and what they needed to satisfy themselves. Now they must be told. Desire, once natural and springing from within, becomes unnatural and imposed from without. Capitalists encourage the confusion of hunger and appetite. If no one were confused, if everyone were able to tell hunger from appetite, capitalism would crack wide open and the fat society would emerge.

The contradictions of capitalism are apparent already in the grostesque, disturbing contrast between the gourmet dieting of the bourgeois world and the famine elsewhere. Though fasting may be paraded as a means to solving the problems of world hunger, the culture of slimming is not magnanimous. Dieters may follow rice diets or sour milk diets, but they do not do so as a gesture of solidarity with the poor of the world confined to such foods. People on diets do not necessarily save money for investment in Third World agriculture, nor do they necessarily insist on massive food aid in the United States. The culture of slimming is based upon a fear of being done in by abundance, of "stuffing ourselves so much we're killing ourselves," not upon a program of international assistance through self-denial.[23]

The image of the fat person as a selfish person is a sly, cruel trick of Late Capitalism. The fat person is not responsible for the fundamental inequities in distribution that make for hunger. This is the doing of capitalists, who may be fat or thin. Blaming fat people for world hunger diverts attention from the real villains who inveigle societies to consume ever more, regardless of consequence. Thin people are capitalism's ideal consumers, for they can devour without seeming gluttonous; they have morality on their side. Fat people are ideal scapegoats; they take food out of the mouths of the starving poor, and they *mean* to do so—else they would summon the will power to keep their weight down and their appetites in check.[24]

Through the culture of slimming, Late Capitalism may have its cake and eat it too. People in the State of Redeucit may think of putting a tax on obesity; they may calculate the fossil fuel savings from a national weight-reduction program. Meanwhile, the sales of desserts may skyrocket; extra-rich ice creams may be the new rage. *American Home* may explain to its readers "How to feed a hungry family while you take off that extra weight!" *Life* may photograph an overweight man in a steel cage inside a tank of water being measured for his percentage of body fat while, on the page opposite, an advertisement displays a roasted turkey in its own wire cage inside the Wear-Ever Oval Roaster. The same magazines that devote pages to diets and exercises may reward their readers with recipes for double-chocolate double-layer cream cakes with icing.[25]

When a society is urged to eat much, eat often, eat sweetly and be slender, fat people are thoroughly victimized. They are victims of the double binds of capitalism, which are sexist, racist and class-biased. Given the primary job as food shoppers, women are persuaded to buy for their families what they are told they should not eat themselves. Informed by science that they are naturally fatter than men, fashion convinces them that they should be naturally thinner. As cooks and hostesses, women must prepare those foods they should not eat and wear those expressions of generosity they must not allow themselves. Fat black women live with worse pressures, for they are not only of a different race but usually of a lower economic stratum. The discrimination against them is so faceted that the society often confuses their fatness with their poverty and both with ignorance. To say in their defense that blacks like fat or that poor people appreciate a bit of extra weight is a forbiddingly neat way to cut them off from the rest of society, to limit their economic and social range.[26]

A fat society would restore natural desire and so ensure equity in the distribution of resources. When people feel thin, they tend to seek dominion over others as proof of their own substantiality. They try to emblazon themselves upon the world by means of conspicuous consumption or conspicuous renunciation. They are hungry for power. Fat people are not concerned about self-aggrandizement; few militarists, murderers or rapists are fat. Fat people in a fat society would be at ease with themselves:

> We were probably the earliest
> civilized, and civilizing, humans,
> the first to win the leisure,
> sweet boredom, life-enhancing sprawl
> that requires style.

Fat people would be diplomatic and judicious:

> Never trust a lean meritocracy
> nor the leader who has been lean;
> only the lifelong big have the knack of wedding
> greatness with balance.

In such a society, sexism, racism and class warfare would be unlikely. Fat people are not intolerant or exploitative. They are not impatient enough to be imperialists. Indeed, "The most effective physiological method of making war impossible in future would be to organize a society for the universal diffusion of adipose."[27]

In a fat society, the National Association to Aid Fat Amercians could disband. Making It Big groups and Weight Worthy groups might be held on occasion for small, wispy people, but fat people would live without guilt or fear. Especially fat women—those who now use their fatness to hold their own in a man's world or to fend off a disabling intimacy. When Fat Power is a reality, the New York City Fat-In of June 1967, with its banners "Buddha Was Fat" and "Think Fat," will no longer seem so revolutionary. Fat people will not simply turn the tables on thin people. Rather, weight and shape will no longer define the personality or confine its expression. People will face each other without calipers or weight charts; they will take each other's measure in more deeply human ways.[28]

The culture of slimming, like capitalism itself, promotes a smallness of character, the "shrink-to-fit permanent identity" of Levi's blue jeans. Dieters and weight-watchers must constantly go against their own best qualities as human beings. They must deny their own inclinations toward generosity, compassion, graciousness and the good humor of laughing with themselves. Diana Trilling, writing of the Scarsdale diet doctor Herman Tarnower, saw precisely how the culture of slimming, as it demeans people, draws toward it the smallest of characters: "Tarnower's was a meagre soul, a spirit without generosity. He would seem to have had an insatiable appetite for small power. . . . He was a small-time emotional imperialist, a respectable middle-class bullyboy of sex. Little wonder he became famous as a diet doctor: he was a glutton for other people's vulnerabilities." He lived, of course, in a suburb called Purchase.[29]

Buying into the culture of slimming is perilous. It means buying into the worst of capitalism and the worst of ourselves: meanness, paranoia, deception. Diet books and diet groups expect people to be weak, unsteady, easily seduced. They anticipate lying and cheating, they sponsor the optical illusions of fashion, they endorse foods that masquerade as the real thing. The dieter's world is not just delusive; it is dishonest. Like capitalism, it warps the best of intentions and the simplest of souls. Capitalism reduces what is real to what is apparent; dieting reduces what we are to our appearances. Capitalism emboldens us to believe that insofar as we deprive ourselves, we can master others. This is also the immorality of dieting. It is as subtle as any hardening of arteries, and as deadly.

The Political Economy of Fat

No single critic has launched such an attack on dieting as I have launched here. I doubt that there is a partisan of Fat Power who would accept without amendment this diatribe. But the protest against the culture of slimming—a protest that began in the 1920s—has become louder over the last two decades, and I have presented that protest at its fullest and fiercest. It would be as wrong to underestimate the appeal of the arguments as to overestimate their cogency. The Fat Society is no less attractive for being utopian.

Like the diatribe, the utopia is a composite. I have pieced it together from poetry and fiction, polemics and farce, pamphlets and fashions. In a sense I have hurried it into being. As a coherent critique of the society it obverts, a utopia matures slowly. The Fat Society, neither a glutton's paradise nor a thin farm, has yet to take shape as a substantial cultural vision.

Recently, however, the Thin Society has found its *1984*—its dystopia. The anorectic girls of *The Golden Cage* and the *Alabaster Chambers* are victims of thinness. Lured into *Competing with the Sylph*, they may perish of their devotion to thinness. "My daughter thinks she's fat. I think she's thin," says a worried father in an advertisement for a hospital program for anorectics. "Actually, she's dying." There are at least a million anorectics in the United States and some 60,000 to 150,000 of them will die of their obsession. An anorectic may be *The Best Little Girl in the World*, but hers is an ultimately fatal world; she has been taught too well by the Thin Society, and she will never be satisfied. In the 1984 thriller *Thinner*, lawyer Billy Halleck, who has dieted and cheated and is still too fat, begins losing 3 to 5 lbs a day no matter what he does. A dieter's dream becomes a Gypsy's potent curse. The world of the anorectic is the dark corner of the Thin Society. It is a world so thin that it cannot endure. Nothing, at last, must come to nothing.[30]

Satirists have often thought to parody those diet menus which reduce the dieter by eliminating everything. "The whole secret," wrote Corey Ford in 1954, "is to *avoid eating during meals.* That's all. No regimens, no restrictions. Order anything you want, but leave the food on your plate and eat around it." (Potato skins, grapefruit rinds, peanut shells, cellophane, doilies were safe.) Comedienne Totie Fields in 1972 conceived of a 2½-calorie-a-day diet: 3 navel orange bellybuttons, 1 doughnut hole, 5 scraped crumbs from burnt toast, 1 can dehydrated coffee, plum pits, eyes of potato, 1 guppy fin, tea steam, butterfly liver, lobster antennas, prime ribs of tadpole *au jus* and boiled-out tablecloth stains. But the startling growth of anorexia in the last generation has drained the humor from such caricature.[31]

Where the humor remains, it is pointed more clearly in the direction of the powerful if petty tyranny of the Thin Society. Humorist Russell Baker during the 1970s put Elizabeth (Betty the Breadbasket) Goolarik on his latest Wanted list of the most despicable people in the United States: "Wanted in thirteen states on charges of being overweight in a public place, and ten counts of failure to look like a bone sack when dressed for dancing. . . . Should be approached with care, as she is skilled with fork, spoon and knife and has, in several cases, lured pursuers into joining her in an order of spaghetti with chicken livers." In 1983, National Public Radio's variety show, "Prairie Home Companion," anticipated the signing into law of an Inhibition Act. Out in Chicago, "Salad Bar to the Cornbelt," Lt. Fred Fettucini leads the Diet Squad in its efforts to stop people from eating food that is bad for them: meat, French fries, junk ("donuts, white bread, you name it") and C's ("the devil's food, Chocolate"). Fettucini books a woman on 504, "Suspicion of Hypoglycemia" while jogging down a big tofu scam at the Tofu Deli and Yogurt Bar-B-Q. He learns of a night delivery by Al Capon's mob of smugglers and confiscates a truckload of tofu in which is sunk a fortune in illicit pastrami, corned beef and C's.[32]

More often than not, such tyrannies have been seen as forms of benevolent despotism. Diet groups, diet authorities and fashion magazines may speak out against the persecution of fat people, but the social pressure is in fact to their advantage, driving people to join their programs, watch their television shows, buy their books and their lines of food and clothing. The editors of *Vogue* wrote in 1953, "Fashion is often reproached for this preoccupation with slimness—and, as a fashion magazine, we mind not at all sharing the accusation. For doctors agree that most women's desire to be slender is a vanity that can pay off in good health and a longer life." And while they may acknowledge the incessant contradiction of a society that demands slimness as it sells sweetness, fast foods and rich ice cream, few diet book authors, diet group executives or fashion editors have been comfortable with questions about social or political action which they might take to get at the root of a national problem. Says Richard Simmons, founder of eighty-five Anatomy Asylums and a diet-and-exercise campaigner on the road three hundred days a year, "I don't even know how to spell 'political.'"[33]

Only with such feminist works as Kim Chernin's *The Obsession* (1981), Marcia Millman's *Such a Pretty Face* (1980) and Susie Orbach's *Fat Is a Feminist Issue* (1978) have some of the politics been spelled out. The fashion and diet industries, wrote Chernin, support a retreat from feminine power: "In the feminist group it is *largeness* in a woman that is sought, the *power* and *abundance* of the feminine. . . . It is always a question of *widening, enlarging, developing and growing*. But in the weight-watching groups the women are trying to *reduce* themselves; and the metaphoric consistency of this is significant: they are trying to make themselves *smaller*, to *narrow* themselves, to become *lightweight*, to lose *gravity*, to *be-little* themselves." The feminist cartoonist Nicole Hollander had a young man ask her heroine Sylvia, "Admit it, Syl. You need us. Can you imagine a world without men?" "No crime," answered Sylvia, "and lots of happy, fat women." Gay women may choose to defy ideal-weight charts as they defy sexual stereotyping. *Not* to be on a diet or watch one's weight can be a woman's assertion of independence from male medicine and commerce and from the self-punishing aspects of women's lives within the Thin Society.[34]

Jane Fonda, long a model and a sex symbol ("Barbarella") in Hollywood, did not see herself as a captive of the Thin Society until she became actively political. Although she had been dieting, taking amphetamines and using diuretics since adolescence, it was her work against the war in Vietnam that brought her face to face—and body to body—with the ferocity of American policy. When she learned that Vietnamese prostitutes were using plastic surgery to build their bodies into stereotypically beautiful American shapes, when she saw a slide of a Saigon billboard with an Asian woman primped and posed like a *Playboy* bunny, she realized that "the women of Vietnam had become victims of the same *Playboy* culture that had played havoc with me." Indeed, these Vietnamese women were torturing themselves to look like her, like Barbarella. "I was shocked into the realization that I myself had played an unwitting role as a movie star and sex symbol in perpetrating the stereotypes that affected women all over the world."[35]

Her response, in part, was to reconceive exercise and diet as ways of taking control of one's own body. In her Workout Studios, *Workout Book* (1981), *Jane Fonda's Workout Record* (1982) and videotapes, she reached more than two million people with the message, "discipline is liberation!" Fitness had become a Liberation Movement. During the workout, Jane Fonda, now an activist woman in her forties, exhorted everyone to "go for the burn." This was no fire next time; it was pyruvate and lactic acid that mounted up as we worked hard and breathed deep. The burn came especially with the buttock tucks, Fonda's favorite, done to Jimmy Buffett's song, "Changes in Latitudes, Changes in Attitudes." The burn was an internal event, the fire *last* time, an expiation through which to achieve a personal transformation.[36]

After the sweat and the burn, we could make our peace with food. Our problem with food, like our problem with the Vietnamese, was that we had mistaken the enemy. "When food becomes the enemy with which we are locked in an obsessive power struggle, then every time we lose the fight we not only gain weight but we lose our self-esteem as well. I know. I've been there." Charles Krauthammer of the *New Republic* accused Fonda of "Adidas socialism," of invading the province of the political right where body worship belongs, but he was too far from the front to understand that Fonda was replaying Vietnam: "instead of focusing your anxieties on food, call off the fight, declare a truce and accept food as a life-giving friend." The diet she proposed, "high-fiber, complex-carbohydrate, low-animal-protein, low-fat," was the diet of the pre-war Vietnamese peasant. She wanted our food to be free of toxins, unadulterated, organic. As we despoiled and defoliated Vietnam, so now we had to expiate at home, drinking bottled water and eating low on the food chain while we cleaned up our own domestic poisons. If our environment was out of whack, "then our individual life-style decisions are mere righteous gestures."[37]

Fonda's utopia was the Fit Society, one that worked out its despairs and disappointments and came to a position of moral strength. If she shared with physicians and breakfast food advertisers a new-found admiration for fiber, this was not just bran but moral fiber, resilience, resolve. The Workout was so successful neither because its exercises were unusual (they were old standards) nor because the sequence of exercises was unique, but because of a moral earnestness in Fonda's tone. It was the tone of the early trade unionist, the labor organizer. The "burn" was the body on strike, a temporary muscle failure. "Going for the burn" was what every worker had to be ready to do to achieve a living wage.

Of course, the Workout was fine for slimming. On Fonda's diet and with Fonda's exercises, losing weight was a good bet. No one needed union rhetoric to do buttock tucks. For all daily purposes the Workout was compatible with the practices of the Thin Society and the profits of Hollywood capitalism. It was entirely possible to go for the burn and not become a social reformer, let alone a political activist.

From Weight to Shape

The impact of the protest against the Thin Society is so far more oblique than direct. However many have deplored the persecution of fat people, comparatively few have embraced a fatter body. But we stand in the mid-1980s in the midst of a change of emphasis from weight-consciousness back to shape-consciousness, and this may be softening the harder edges of the culture of slimming. Now it is muscle tone, skin tone, and "being in shape" rather than an insistent call to the scale. Public concern with anorexia is nudging fashion away from ultra-thin models.[38] Most notably, Metropolitan Life in 1983 revised its weight tables to the advantages of its heavier clients.

Since the 1920s, as insurance companies insisted on progressively lower ideal weights, the average weights of American adults have been growing. For the overall adult population between 1912 and 1962, men had gained 1 to 5 lbs and woman 2 to 6 lbs. These were worrisome statistics only in a Thin Society, for men and women were both adding at least an inch to their average heights. Data for the 1960s, however, showed that within each height category, weights were increasing—by 3 to 7 lbs, for example, for ages 25–34. Data for the 1970s showed a similar trend. "Obviously," wrote Letitia Brewster and Michael F. Jacobson in *The Changing American Diet* (1978), "all the cyclamate, saccharin, and other miracle weight-loss aids used in the last twenty years did not result in any miracles." They reported a 6 percent increase in the caloric intake of the average American since 1950.[39]

There were other signs that the culture of slimming might be a physiological failure. The National Bureau of Standards in 1971 found that bust, hips and waist measurements for clothing were all expanding. The size 12 for women in 1939 was proportioned as 34-25-36, while in 1971 it was 35-26-37. The 1939 junior size 9 was proportioned at 32-23½-33½, while in 1971 it was 33-23½-35. For men, the seats at the Los Angeles Coliseum during the 1960s were given a broader base, and in 1984 the American Seating Company was finding that "where chair sizes of 18″ and 19″ seat width were common during the 40's and 50's, it is now most uncommon to furnish anything smaller than a 20″ chair size." For captains of industry, corporation auditorium seating is 22 inches wide, often 23 inches, sometimes 24 inches.[40]

After the 1959 *Build and Blood Pressure Study*, Metropolitan Life actuaries revised the company's weight tables—downward. After the new 1979 *Build Study* by the Society of Actuaries, the company in 1983 revised its tables—upward. That is, evidences for lowest mortality were compatible with higher ideal weights. Substantially higher: 6 to 10 to 15 lbs, depending on frame size as determined by elbow width. Compare these ideal weights for the average-height American adult woman and man:

		Small Frame	Medium Frame	Large Frame
Woman 5′4″	1960	108–116	113–126	121–138
	1983	114–127	124–138	134–151
Man 5′9″	1960	136–145	142–156	151–170
	1983	142–151	148–160	155–176

(The lesser latitudes for men reflect the greater association between heart attacks and overweight among older males.) In the two years after the issuance of the new tables, Metropolitan Life received more than ten thousand requests for them.[41]

Weight Watchers, however, will have nothing to do with the higher ideal weights. Nor will Diet Workshop. Nor the American Heart Association, which argues that fatter people have higher inci-

dences of chronic disease, and that if they now live longer, the credit
may belong to earlier or more effective medical intervention. Nor
the American Cancer Society, which suspects that the unfactored
presence of smokers may have warped the data; since smokers tend
to weigh less and die earlier, of course the tables will show a higher
optimal weight.[42]

This resistance to the new tables is indicative of the vitality of the
culture of slimming. It is not at all clear whether the new tables will
utlimately have the same authority as the old tables or whether, indeed, any such table will ever again have the same cultural bearing
as those tables at midcentury. As the Thin Society moves to emphasize shape over weight, people will not necessarily believe that they
should be heavier, but they may look for signs of leanness elsewhere
than on the scale.[43]

If over*weight* no longer seems quite so fatal, and if absolute thinness seems more fatal and more prevalent by the month, then Americans in the coming years may be more responsive to the vision of a
Fat Society. At present, the Fat Society is only a sliver of what it
might be, but "Inside every diet doctor," writes Richard Smith in
The Bronx Diet, "is a pastry chef screaming to get out."[44]

We Eat What We Are

It may be that the desire to be slim is merely a response to a climatic
change; since the late 17th century, the Northern Hemisphere has
become progressively warmer and our layers of fat more burdensome. We are in for a cold spell now, it seems, and perhaps all the
dieting will stop.[45]

It may be that fuel shortages, with or without a colder climate,
will force us to take on the fat once again. Or that food shortages
will force us to reevaluate our basic foods. Or that, with fuel and
food shortages, people will exert their bodies more and consume
less, so that dieting will become unnecessary or foolish.

If it be as simple as that, if we will return to fatness or be driven
to thinness by ecological circumstance, then the political economy
of fat may be dismissed as ultimately trivial. But thinness was also
desirable in the late gothic period during Europe's Little Ice Age,
and the Gurage of southwest Ethiopa, who until recently had never
known famine, had nonetheless a long-standing conviction of scarcity and an intense dislike for those who overate.[46] Our bodies and

our foods are as much social constructs as they are proteins, carbohydrates, fats (themselves, of course, another system of inventions).
We are *not* what we eat. We eat what we are. And how we are.[47]

We are, still, dazed by appetite, disturbed by hunger, and dis-
trustful of both. Not that we are haunted by a malign Puritanism
which sours all pleasures, curdles all judgments. Rather we have so
far failed to make good on that sense of stewardship by which some
Puritans managed a separate peace with the bewildering richness of
the New World.

We are, still, fearful of abundance. As long as that fear remains,
we will eat cautiously, pinch an inch, watch our weight. Our desires
will confuse us. The best diet, wrote satirist Jean Kerr in 1957, is to
"eat as much as you want of everything you don't like. And if you
should be in a hurry for any reason . . ., then you should confine
yourself to food that you just plain hate."[48]

There is a bitterness to such humor, like the bitter aftertaste of
saccharin. It is best to end this book here, a little taken aback, and
never satisfied.

Grace

IN MY TRADITION, one says grace after the meal. This is most appropriate here, for even as the book goes to press, diet brochures are still being squeezed through my mail slot (the latest, the Great Body Grapefruit Diet, assures me that "Great Bodies are made . . . not born"), and family and friends are relentless as my international clipping service. The pursuit of the history of slimming, it seems, must be nearly as perpetual as slimming itself.

It is always more difficult to acknowledge constant acts of kindness and intuition, wherefore archivists and librarians remain anonymous in their benevolence. I wish especially to thank the staffs of the Academy of Food Marketing (St. Joseph's College, Philadelphia), the American Antiquarian Society, the Boston Public Library, the Chicago Historical Society, the National Library of Medicine (History of Medicine Division), the New York Academy of Medicine, the Schlesinger Library (Radcliffe College), the University of California at San Diego libraries, the University of Vermont Library (Special Collections), Watkins Library (Trinity College, Hartford), and the Wisconsin State Historical Society.

For more particular kindnesses, I am indebted to the world of scale manufacturers and scale collectors, all of whose efforts on my behalf have not yet convinced me to buy a scale, but whose interest and assistance have considerably enriched this book. I am especially thankful for the help of Mack Rapp of the Detecto Scale Company, Hyland B. Erickson of the

341

Borg-Erickson Corporation, Jean Dominic and Mike Tunney of the Hanson Scale Company, Ray Farr of the Farr Weighing Machine Company, and Gerald "Red" Meade of the Antique Penny Scale Company.

Janice F. Jiggetts of the Metropolitan Life Insurance Company was kind enough to arrange for me to see two movies produced by the company, "Losing to Win" (1951) and "A Song of Arthur, or How Arthur Changed His Tune and Solved a Weighty Problem" (1967), the latter a marvelous film with music and lyrics by Stan Freeman and starring Madeline Kahn and Steve Roland, who do an impressive dance in the kitchen to the tune, "Love and Goulash."

Wayland Hand of the Folklore Center at UCLA, editor of the Dictionary of American Popular Beliefs and Superstitions, gave me access to the in-process files of his enormous project. Harvey Green of the Margaret Woodbury Strong Museum in Rochester (NY) told me of the whereabouts of the Horace Fletcher Correspondence, and the rest of the staff of the museum was equally helpful.

W. Stewart Agras and Janet Polivy shared prepublication copies of their work with me. Laurel T. Ulrich supplied me with some invaluable references. Rozanne S., founder of Overeaters Anonymous, and Lois L. Lindauer, founder of Diet Workshop, Inc., were most thoughtful respondents in our interviews.

The manuscript was read at various stages by David Kunzle, Jane Laurent, David G. Roskies, Bobbi Sandberg, Pat Schmidt, Michael Schudson, Sue Schudson, Laura Shapiro, Gene VanBrook, Ferdinand van der Veen, Jay Vanos and Jeanie Vanos. It was also read all along the line by Sidney Blumenthal, who suggested this topic to me more years ago than I care to admit.

Let it be known that I myself took this book through all its versions on an old Olympia manual typewriter. It has recently been calcuated that, *ceteris paribus*, the substitution of an electronic typewriter or word processor for a manual typewriter will put an extra 3 lbs of fat per year on an historian. I may have spent a small fortune on correction fluid and liquid thinner, but I am some 10 lbs lighter for the exercise.

Hillel Schwartz
Encinitas, Calif.
March 1986

Notes

Abbreviations

All second and subsequent citations within a chapter have been short titled. Many subtitles have been dropped. The original date of publication has been inset in brackets where a later edition was used and the chronological argument in the text demands precise dating of the first edition. The following abbreviations of recurrent words in titles of many journals and books in series have been used:

Amer   America, American
Assoc   Association
Educ   Education, Educational
Int   International
J   Journal
Med   Medical, Medicine
NY   New York
Proc   Proceedings
Psych   Psychology, Psychological
Q   Quarterly
R   Review, Reviews
Soc   Society
St   State
Tr   Transactions
Univ   University

The most commonly cited publications have been reduced to acronyms:

AA	*Advertising Age*
AAPT	*Association of American Physicians Transactions*
ADC	*Archives of Disease in Childhood*
AHR	*American Historical Review*
AIM	*Annals of Internal Medicine*
AJCM	*American Journal of Clinical Medicine*
AJCN	*American Journal of Clinical Nutrition*
AJDC	*American Journal of the Diseases of Children*
AJMS	*American Journal of the Medical Sciences*
AJOG	*American Journal of Obstetrics and Gynecology*
AJPA	*American Journal of Physical Anthropology*
AJPH	*American Journal of Public Health*
APER	*American Physical Education Review*
ARIM	*Archives of Internal Medicine*
BHM	*Bulletin of the History of Medicine*
BMJ	*British Medical Journal*
BMSJ	*Boston Medical and Surgical Journal*
BNYAM	*Bulletin of the New York Academy of Medicine*
CSSH	*Comparative Studies in Society and History*
DAB	*Dictionary of American Biography*
DNB	*Dictionary of National Biography*
DSB	*Dictionary of Scientific Biography*
FE	*Food Engineering*
FPD	*Food Products Development*
GH	*Good Housekeeping*
GJHL	*Graham Journal of Health and Longevity*
IJO	*International Journal of Obesity*
JADA	*Journal of the American Dietetic Association*
JAH	*Journal of American History*
JAMA	*Journal of the American Medical Association*
JHE	*Journal of Home Economics*
JHM	*Journal of the History of Medicine and Allied Sciences*
JNMD	*Journal of Nervous and Mental Disease*
JP	*Journal of Pediatrics*
JSH	*Journal of Social History*
LHJ	*Ladies' Home Journal*
MCNA	*Medical Clinics of North America*
MLIC	*Metropolitan Life Insurance Company Statistical Bulletin*
NCAB	*National Cyclopaedia of American Biography*
NEJM	*New England Journal of Medicine*
Nostrums I, II, III	American Medical Association,
	Nostrums and Quackery (Chicago, 1911) as I;

            Nostrums and Quackery (Chicago, 1921) as II;
            Nostrums and Quackery and Pseudo-Medicine (Chicago,
1936) as III.
            Volumes II and III edited by Arthur J. Cramp

NYDT	*New York Daily Tribune*
NYT	*New York Times*
OED	*Oxford English Dictionary*
PM	*Parents' Magazine*
PMS	*Perceptual and Motor Skills*
RD	*Readers' Digest*
SEP	*Saturday Evening Post*
WCJ	*Water-Cure Journal*
WHC	*Woman's Home Companion*
WW	*Weight Watchers Magazine*

Certain manuscript and pamphlet collections have also been short-titled, as follows:

Chittenden Papers	Russell Chittenden Papers, Yale University Library
Dignam Papers	Dorothy Dignam Papers, Wisconsin State Historical Society
Fairbanks Papers	Fairbanks Scale Company Papers, Special Collections, University of Vermont Library
Fletcher Correspondence	Horace Fletcher MSS, bMS Am791 Houghton Library, Harvard University
Graham MSS	Sylvester Graham MSS, American Antiquarian Society Worcester, Massachusetts
Howe Papers	Howe Scale Company Records Special Collections, University of Vermont Library
Landauer	Bella C. Landauer Collection, Print Department, New York Historical Society
LPI	Records of the Meetings of the Ladies Physiological Institute of Boston and Vicinity, Schlesinger Library Radcliffe College
Warshaw	Warshaw Collection of Business Americana, Museum of National History, Smithsonian Institution

CHAPTER ONE
Prologue

1. Leon Rooke, *Fat Woman* (NY, 1981) 38–39, quoted with permission of Alfred A. Knopf, Inc.

2. Thoughtful work has been done by Anne Hollander in "A lust for leanness," *Times Literary Supplement* (June 23, 1978) 691–92, and *Seeing Through Clothes* (NY, 1978) esp. 337–38. Kim Chernin in *The Hungry Self* (NY, 1985) attempts an historical analysis of eating disorders, but her chronology is far less cogent than her psychology.

3. Judith Thurman, "Never too thin to feel fat," *Ms.* 6 (Sept 1977) 48–50, 82–84, quote on 48.

4. *Science News Letter* 68 (Nov 19, 1955) 324; Peter Wyden, *The Overweight Society* (NY, 1965) ch. 12 on "Regimen"; and series of articles in *AA* 36 (March 1–May 10, 1965).

5. On the fluctuating reputation of PPA (= PPH), see House of Representatives, Comm. on Government Operations, *False and Misleading Advertising (Weight-Reducing Preparations)* (Washington, D.C., 1957) 31–36, 150–52; "PPA diet pills get clearance from FDA panel," *Drug Topics* 126 (March 15, 1982) 40; and "Weight control drug products for over-the-counter human use," *Federal Register* 47,39 (1982) 8466–84.

6. Wilhelm Ebstein, *Corpulence and Its Treatment*, trans. Emil W. Hoeber (NY, 1884) 18–19; Vilhjalmur Stefansson, *Not by Bread Alone* (NY, 1946); Elizabeth Woody, "The eat-all-you-want reducing diet," *Holiday* 9 (Feb 1951) 64–66 + ; Alfred W. Pennington, "A reorientation on obesity," *NEJM* 248 (1953) 959–64; Herman Taller, *Calories Don't Count* (NY, 1961); Sidney Petrie, *Martinis and Whipped Cream* (NY, 1966); Gardner Jameson and Elliott Williams, *The New Drinking Man's Diet and Cookbook*, ed. Robert W. Cameron (NY, 1974); and Carol Guilford, *The Diet Book* (NY, 1973), an inaccurate survey of high-fat diets.

7. For ratings, see Guilford, *The Diet Book*; Nikki Goldbeck and David Goldbeck, *The Dieter's Companion* (NY, 1975); Larry Goldberg, *Goldberg's Diet Catalog* (NY, 1977); and Theodore Berland, *Rating the Diets* (NY, 1979).

8. Françoise Loux, *Le corps dans la société traditionnelle* (Paris, 1979) 76; Hans Hinrichs, *The Glutton's Paradise* (Mount Vernon, N.Y., 1955); and René Carel, "L'obésité dans l'histoire et la littérature," *Aesculape* n.s. 29,2 (1939) 26–32 and 29,3 (1939) 58–64.

9. Morton Bloomfield, *The Seven Deadly Sins* (East Lansing, Mich., 1952); Ruth E. Messenger, *Ethical Teachings in the Latin Hymns of*

Medieval England (NY, 1967); R. F. Yeager, "Aspects of gluttony in Chaucer and Gower," *Studies in Philology* 81 (Winter 1984) 42–55; Alan E. Knight, "The condemnation of pleasure in late medieval French morality plays," *French R* 57 (1983) 1–9; John T. McNeill and Helen M. Gamer, *Medieval Handbooks of Penance* (NY, 1938) esp. 101. Cf. Stephen Mennell, *All Manners of Food* (Oxford, 1985) ch. 2.

10. Lewis Cornaro, *A Treatise of the Benefits of a Sober Life*, trans. into Latin by Leonard Lessius, thence into English by Timothy Smith (London, 1743)—the first English edition of Cornaro's *Trattato de la vita sobria* (1558), often entitled *Discorsi della vita sobria*. Quotes on 5, 12. Cf. Gertrude B. Richards, "A Renaissance regimen," *BHM* 7 (1939) 1170–80.

11. Santorio Santorio (= Sanctorius Sanctorius), *Medicina Statica: or, Rules of Health, in Eight Sections of Aphorisms*, trans. J.D. (London, 1676)—first English edition of the *De Statica Medicina* (1614).

12. *Ibid.*, 2, 3, 9, 22, 171, and throughout.

13. Cornaro's work has had at least 3 Swedish editions, 4 Dutch, 4 German, 7 Latin, 11 French, 12 Italian; it reached its 53d English edition by 1826 and has had 33 American editions.

14. Cf. Eric J. Trimmer, *Rejuvenation: The History of an Idea* (London, 1967); Gerald J. Gruman, *A History of Ideas About the Prolongation of Life* (Philadelphia, 1966). Cornaro has often been credited with a centenarian life, though modern authorities now agree that he was born in 1475 and died in 1566.

15. See Mary P. Perry, "On the psychostasis in Christian art," *Burlington Mag* 22 (1912–13) 94–105, 208–18; Leopold Kretzenbacher, *Die Seelenwaage* (Klagenfurt, 1958).

16. Cf. Jerome J. Bylebyl, "Nutrition, quantification and circulation," *BHM* 51 (1977) 377–78.

17. Santorio, *Medicina Statica*, 173.

18. George Cheyne, *The English Malady* (London, 1733) 222–41, some of which is rehashed in Bryan S. Turner, "The discourse of diet," *Theory, Culture and Society* 1 (1982) 23–32.

19. Cheyne, *English Malady*, 249.

20. George Cheyne, *An Essay of Health and Long Life*, 4th ed. (London, 1725 [1724]) 39.

21. Leonard W. Labaree, ed., *Papers of Benjamin Franklin* (New Haven, 1960) II, 339–40, and (1963) VI, 325.

22. "Extracts of two letters from Dr. John Lining . . .," *Philosophical Tr of the Royal Soc of London* 42 (1742–43) 491–509, quotes on 495,

496, and "A letter from Dr. John Lining," *ibid.* 43 (1744–45) 318–30; Franklin C. Bing, "John Lining (1708–1760)," *DAB* VI, 280–81.

23. Thomas Moffett, *Health's Improvement,* ed. Christopher Bennet (London, 1655). Moffett (also Muffett, Moffet) lived from 1553 to 1604; see John Ritchie, "Moffet's *Health's Improvement,*" *Caledonian Med J* 15 (1935) 411–16.

24. Thomas Vicary, *Anatomie of Man's Body* (London, 1548) 232.

25. Pan S. Codellas, "The Epimonidion pharmacon of Philon the Byzantine," *BHM* 22 (1948) 630–34.

26. Paul Ghalioungui, *Magic and Medical Science in Ancient Egypt* (London, 1963) 72–73.

27. James MacKenzie, *The History of Health and the Art of Preserving It,* 2d ed. (Edinburgh, 1759) 377, an invaluable anthology (quote is evidently from MacKenzie himself). Cf. "Corpulency," *A New and Complete Dictionary of Arts and Sciences* (London, 1754) I, 758.

28. Bruno Kisch, "The medical use of scales," *Amer J of Cardiology* 5 (1960) 262 on the European vogue; Robert W. Allen, *Number Three Saint James's Street: A History of Berry's, the Wine Merchants* (London, 1950); Berry Brothers & Rudd, "History in the Weighing," *Number Three Saint James's Street* 56 (Spring 1982) 15–24; Edward V. Lucas, "Signs and avoirdupois," *Giving and Receiving* (NY, 1922) 105–15; Ivo Geikie-Cobb, "Obesity: then and now," *Practitioner* 167 (1951) 174; and letter from Anthony Berry, Sept 4, 1984.

29. Ralph Nevill, *The Sport of Kings* (London, 1926) 21, 37–38; Joe H. Palmer, *This Was Racing,* ed. Red Smith (NY, 1953) 22, 117–20; and Bob Champion and Jonathan Powell, *Champion's Story* (NY, 1981) 46–55 for an extreme modern example.

30. William Kitchiner, *The Art of Invigorating and Prolonging Life,* 3d ed. (London, 1822) 3n.

31. This argument has been made by David Kunzle, *Fashion and Fetishism* (Totowa, N.J., 1982). Contrast Valerie Steele, *Fashion and Eroticism* (NY, 1985) ch. 9.

32. That clothing styles neither create nor exaggerate the demand for a slimmer body can best be seen in Patricia Weeden, "Study patterned on Kroeber's investigation of style," *Dress* 3 (1977) 9–19. Though the desire for a slimmer body has increased steadily over the last sixty years, fashionable waist widths and other costume proportions have fluctuated seriously during the same period.

CHAPTER TWO

The Thin Body and the Jacksonians

1. Sylvester Graham, "To the citizens of Boston and the public in general," *Boston Courier* (March 17, 1837) 1:2–3, (March 21, 1837) 1:2–

3, and (March 24, 1837) 1:1; Graham MSS, Science of Life, folio volume, last page, verso.

2. John S. Bartlett, "Medical impeachment," *BMSJ* 14 (June 8, 1836) 282.

3. *Ibid.*, quote on 282; *Boston Courier* (April 6, 1837) 1:1–2.

4. *Boston Courier* (April 6, 1837) 2; *Boston Post* (March 4, 1837) 2 and (March 6, 1837) 2; *Daily Evening Transcript* (March 3, 1837) 2:1; *Liberator* (March 11, 1837) 3; Rare Book Room, Boston Public Library, MS A.9.2.8.15, letter from Lucia Weston to Debora Weston, March 3, 1837 (misdated 1836), and MS A.9.2.9.15, letter from Caroline Weston to same, March 3, 1837.

5. *Boston Courier* (March 15, 1837) 2:2.

6. *Means Without Living* (Boston, 1837) 62, a thinly veiled description of Graham by an anonymous satirist.

7. Charles Caldwell, "Excess in quantity of food," *Transylvania J of Med* (Sept 1832) 313, reprinted in *GJHL* 1 (1837) 68–69; William A. Alcott, "Gluttony," *Library of Health* 6 (1842) 293; idem, "July and Independence," *Moral Reformer* I (1835) 198; Sylvester Graham, "Excessive alimentation," *GJHL* 2 (1838) 161.

8. Sylvester Graham, *Treatise on Bread and Bread-Making* (Boston, 1837) quote on 97. Cf. Stephen Nissenbaum, *Sex, Diet, and Debility in Jacksonian America: Sylvester Graham and Health Reform* (Westport, Conn., 1980) 5–8. For an example of Grahamite childrearing, see A.W., "Graham system adapted to infancy," *GJHL* 1 (1837) 177–78.

9. Sylvester Graham, *A Lecture to Young Men* (Providence, 1834) 16–19, 35, often republished under the title, *Chastity*.

10. If yeast were used, newly baked bread should not be eaten for at least twenty-four hours until the last of the alcohol in the bread had evaporated, whence the liking for healthful stale breads. Graham, *Treatise on Bread*, 100–101. On the context for Graham's vision of the domestic world, see Barbara L. Epstein, *The Politics of Domesticity: Evangelism and Temperance in Nineteenth-Century America* (Middletown, Conn., 1981); Mary P. Ryan, *The Empire of the Mother: American Writing about Domesticity, 1830–1860* (NY, 1982); Carole Shammas, "The domestic environment in early modern England and America," *JSH* 14 (1980–81) 3–24; and Sarah F. McMahon, "A comfortable subsistence: changing composition of diet in rural New England, 1620–1840," *William & Mary Q* 42 (1985) 26–65.

11. Sylvester Graham, *A Lecture on the Responsibleness of Human Beings in the Exercise of their Moral Power* (Northampton, Mass., 1841) quote on 42, and idem, *The Philosophy of Sacred History Considered in Relation to Human Aliment and the Wines of Scripture*, ed. Henry S. Clubb (NY, 1855) esp. 551, quote on 556.

12. "Dietetic charlatanry—new ethics of eating," *New-York R* 1 (1837) 336–51, quote on 341. For a more accurate description, see "A Graham dinner," *Botanico-Medical Recorder* 8 (Jan 25, 1840) 141–42.

13. [Thomas C. Haliburton], "The Clockmaker; or, the Sayings and Doings of Samuel Slick, of Slickville. Ch. XVIII. The Grahamite and the Irish Plot," *Brown's Literary Omnibus* 2 (Jan 12, 1838) 3.

14. For a summary of the Graham system in popular practice, see *GJHL* 1 (1837) 17.

15. Sylvester Graham, *The Aesculapian Tablets of the Nineteenth Century* (Providence, 1834) 46–50, 56, 65–66, 70–73; *GJHL* 1 (1837) 3, 14–15, 30, 42, 118.

16. Phineas T. Barnum, *Selected Letters*, ed. A. H. Saxon (NY, 1983) 18, 21, 28.

17. "Mr. G's lectures on Temperance," *Genius of Temperance* 5 (June 29, 1831) 2.

18. Russell T. Trall, "Biographical sketch of Sylvester Graham," *WCJ* 12 (1851) 110, and "Doctor Bran—his dignity and consistency," *Northampton Courier* (Aug 12, 1851) 2:5.

19. On Graham's life I have used Helen Graham Carpenter, *The Rev. John Graham of Woodbury, Connecticut and His Descendants* (Chicago, 1942); Edith W. Cole, "Sylvester Graham, Lecturer on the Science of Human Life," Ph.D. thesis, Indiana Univ, 1975, 6–18; and Nissenbaum, *Sex, Diet and Debility*.

20. Carpenter, *The Rev. John Graham*, 188.

21. Sylvester Graham, "Dr. Graham's sickness and apology," *Northampton Courier* (July 29, 1840) 2:3–4; (Aug 19, 1840) 2:3–4; and (Sept 2, 1840) 1:4–5 and 2:1–2.

22. Xavier Bichat, *Physiological Researches on Life and Death*, trans. F. Gold (Boston, 1827) 10, 11, 100; Mildred Naylor, "Sylvester Graham, 1794–1851," *Annals of Med History* ser. 3, 4 (1942) 236–40; James C. Whorton, *Crusaders for Fitness* (Princeton, N.J., 1982) 40–42; and Nissenbaum, *Sex, Diet and Debility*, 20–21, 57–64. On Bichat and Broussais, see John E. Lesch, *Science and Medicine in France: The Emergence of Experimental Physiology 1790–1855* (Cambridge, Mass., 1984) esp. ch. 3; Geoffrey Sutton, "The physical and chemical path to vitalism," *BHM* 58 (1984) 53–71.

23. See E. Benton, "Vitalism in nineteenth-century scientific thought," *Studies in the History and Philosophy of Science* 5 (1974) 17–48.

24. William Beaumont, *Experiments and Observations on the Gastric Juice and the Physiology of Digestion* (Plattsburgh, N.Y., 1833); J. J. Bylebyl, "William Beaumont, Robley Dunglison and the 'Philadelphia Physiologists,'" *JHM* 25 (1970) 3–21; and Frederic L. Holmes,

Claude Bernard and Animal Chemistry (Cambridge, Mass., 1974) ch. 7.

25. Graham, *Lectures on the Science of Human Life* I, 311–12 (quote), and idem, *A Lecture on Epidemic Diseases Generally, and Particularly the Spasmodic Cholera*, new ed. (Boston, 1838) 110–11.

26. Jesse S. Myer, *Life and Letters of Dr. William Beaumont* (St. Louis, 1939) 138, 153; Lewis Cornaro, *Discourses on a Sober and Temperate Life. With Introduction and Notes by Sylvester Graham* (NY, 1832) 52n–53n. Cf. John A. Paris, *A Treatise on Diet* (NY, 1828) 136, criticizing Cornaro; Graham owned a copy of this book.

27. Graham, *Lectures on Epidemic Diseases*, 9, 10, 11, 13; *GJHL* 1 (1837) 214–15.

28. François J. V. Broussais, *Principles of Physiological Medicine*, trans. Isaac Hays and R. Eglesfield Griffith (Philadelphia, 1832) 204, 523, 525; *Boston Daily Advertiser* (July 4, 1834) 2; "The dyspeptic," *GJHL* 2 (1838) 312–13 and also 373, and cf. 1 (1837) 254, a British visitor saying, "I never saw a Yankee that did not bolt his food whole, like a boa constrictor."

29. John Graham, *The Duty of Renewing Their Baptismal Covenant Proved and Urged Upon the Adult Children of Professing Parents* (Boston, 1734) 3.

30. I have been inspired here by Karen Halttunen, *Confidence Men and Painted Women: A Study of Middle-Class Culture in America, 1830–1870* (New Haven, 1982).

31. Xavier Bichat, *General Anatomy*, trans. George Hayward (Boston, 1822) I, 26; Graham, *Aesculapian Tablets*, 19; "Future longevity of man," *Library of Health* 1 (1837) 376; Graham, *Lectures on the Science of Human Life* I, 450; and Graham MSS, unpublished lecture notes (1831–1847), 9th lecture, f. 10v., notes by an auditor, "I should think that he thought the average of a 100 years & upward might be reached by all, yet he was not very definite on that subject." On buoyancy, see the 10th lecture, f. 11, and Graham, *Aesculapian Tablets*, 16, 50.

32. Graham MSS, Science of Life, folio volume, p. 22, clipping from *NY Tribune* (June 22, 1844), and Graham, *Treatise on Bread*, 52.

33. On the Bank I have used Ralph C. H. Catterall, *The Second Bank of the United States* (Chicago, 1902) esp. 351; John M. McFaul, *The Politics of Jacksonian Finance* (Ithaca, N.Y., 1972); Ronald P. Formisano, "Toward a reorientation of Jacksonian politics," *JAH* 63 (1976–77) 43–65; Sean Wilentz, "On class and politics in Jacksonian America," *R in Amer History* 10, 4 (1982) 45–63; and Robert H. Wiebe, *The Opening of American Society* (NY, 1984) 151, 220–21, 238–41. See also notes below.

34. Robert V. Remini, *Andrew Jackson and the Bank War* (NY, 1967) esp. 118–20; Michael Paul Rogin, *Fathers & Children: Andrew Jackson and the Subjugation of the American Indian* (NY, 1975) ch. 9; and Frank O. Gatell, ed., *The Jacksonians and the Money Power, 1829–1840* (Chicago, 1967) esp. 5.

35. Remini, *Andrew Jackson and the Bank War*, 34, and Rudolph Marx, *The Health of the Presidents* (NY, 1960) 108, 113–15.

36. Thomas C. Cochran, *Two Hundred Years of American Business* (NY, 1977) 98, and Martin Van Buren, message to Congress, Sept 4, 1837, reprinted in Gatell, *Jacksonians and the Money Power*, 40. Cf. Rogin, *Fathers & Children*, 285–86, on Jacksonian cultural psychology relating the debt to gluttony.

37. Richard Selden, *Newest Keep-Sake for 1839* (Boston, 1839) 120–21.

38. Charles Ogle, *The Regal Splendor of the President's Palace* (Boston, 1840) 1, 17, menu on 21. "Locofoco" referred to the more radical faction of New York City Democrats.

39. *Congressional Globe* 8 (Dec 9, 1839–July 21, 1840) 26th Congress, 1st Session, April 14, 1840, p. 327; Robert G. Gunderson, *The Log-Cabin Campaign* (Lexington, Ky., 1947) 105, 114; Marx, *Health of the Presidents*, 123, 127–28; John Niven, *Martin Van Buren* (NY, 1983) 462; and James Fenimore Cooper, *The Pathfinder* (NY, 1953 [1840]) 37–39.

40. "Song," *Boston Daily Advertiser* (July 7, 1834), and "Dietetic charlatanry," *New-York R* 1 (1837) 342. Graham, like many of those working in benevolent societies, was anti-Jacksonian; see Clifford S. Griffin, *Their Brothers' Keeper: Moral Stewardship in the United States, 1800–1850* (New Brunswick, N.J., 1960) 57.

41. Benjamin Labaree, *A Sermon on the Death of General Harrison* (Middlebury, Vt., 1841).

42. Lois W. Banner, *American Beauty* (NY, 1983) ch. 3; Halttunen, *Confidence Men and Painted Women*, 74–75, 79; and A Reformed Dandy of the Eighteenth Century, "Fashion," *New England Mag* 4 (1833) 345–60.

43. Banner, *American Beauty*, 47, 61–62; Leslie A. Marchand, *Byron: A Portrait* (NY, 1970) 43, 109, 243, 386 (quote), 397, 399—and on the lobster salad, 133; idem, ed., *Byron's Letters and Journals* (Cambridge, Mass., 1978) VIII, 165; Wilma Paterson, "Was Byron anorexic?" *World Med* 17 (May 15, 1982) 35–38; Alison Gernsheim, *Fashion and Reality 1840–1914* (London, 1963) 27; and a Native of the United States, *American Sketches* (London, 1827) 391–92, reproduced in Clifton J. Farness, *The Genteel Female* (NY, 1931) 222.

44. "The higher circles and the lower circles," *Graham's Lady's and Gentleman's Mag* 24 (1844) 296—this Graham was unrelated to Sylves-

ter; Banner, *American Beauty*, 63–64; Wendy W. Reaves, "Portraits for every parlor: Albert Newson and American portrait lithographs," in *American Portrait Prints*, ed. Reaves (Charlottesville, Va., 1983) 85, 107; Jonathan L. Fairbanks and Elizabeth B. Bates, *American Furniture, 1620 to the Present* (NY, 1981) esp. 254; and *American Art-Union Tr* (1850) frontispiece and 24.

45. The Newark paper is quoted in *GJHL* 2 (1838) 319. See also "National postures," *New England Mag* 7 (1834) 230; Claudia B. Kidwell and Margaret C. Christman, *Suiting Everyone: The Democratization of Clothing in America* (Washington, D.C., 1974) 37–52; G. J. Cowles, "Spinal endermic medication," *Western J of the Med and Physical Sciences* 2 (1837) 192–98; Francis Schiller, "Spinal irritation and osteopathy," *BHM 45 (1971) 250–66;* and Alfred R. Shands, *Early Orthopedic Surgeons of America* (St. Louis, 1970).

46. Arthur M. Schlesinger, Sr., "A dietary interpretation of American history," *Massachusetts Historical Soc Proc* 73 (1944–47) 210, citing Thackeray; Thomas Colley Grattan, *Civilized America* (London, 1859) II, 55–56; Banner, *American Beauty*, 57–58. Meanwhile, in 1836 Charles Dickens was introducing Joe the fat boy to English readers of his *Pickwick Papers*, whence the "Pickwickian syndrome" as a diagnosis for obese, sleepy people.

47. Kenneth L. Sokoloff and Georgia C. Villaflor, "The early achievement of modern stature in America," *Social Science History* 6 (1982) 453–81, and Robert W. Fogel et al., "Secular changes in American and British stature and nutrition," *JIH* 14 (1983) 445–81. For blacks, see David Eltis, "Nutritional trends in Africa and the Americas: heights of Africans, 1819–1839," *JIH* 12 (1981) 453–75. There are no good data on women for this period; I am assuming that their comparative tallness at the end of the century held for the beginning as well. For later data, see Milicent L. Hathaway and Elsie Foard, *Heights and Weights of Adults in the United States*, Home Economics Research Report No. 10 (Washington, D.C., 1960) 4.

48. Daniel Drake, *A Systematic Treatise* (Cincinnati, 1850; rept. 1971) I, 650–52, and John Hutchinson, "On the capacity of the lungs . . .," *Royal Med and Chirurgical Soc of London Tr* 29 (1846) 167–68.

49. Cooper, *Pathfinder*, 53, with illustrations by F. O. C. Darley reproduced in this 1953 edition opp. pp. 400, 500.

50. Sokoloff and Villaflor, "Modern stature," 460; Fogel et al., "Secular changes," 464; and Gunderson, *Log-Cabin Campaign*, 138. On the variety in the diet, see Waverly Root and Richard D. Rochemont, *Eating in America: A History* (NY, 1976).

51. William Cobbett, *A Year's Residence in America* (Boston, 1929 [1819]) 156; Anthony F. M. Willich, *Lectures on Diet and Regimen*

(Boston, 1800, from 2d London ed.) editor's note, vii; and A Gentleman, *The Laws of Etiquette*, 2d ed. (Philadelphia, 1838) 164 and cf. 152.

52. Root and Rochemont, *Eating in America*, 134; Sophia Smith Collection, Smith College, Garrison Family MSS, Box 64, Cookbooks 1694–1832, Cookbook No. 2, c. 1810, p. 12 (cited with permission from John Bright Garrison), and *The Cook Not Mad, or Rational Cookery* (Watertown, N.Y., 1830) iii, 9.

53. Root and Rochement, *Eating in America*, 139; Richard O. Cummings, *The American and His Food* (Chicago, 1940) 12; Sam B. Hilliard, *Hog Meat and Hoecake: Food Supply in the Old South, 1840–1860* (Carbondale, Ill., 1972) 41; Drake, *Systematic Treatise*, I, 655; and John Drury, *Rare and Well Done: Some Historical Notes on Meat and Meatmen* (Chicago, 1966) 96.

54. Luther V. Bell, "Boylston Prize Dissertation for 1835," *BMSJ* 13 (1835) 261, quoting C. F. Volney in the text and another Frenchman in the footnote, the latter on melted butter; Constantin François Chassebeuf, Comte de Volney, *A View of the Soil and Climate of the United States of America*, trans. C. B. Brown (Philadelphia, 1804) 257; and Drake, *Systematic Treatise*, I, 655, 657.

55. "What we eat," *Lady's Home Mag* 13 (1859) 316 (quote); Root and Rochemont, *Eating in America*, 41, 136–37; David Macrae, *The Americans at Home*, rev. ed. (Glasgow, 1875 [1860]) 29–30; and Richard J. Hooker, *Food and Drink in America* (Indianapolis, 1981) 248, quoting C. W. Gesner, "Concerning restaurants," *Harper's New Monthly Mag* 32 (1866) 591–92. My count of pages devoted to sweet foods yielded a range of 27–63 percent for American cookbooks 1796–1857, and a range of 10–30 percent for English cookbooks of the same period.

56. Thomas Carlyle, *Correspondence of Thomas Carlyle and Ralph Waldo Emerson*, ed. C. E. Norton (Boston, 1883) II, 177, quoted in Cummings, *American and His Food*, 76.

57. Aleksander B. Lakier, *A Russian Looks at America: The Journey of Aleksander Borisovich Lakier in 1857* (Chicago, 1979) 61–62; [Robert Tomes], "Why we get sick," *Harper's New Monthly Mag* 13 (1856) 645; Gottfried Duden, *Report on a Journey to the Western States of North America*, trans. James W. Goodrich et al. (Columbia, S.C., 1980 [1829]) 28–29; James E. Gross, "Dyspepsia among farmers," *Water-Cure Monthly* 3 (July 1860) 15; and Macrae, *Americans at Home*, 25.

58. Hooker, *Food and Drink*, 147, 254; Schlesinger, "Dietary interpretation," 209–10 on bad teeth; and [Tomes], "Why we get sick," 645 (quote).

59. Leslie Dorsey and Janice Devine, *Fare Thee Well* (NY, 1964) 33, 36; S. W. Avery, *Dyspeptic's Monitor*, 2d ed. (NY, 1830) 69, on boarding-houses, and Médéric-Louis-Elie Moreau de St. Méry, *Moreau de St. Méry's American Journey (1793–1798)*, trans. and ed. Kenneth Roberts and Anna M. Roberts (Garden City, N.Y., 1947) 265.

60. I draw Harry Hurry out of James Fenimore Cooper's *Deerslayer* (1841). Cooper himself called Americans "gross feeders" who ate too much greasy food. See Chris Chase, *The Great American Waistline* (NY, 1981) 22. On forks, see Hooker, *Food and Drink*, 97. On small bites and gentility, see A New Contributor, "Giving a dinner," *Graham's Mag* 44 (1854)—again, no relation to Sylvester.

61. Hooker, *Food and Drink*, 96

62. For a full statement of this theory, see C. Drake's review of Avery's *Dyspeptic's Monitor* in *AJMS* 7 (1830) 206.

63. Robert S. Fletcher, "Bread and doctrine at Oberlin," *Ohio St Archaeological and Historial Q* 49 (1940) 65; "Hints toward the formation of a Society for the Suppression of Eating," *New England Mag* 2 (1832) 315; and Timothy Titterwell (= Samuel Kettell), *Yankee Notions* (Boston, 1838) 105, 169, 171.

64. W* W*, "Some facts and logic respecting dietetics," *BMSJ* 14 (1836) 167, 171 on buoyancy; Fletcher, "Bread and doctrine at Oberlin," 66; Alcott, "July and Independence," 198; O.P.Q., "Effects of gluttony," *Library of Health* 5 (1841); and *Means Without Living*, 18. On Alcott, see Martin C. Van Buren, "The Indispensable God of Health: A Study of Republican Hygiene and the Ideology of William Alcott," Ph.D. thesis, UCLA, 1977. On other contemporaries troubled by abundance, see Harvey Green, *Fit for America* (NY, 1986) 15–16.

65. Fletcher, "Bread and doctrine at Oberlin."

66. Cf. Jayme A. Sokolow, *Eros and Modernization: Sylvester Graham, Health Reform and the Origins of Victorian Sexuality in America* (Rutherford, N.J., 1983) 122, and Whorton, *Crusaders for Fitness*, 44. Quote from W* W*, "Some facts and logic," 168 (italics removed from the original).

67. Arthur W. Brayley, *Bakers and Baking in Massachusetts* (Boston, 1909) 135; Fogel et al., "Secular changes," 472; and Sokolow, *Eros and Modernization*, 116.

68. A. B. Norton, *The Great Revolution of 1840: Reminiscences of the Log Cabin and Hard Cider Campaign* (Mt. Vernon, Vt., 1888) 88–89; Gunderson, *Log-Cabin Campaign*, 219–20, 241; and Naylor, "Sylvester Graham," 239. See also David E. Shi, *The Simple Life* (NY, 1985) ch. 5 on Jacksonian conflicts about plain living.

CHAPTER THREE
The Buoyant Body in Victorian America

.1. Patent 3480, March 13, 1844. On the Millerites, see Edwin S. Gaustad, ed., *The Rise of Adventism* (NY, 1974) essays by David T. Arthur and Jonathan M. Butler, 154–206.

2. Edward Hitchcock, *Dyspepsy Forestalled and Resisted* (Amherst, Mass., 1830) 74, 213, 327, 339–40, 344. Cf. Gert H. Brieger, "Dyspepsia: the American disease," in *Healing and History*, ed. Charles E. Rosenberg (NY, 1979) 179–90.

    A complete list of symptoms appears in William Sweetser, *A Treatise on Digestion* (Boston, 1837) 168–81. The *Encyclopedia Americana* (Philadelphia, 1830) IV, 356, described dyspepsia as a common ailment "which, formerly, was termed *liver disease, bilious disorder,* &c." The prevalence of dyspepsia was due in part to a nosological shift.

3. Oliver Halsted, *A Full and Accurate Account of the New Method of Curing Dyspepsia* (NY, 1830) 113, 118, 119; "Halsted on dyspepsia," *Amer Q R* 9 (1831) 241–42, and cf. Nathaniel Chapman, "On dyspepsia, or indigestion," *Amer J of Med Sciences* 25 (1839) 332.

4. Médéric-Louis-Elie Moreau de St. Méry, *American Journey (1793–1798)*, trans. and ed. Kenneth Roberts and Anna M. Roberts (Garden City, N.Y., 1947) 287.

5. Peter Puckerbrodt, "Improved dyspepsia bread," *NY Constellation* 3 (July 14, 1832) 276.

6. John B. Blake, "Mary Gove Nichols, prophetess of health," *Amer Philosophical Soc Proc* 106 (1962) 219–34, quote on 219; Mary S. Gove, *Lectures to Women on Anatomy and Physiology with an Appendix on Water Cure* (NY, 1846) 187 (quote), 244; and *WCJ* 1,5 (1846) 93. I have also used Janet H. Noever, "Passionate Rebel: The Life of Mary Gove Nichols, 1810–1884," Ph.D. thesis, Univ of Oklahoma, 1983; John B. Blake "Nichols, Mary Sargeant Neal Gove," *Notable American Women 1607–1950* (Cambridge, Mass., 1971) II, 627–29; and H. E. Hoff and J. F. Fulton, "Centenary of the First American Physiological Society," *BHM* 5 (1937) 702–3.

7. See Thomas N. Haviland and Lawrence C. Parish, "A brief account of the use of wax models in the study of medicine," *JHM* 25 (1970) 52–75.

8. E. J. Pyke, *Biographical Dictionary of Wax Modellers* (Oxford, 1973) 29, 78, 126–27; Charles C. Sellers, *Patience Wright* (Middletown, Conn., 1976) 34–38, 41; and Neil McKendrick, "Commercialization and the economy," in *The Birth of a Consumer Society*, eds. McKendrick et al. (Bloomington, Ind., 1982) 43–47.

9. On the new manikins, see *GJHL* 3 (1839) 263; *Library of Health* 6 (1842) 39; and James C. Mohr, *Abortion in America* (NY, 1978) 69. On lightly-framed structures, Daniel Calhoun, *The Intelligence of a People* (Princeton, N.J., 1973) 118, 232–33, 295–300, 306–7; and Thomas Low Nichols, *Forty Years of American Life*, 2d ed. (London, 1874) 68. On the models, see LPI, Secretary's Reports, Box 1, lv (Nov 29, 1850) pp. 118–19, 3v (1851–64) p. 42, 4v (May 1854–57) f. 18v (quote).

10. Daniel Irwin, "Historical development of terrain representation in American cartography," *Int Yearbook of Cartography* 16 (1976) 70–75.

11. *WCJ* 21 (June 1856) 143, personal #223 (quote). On phrenology see John D. Davies, *Phrenology, Fad and Science* (New Haven, 1955); David di Giustino, *Conquest of Mind: Phrenology and Victorian Social Thought* (London, 1975); and Anthony A. Walsh, "Phrenology and the Boston medical community in the 1830s," *BHM* 50 (1976) 261–73.

12. Madeleine B. Stern, *Heads and Headlines: The Phrenological Fowlers* (Norman, Okla., 1971); Carl Carmer, "That was New York: the Fowlers, practical phrenologists," *New Yorker* (Feb 13, 1937) 22–27; and Orson Squire Fowler, "Phrenology and physiology applied to education and self-improvement," *Amer Phrenological J* 5 (1843) 185.

13. *Amer Vegetarian and Health J* 3 (1853) 198 on Hite; Davies, *Phrenology*, 38; and LPI, Box 1, 3v, Fourth Annual Report (by Frances Atherton Buffum, May 5, 1852) p. 137.

14. William T. Shreve, *The Venus of Milo* (Boston, 1878); Lois Banner, *American Beauty* (NY, 1983) 59–60; and Nichols, *Forty Years*, 115 on Powers.

15. Alan Thomas, *Time in a Frame: Photography and the Nineteenth-Century Mind* (NY, 1977) 7, 14, 17; William Welling, *Photography in America: The Formative Years 1839–1900* (NY, 1976) esp. 57, 71; Peter C. Marzio, *The Art Crusade: An Analysis of American Drawing Manuals 1820–1866* (Washington, D.C., 1976); and Karen Halttunen, *Confidence Men and Painted Women* (New Haven, 1982).

16. "Fleshiness," *The Letter Box* 2 (Sept 1859) 73.

17. Banner, *American Beauty*, 63–64 (ballerinas); Calhoun, *The Intelligence of a People*, 232–33, 247–50 (ships); *Boston Daily Advertiser* (June 21, 1834) 2 on balloons; Tom D. Crouch, *The Eagle Aloft* (Washington, D.C., 1983) 119–24, 162 *et passim* on balloon mania; Gerald Bordman, *American Musical Theatre* (NY, 1978) 11; and "Animal magnetism," *BMSJ* 13 (1836) 418–19.

18. Albert R. Eaches, "Scales and weighing devices," *History News* 27 (1972) 53–64; David Kunzle, *Fashion and Fetishism* (Totowa, N.J.,

1982) esp. 128–29; Gove, *Lectures to Women*, 47; and Halsted, *Full and Accurate Account*, 35.

19. Charles N. Gattey, *The Bloomer Girls* (NY, 1968) quote on 112; Banner, *American Beauty*, 86–88, 94–97; Stella Mary Newton, *Health, Art and Reason: Dress Reformers of the Nineteenth Century* (London, 1974) 4; and Mrs. S. C. Hall, "Nelly Nowlan on Bloomers," *Graham's Mag* 41 (1852) 207. Cf. Valerie Steele, *Fashion and Eroticism* (NY, 1985) 145–50.

20. Gattey, *Bloomer Girls*, 59, 147 (quotes), and Lola Montez, *The Arts of Beauty* (NY, 1858) 71.

21. Elizabeth Ewing, *Dress and Undress: A History of Women's Underwear* (London, 1978) 74; *The Sibyl* 1 (July 1, 1856) 3, quoting the *NYT* on flounces and crinolines, and see also 3 (Dec 1, 1859) 659 on decline of tight-lacing; and cartoon in *Harper's Weekly* (Nov 21, 1857).

22. David Macrae, *The Americans at Home*, rev. ed. (Glasgow, 1875 [1860]) 29.

23. Howe Papers, Scrapbook, part I, f. 5, clipping from the *Boston Journal* circa 1859, and f. 6, from the *Boston Transcript*; Thomas King Chambers, "On corpulence," *Lancet* 2 (1850) 345, refusing to set weight standards; Richardson L. Wright, *Hawkers and Walkers in Early America* (NY, 1927) 180, 191; *The Life of That Wonderful and Extraordinarily Heavy Man, Daniel Lambert* (NY, 1815); "Miss Susan Barton The Mammoth Lady as Exhibited at Barnum's American Museum"—poster printed by N. Currier (NY, 1849); "Obesity," *BMSJ* 47 (1852) 124; "Extraordinary obesity," *AJMS* ser 2, 34 (1857) 560; C. J. B. Williams, "Obesity," *Cyclopaedia of Practical Medicine*, eds. John Forbes et al. (Philadelphia, 1845) III, 404 on buoyancy; John C. Greene, "Science and the public in the Age of Jackson," *Isis* 49 (1958) 20, quoting the *Med Repository* 2 (1808) 320; and *The Sibyl* 1 (Oct 1, 1856), "Singular night scene," quoting *St. Louis Herald*.

24. Banner, *American Beauty*, 88–89, and Halttunen, *Confidence Men and Painted Women*, 159, 167.

25. Gattey, *Bloomer Girls*, 16, and *WCJ* personals (in order as quoted): 19 (April 1855) 89 #75; 19 (Jan 1855) 18 #52; 19 (May 1855) 113 #84; 22 (Dec 1856) 138 #253; 20 (Aug 1855) 42 #136; 21 (June 1856) 143 #223; 17 (March 1854) 60; 18 (July 1854) 17 #6. For average weights at fairs, see Howe Papers, note 23 above.

26. Marshall S. Legan, "Hydropathy in America," *BHM* 45 (1971) 275; William Leach, *True Love and Perfect Union* (NY, 1980) 244–46; and *WCJ* 21 (Jan 1856) 23 #186.

27. Mark E. Lender and James K. Martin, *Drinking in America* (NY, 1982) 4–9, 14, 30–33; E. S. Turner, *Taking the Cure* (London, 1967);

and Carl Bridenbaugh, "Baths and watering places in colonial America," *William & Mary Q* 3 (1946) 151–81.

28. James Allin, *Serious Advice to Delivered Ones from Sickness* (Boston, 1679) 1; Harold D. Eberlein, "When society first took a bath," *Pennsylvania Mag of History* 67 (1943) 30–48, quote on 42; Charles E. Rosenberg, *No Other Gods* (Baltimore, 1976) 121; and *Yankee Notions* 1 (1852) 362–63, baths caricatured.

29. Joseph Rodman Drake, "The Culprit Frog" (c. 1816) stanza XIV, in Alphonso G. Newcomer et al., eds., *Three Centuries of American Poetry and Prose* (Chicago, 1917) 292; J. Frost, *The Art of Swimming*, new ed. (London, 1815) reprinting Ben Franklin's *Advice to Swimmers*, 25 ff., quote on 27; and James Arlington Bennet, *The Art of Swimming* (NY, 1846) 6–8.

30. Gove, *Lectures to Women*, 249; Blake, "Mary Gove Nichols," 223; Ronald L. Numbers, "Do-it-yourself the sectarian way," in *Medicine Without Doctors*, eds. G. B. Risse et al. (NY, 1977) 49–72; Harry B. Weiss and Howard R. Kemble, *The Great American Water-Cure Craze* (Trenton, 1967) 72–90; and A Water Patient (= H. F. Phinney), *The Water-Cure in America* (NY, 1848) 25–26.

31. Weiss and Kemble, *Water-Cure Craze*, 7, 8, 11, 12, 42; Turner, *Taking the Cure*, 154, 166–67; Francis J. Grund, "Reminiscences of watering-places," *Graham's Mag* 31 (1847) 219; Richard J. Lane, *Life at the Water Cure* (London, 1846) 25; and "Diet at Grafenburg," *WCJ* 1 (Jan 1, 1846) 40.

32. Phinney, *Water Cure in America*, esp. 43–45; P. H. Hayes, *Report of the Wyoming Water-Cure Institute* (Buffalo, 1853); and *WCJ* 2 (1846) 30, 59, and 17 (1854) 19 on virtues of low diet, and 20 (Oct 1855) 95, #160 Amarintha.

33. Weiss and Kemble, *Water-Cure Craze*, 18, 41, 44, and Blake, "Mary Gove Nichols," 233. On the position of women as healers in the 19th century, see Regina M. Morantz, "19th-century health reform and women," in *Medicine Without Doctors*, 73–94; Ann Douglas, *The Feminization of American Culture* (NY, 1977) ch. 3; and Mary Roth Walsh, *"Doctors Wanted: No Women Need Apply": Sexual Barriers in the Medical Profession, 1835–1975* (New Haven, 1977).

34. Phinney, *Water Cure in America*, 176, and *The Letter Box* 2 (Nov 1859) 98 for statistics.

35. Gove, *Lectures to Women*, 234, 241; *WCJ* 2 (1846) 60; *Botanico-Medical Recorder* 8 (Jan 25, 1840) 142; and Harriet Beecher Stowe, *The Chimney-Corner* (Boston, 1868) 146. The water cure had American parallels with Thomsonian steamopathy and homeopathic desires to stimulate a therapeutic crisis. Like Thomsonian and homeopathic medicine, the water cure appealed especially to women.

36. Kathryn Kish Sklar, *Catharine Beecher* (NY, 1973) 206–7; Linda Gordon, *Woman's Body, Woman's Right: A Social History of Birth Control in America* (NY, 1976), 51–57; James C. Mohr, *Abortion in America*, esp. 3–18, 48–50, 67; and Carl Degler, *At Odds: Women and the Family in America from the Revolution to the Present* (NY, 1980) 228, 231, 236, 240, 246.

37. Sklar, *Catharine Beecher*, 184–85, 204, 206; Mary P. Ryan, "The power of women's networks: a case study of female moral reform in antebellum America," *Feminist Studies* 5 (1979) 66–85; idem, *The Empire of the Mother* (NY, 1982) esp. 33, 106, 113; Marie Louise Shew, *Water-Cure for Ladies* (NY, 1844); and *WCJ* 1 (March 1, 1846) 103. Santorio quotation is from James MacKenzie, *History of Health and Art of Preserving It*, 2d ed. (Edinburgh, 1759) 266.

38. See Beatrice Farwell, "Courbet's 'Baigneuses' and the rhetorical feminine image," in *Woman as Sex Object: Studies in Erotic Art, 1730–1970*, eds. Thomas B. Hess and Linda Nochlin, (NY, 1972) 65–79.

39. John B. Blake, "Health reform," in *The Rise of Adventism*, 30, and also essay by Butler, 173–206; R. W. Schwarz, *John Harvey Kellogg, M.D.* (Nashville, 1970) 10–12, 17, 24–25; Blake, "Mary Gove Nichols," 231; and Weiss and Kemble, *Water-Cure Craze*, 78.

40. "The dyspeptic," *Journal of Health* 1, 17 (1830) 272; R. P. Basler, ed., *Collected Works of Abraham Lincoln* (New Brunswick, N.J., 1953) II, 461; Ralph Waldo Emerson, *Journals*, (Boston, 1913) IX, 324–26 (May 3, 1861), excerpted in Jack Lindeman, ed., *Conflict of Convictions* (Philadelphia, 1968) 11–12; George M. Fredrickson, *The Inner Civil War* (NY, 1965) 48, 75, and ch. 11; and James H. Moorhead, *American Apocalypse: Yankee Protestants and the Civil War, 1860–1869* (New Haven, 1978).

41. Leonard W. Labaree, ed., *Papers of Benjamin Franklin* (New Haven, 1960) II, 340; "Calisthenic exercises," *Graham's Mag* (= *Atkinson's Casket*) 7 (1832) 186–87; "Gymnastics," *Amer Q R* 3 (1828) 126–50; Almira H. Lincoln Phelps, *The Female Student*, 2d ed. (NY, 1836) 61–92; Gilbert H. Barnes and Dwight L. Dumond, eds., *Letters of Theodore Dwight Weld . . .* (Gloucester, Mass., 1965) II, 532 (Feb 8, 1838); Gove, *Lectures to Women*, 44–45, 218; Catharine E. Beecher, *Letters to the People on Health and Happiness* (NY, 1855) 187; and Ryan, *Empire of the Mother*, 55. See also John R. Betts, "Mind and body in early American thought," *JAH* 54 (1968) 787–805, and idem, "American medical thought on exercise as the road to health," *BHM* 45 (1971) 138–52.

42. *WCJ* 1 (March 1, 1846) 119; An Aged Physician (= William A. Alcott), *Forty Years in the Wilderness of Pills and Powders* (Boston, 1859) 232; Andrew Combe, *Principles of Physiology* (NY, 1837) 38–

39; William Turnbull, *Manual on Health*, 2d ed. (NY, 1835) 64 (quote), 67n; Gove, *Lectures to Women*, 26; Joel Shew, "Insensible perspiration," *WCJ* 16 (1853) 1–2; John H. Griscom, *First Lessons in Human Physiology*, 2d ed. (NY, 1846) 45–46, 83; and Beecher, *Letters to the People*, quote on 72.

43. George H. Taylor, *Illustrated Sketch of the Movement Cure* (NY, 1866), and Andrew Combe, *Physiology of Digestion* (Boston, 1836) 225. See also Harvey Green, *Fit for America* (NY, 1986) 85, 91–94, 100.

44. Dio Lewis, *Our Girls* (NY, 1871) esp. 85–88, 91–92, 357. On Lewis see Mary F. Eastman, *The Biography of Dio Lewis, A.M., M.D.* (NY, 1891); Henry R. Viets, "Lewis, Dioclesian," *DAB* VI, 209; and Norma Schwendener, *A History of Physical Education in the United States* (NY, 1942) ch. 6.

45. Dio Lewis, *The New Gymnastics*, 18th ed. (Boston, 1881 [1862]) esp. 7–15; Lewis, *Our Girls*, 21, 345–47; and Fred E. Leonard, "The 'New Gymnastics' of Dio Lewis," *APER* 11 (1906) 83–95, 187–98.

46. "Muscle-mania," *Amer Phrenological J* 32 (Dec 1860) 84; Lewis, *The New Gymnastics*, 72, 79, 82; Lewis, *Our Girls*, 69 (quotes), 191, 239; and Dio Lewis, *Our Digestion* (Philadelphia, 1872) 28, 131 (quote), 192 (quote).

47. Lewis, *Our Digestion*, 32, 85–92; Lewis, *Our Girls*, 85–92, 305–7; and "Fleshiness," *Letter Box* 2 (Sept 1859) 73.

48. Lewis, *The New Gymnastics*, 16; Lewis, *Our Girls*, 226, 37–44, 284–86; Institute for Physical Education (Boston), *Physical Education* (Boston, 1862?) 211–60 on the Schreber Pangymnastikon, and cf. Morton Schatzman, *Soul Murder* (NY, 1973) ch. 4.

49. Lewis, *The New Gymnastics*, 124–51, 207–19.

50. Page Smith, *Trial by Fire* (NY, 1982) 63; Bruce Catton, *Mr. Lincoln's Army,* (NY, 1962) 179–84; and W. W. Hall, *Soldier-Health Army Edition* (NY, 1861) esp. 14, 15, 23.

51. Oliver Wendell Holmes, "My hunt after the Captain," *Pages from an Old Volume of Life* (Boston, 1904) and *Life and Letters*, ed. John T. Morse, Jr. (Boston, 1896) II, 167, letter of Aug 29, 1862, both excerpted in Lindeman, *Conflict of Convictions*, 106, 94, and Hitchcock, *Dyspepsy Forestalled*, 360. For the poetic snippets, see Walt Whitman, "The Wound Dresser," Margaret J. Preston, "The Shade of the Trees," and James B. Hope, "Under One Blanket," in Newcomer et al., *Three Centuries of American Poetry and Prose*, 761, 816–17, 820.

52. George M. Beard, "Neurasthenia, or nervous exhaustion," *BMSJ* 80 (1869) 217–19; idem, "Other symptoms of neurasthenia," *JNMD* 6

(1879) 246–61; idem, *Practical Treatise on Nervous Exhaustion (Neurasthenia)*, ed. A. D. Rockwell, 5th ed. (NY, 1905 [1880]); and idem, *American Nervousness* (NY, 1881) 78. Brieger, "Dyspepsia: the American disease?" 184, also notes the shift from dyspepsia to neurasthenia. On Beard I have used G. Alder Blumer, "Beard, George Miller," *DAB* I, 92–93; Barbara Sicherman, "The paradox of prudence: mental health in the Gilded Age," *JAH* 62 (1976) 890–912; and Charles E. Rosenberg, "George M. Beard and American nervousness," *No Other Gods*, ch. 5.

53. Charles Caldwell, *Thoughts on Physical Education* (Boston, 1834) quote on 94; Samuel Tissot, *Remarks on the Disorders of Literary Men* (Boston, 1825 [1758]) 11, 60; *Amer Art-Union Tr* (1844) quote on 7; and John H. Griscom, *Sanitary Condition of the Laboring Population of New York* (NY, 1842) 20.

54. *Health Reformer* 3,9 (1869) 174, correspondence column; James H. Robbins, "American dyspepsia," *BMSJ* 107 (1882) 132–34 is nicely transitional, and cf. Edward Wakefield, "Nervousness: the national disease of America," *McClure's Mag* 2 (Feb 1894) 302–7. The transition was slow; Mary Newton Henderson in *The Aristocracy of Health* (NY, 1906) 43, would still describe "Americanitis" as "a very disrespectful name given to a compound illness composed of dyspepsia and nervous conditions."

55. John Higham, *Strangers in the Land: Patterns of American Nativism, 1860–1925*, 2d ed. (NY, 1965); Robert P. Hudson, "The biography of disease: lessons from chlorosis," *BHM* 51 (1977) 448–63; Joan J. Brumberg, "Chlorotic girls, 1870–1920," in *Women and Health in America*, ed. Judith W. Leavitt (Madison, Wisc., 1984) 186–95; Degler, *At Odds*, 180–83; Ellen K. Rothman, *Hands and Hearts: A History of Courtship in America* (NY, 1984) 249, 265, and cf. a modern study with a peculiarly 19th-century tone, Mel Davies, "Corsets and conception: fashion and demographic trends in the 19th century," *CSSH* 24 (1982) 611–41.

56. Gerald N. Grob, *Mental Illness and American Society, 1875–1940* (Princeton, N.J., 1983) 8; [Robert Tomes], "Why we get sick," *Harper's New Monthly Mag* 13 (1856) 644; Blumer, "Beard, George Miller"; and Francis G. Gosling, III, "American Nervousness: A Study in Medical and Social Values in the Gilded Age, 1870–1900," Ph.D. thesis, Univ of Oklahoma, 1976.

57. Beard, *A Practical Treatise*, 40–43, 54, 58, 61; Holmes, "Dread and the newspapers," *Pages from an Old Volume of Life*, excerpted in Lindeman, *Conflict of Convictions*, 45; Nichols, *Forty Years*, 210–11; Frank S. Presbrey, *History and Development of Advertising* (Garden City, N.Y., 1929) 210; and S. P. Fullinwider, "Neurasthenia: the

genteel caste's journey inward," *Rocky Mountain Social Science J* 11, 2 (1974) 1–9 on attention.

58. David H. Fischer, *Growing Old in America* (NY, 1977) 80, 91, 122, 130, 224–28; Carole Haber, *Beyond Sixty-Five* (Cambridge, 1983) 62–64, ch. 6; and W. Andrew Achenbaum, *Old Age in the New Land* (Baltimore, 1978) ch. 3.

59. Augustus Hoppin, *A Fashionable Sufferer* (Boston, 1883) quote on 13; Beard, *A Practical Treatise*, 192–207; and T. J. Jackson Lears, *No Place of Grace: Antimodernism and the Transformation of American Culture 1880–1920* (NY, 1981) 51–56.

60. Anna R. Burr, *Weir Mitchell* (NY, 1929) esp. 32, 104–7, 121; Richard D. Walter, *S. Weir Mitchell, M.D., Neurologist* (Springfield, Ill., 1970) 47–61, 91; and W. Bruce Fye, "S. Weir Mitchell, Philadelphia's 'lost' physiologist," *BHM* 57 (1983) 188–202.

61. There was a change at midcentury from feeding down to feeding up the sick person, so that an increase in weight was a good sign in both the tubercular patient and the neurasthenic. Dr. George S. Keith dated this change circa 1845 in his *Plea for a Simpler Life* (London, 1901) xx, 4. Cf. Lorna Duffin, "The conspicuous consumptive: woman as an invalid," in *The Nineteenth-Century Woman*, eds. Sara Delamont and Lorna Duffin (London, 1978) 26–56.

62. On neurasthenia among men and the working class, see "A feminine rebellion," *Insurance Monitor* 31 (1883) 346; Stow Persons, *Decline of American Gentility* (NY 1973) 285; James B. Gilbert, *Work Without Salvation: America's Intellectuals and Industrial Alienation, 1880–1910* (Baltimore, 1977) 31–36; and Barbara Sicherman, "The uses of a diagnosis: doctors, patients, and neurasthenia," *JHM* 32 (1977) 33–54.

63. On the charismatic and authoritarian nature of the rest cure, see esp. T. W. Fisher, "Neurasthenia," *BMSJ* 86 (1872) 72; J. S. Green, "Neurasthenia: its causes and home treatment," *BMSJ* 109 (1883) 75–78; Charlotte Perkins Gilman, "The Yellow Wall-Paper" (1892) in Ann J. Lane, ed., *The Charlotte Perkins Gilman Reader* (NY, 1980) 3–20; Burr, *Weir Mitchell*, 185; and Suzanne Poirier, "The Weir Mitchell rest cure: doctor and patients," *Women's Studies* 10 (1983) 15–40. Mitchell quote is from his *Characteristics* (1892) in his *Works* (NY 1915) III, 219.

64. Sicherman, "Uses of a diagnosis," 32 (quoting Margaret Cleaves), 34; Edwin L. Bynner, "Diary of a nervous invalid," *Atlantic Monthly* 71 (Jan 1893) 33–46; and Margaret A. Cleaves, *Autobiography of a Neurasthene* (Boston, 1910) esp. 96.

65. S. Weir Mitchell, *The Early History of Instrumental Precision in Medicine* (New Haven, 1892) 18–21, 32–42.

CHAPTER FOUR
The Balanced Body at Century's Turn

1. Tom D. Crouch, *A Dream of Wings: Americans and the Airplane, 1875–1905* (NY, 1981) quotes on 113–14, 213. I am heavily indebted to this book for the material on flight in the following pages.

2. Albert F. Hill, "Bicycle," *Encyclopaedia Britannica*, 9th ed. (NY, 1886) Supp. I, 515–16 (quote), and Crouch, *Dream of Wings*, 162, 229 (quotes), 230, 290, 295.

3. Crouch, *Dream of Wings*, 13–15.

4. *Ibid.*, 235, 252.

5. Genevieve Stebbins, *Delsarte System of Expression*, 6th ed. (NY, 1902 [1885]); Claude L. Shaver, "Steele MacKaye and the Delsartian tradition," in *History of Speech Education in America*, ed. Karl R. Wallace (NY, 1954) 202–18; Nancy Lee Ruyter, *Reformers and Visionaries: The Americanization of the Art of Dance* (NY, 1979) ch. 2; and Wisconsin State Historical Society (Madison), Homeopathic Medical Society of the State of Wisconsin, MSS 14 PB/4, Minutes, Oct 18, 1865–May 19, 1910, vol. one, 282–83 (= 1892 Transactions), comment by Dr. E. H. Pratt.

6. Charles W. Emerson, *Physical Culture*, 2d ed. (Boston, 1891) 14, 42 (quote), 82 (quote); John F. Bovard and Frederick W. Cozens, *Tests and Measurements in Physical Education* (Philadelphia, 1930), a good overview; and Isabel Chapin Barrows, ed., *Physical Training* (Boston, 1890).

7. Elizabeth Kendall, *Where She Danced: The Birth of American Art-Dance* (NY, 1979) Part 1; Ruyter, *Reformers and Visionaries*, 23, 35; and Crouch, *Dream of Wings*, 230.

8. Joseph J. Corn, *The Winged Gospel: America's Romance with Aviation, 1900–1950* (NY, 1982) esp. 72.

9. Daniel Nelson, *Frederick W. Taylor and the Rise of Scientific Management* (Madison, Wisc., 1980); Alfred D. Chandler, *The Visible Hand: The Managerial Revolution in American Business* (Cambridge, Mass., 1977) 272–83, 438, 445; Dan Clawson, *Bureaucracy and the Labor Process* (NY, 1980) 30–33, 153–56, 201–53; and Harry Braverman, *Labor and Monopoly Capital* (NY, 1974) ch. 4.

10. Frederick W. Taylor, *Principles of Scientific Management* (NY, 1911) 5, 117, and Nelson, *Frederick W. Taylor*, 102.

11. Nelson, *Frederick W. Taylor*, 131–36; Edna Yost, *Frank and Lillian Gilbreth* (New Brunswick, N.J., 1949); and Siegfried Giedion, *Mechanization Takes Command* (NY, 1969) 17–29, 96–106.

12. On dance and movement instruction, see Hillel Schwartz, "The zipper and the child," in *Notebooks in Cultural Analysis, Volume II*, eds. Norman F. Cantor and Nathalia King (Durham, N.C., 1985) 1–28.

13. Bettina Berch, "Scientific management in the home: the Empress's new clothes," *J of Amer Culture* 3 (1980) 442. On the pervasiveness of scientific management, see Samuel Haber, *Efficiency and Uplift: Scientific Management in the Progressive Era, 1890–1920* (Chicago, 1964).

14. Adelaide Hechtlinger, *The Seasonal Hearth* (Woodstock, N.Y., 1977) quote from Ellet on 40; Schlesinger Library, Radcliffe College, MSS B-14, Mothers' Club of Cambridge, Records 1881–1942, vol. one, Meetings 1881–86, 10th Meeting, March 1, 1882; and Marion Harland (= Mary Virginia Terhune), *Eve's Daughters* (NY, 1882) 325.

15. On women's work I have used Susan E. Kennedy, *If All We Did Was to Weep at Home* (Bloomington, Ind., 1979) and Alice Kessler-Harris, *Out to Work* (NY, 1982). On the redesigned and influential typewriter, see Yost, *Gilbreth*, 261, and Margery W. Davies, *Woman's Place Is at the Typewriter: Office Work and Office Workers, 1870–1930* (Philadelphia, 1982) ch. 6. On home economics education, see Isabel Bevier and Susannah Usher, *The Home Economics Movement* (Boston, 1906) with chronology on 94–95, and Emma S. Weigley, "It might have been euthenics: the Lake Placid Conference and the Home Economics Movement," *Amer Q* 26 (1974) 80.

16. René Bache, "Women as inventors," *Technical World Mag* (Aug 1906) 617; Jonathan L. Fairbanks and Elizabeth B. Bates, *American Furniture, 1620 to the Present* (NY, 1981) 366–69, 413; Robert Bishop, *Centuries and Styles of the American Chair 1640–1970* (NY, 1972) 419; and Giedion, *Mechanization*, 473.

17. Landauer, Green Box (Clothing—Women's), Chicago Corset Company Mother Goose Picture Book, 1894, p. 3; William Leach, *True Love and Perfect Union* (NY, 1980) 259; and Reduso ad in *Delineator* 73 (April 1909) 519.

18. Giedion, *Mechanization*, 528–36, 554–55; idem, *Space, Time and Architecture* (Cambridge, Mass., 1947) 287–89; Kathleen A. Smallzried, *The Everlasting Pleasure: Influences on America's Kitchens . . .* (NY, 1956) 94–101, 115, 120–22; Kimberley W. Carrell, "The Industrial Revolution comes to the home: kitchen design reform and middle-class women," *J of Amer Culture* 2 (1979) 488–99; Gwendolyn Wright, *Moralism and the Modern Home* (Chicago, 1980) 37, 239, 244; Roger L. Welsch, "An interdependence of foodways and architecture," in *Food in Perspective*, eds. A. Fenton and

T. M. Owen (Edinburgh, 1981) 365–75; and Susan Strasser, *Never Done: A History of American Housework* (NY, 1982) 41, 46, 61, 63.

19. David P. Handlin, *The American Home: Architecture and Society, 1815–1915* (NY, 1978) 404–25, esp. 417–19 on Mary Pattison's 1915 book, *Principles of Domestic Engineering;* Christine Frederick, *Household Engineering: Scientific Management in the Home* (Chicago, 1919); Giedion, *Mechanization,* 516–21; Caroline L. Hunt, *Life of Ellen Richards* (Boston, 1912) 183; Elizabeth S. Kirkland, *Six Little Cooks* (Chicago, 1877) 32, 34, 65; and Bruce M. Watson and Charles E. White, *Intermediate Arithmetic* (Boston, 1910). For a recent assessment of the domestic scientists, see Laura Shapiro, *Perfection Salad* (NY, 1986).

20. *Six Hundred Dollars a Year: A Wife's Effort at Low Living Under High Prices* (Boston, 1867); Bevier and Usher, *Home Economics Movement,* 45; Christine Terhune Herrick, *Liberal Living upon Narrow Means* (Boston, 1890); Hunt, *Ellen Richards,* 223, 225; and Mary J. Lincoln, "Poverty suppers," *Amer Kitchen Mag* 4 (1896) 172–75.

21. Weigley, "It might have been euthenics," 86; Dee Garrison, *Apostles of Culture: The Public Librarian and American Society 1876–1920* (NY, 1979) 119; and Ellen H. Richards, *The Cost of Food,* 2d ed. (NY, 1910) 9.

22. Mary L. Wade, "Healthful and economical foods," *Amer Kitchen Mag* 5 (1896) 33 and see Harvey Levenstein, "The New England Kitchen and the origins of modern American eating habits," *Amer Q* 32 (1980) 369–86.

23. See Samuel P. Hays, *Conservation and the Gospel of Efficiency: The Progressive Conservation Movement 1890–1920* (NY, 1959).

24. Weigley, "It might have been euthenics," 80; Donald B. Meyer, *The Positive Thinkers* (Garden City, N.Y., 1965) esp. 78; Dio Lewis, *The New Gymnastics,* 18th ed. (Boston, 1881) 82; Anna C. Brackett, "Physical education, or, the culture of the body," in *The Education of American Girls,* ed. Brackett (NY, 1886) 29; and David M. Potter, *People of Plenty: Economic Abundance and the American Character* (Chicago, 1954). Ruth Schwartz Cowan warns against a too-ready acceptance of the idea that the modern household is no longer a productive unit; *More Work for Mother* (NY, 1983) ch. 4.

25. Diane Lindstrom, "Macroeconomic growth: the U.S. in the 19th century," *JIH* 13 (1983) 679–705; Amasa Walker, *The Science of Wealth,* 3rd ed. (Boston, 1866) 383, 391; David A. Wells, *Recent Economic Changes* (NY, 1889) excerpted in *The Transformation of American Society, 1870–1890,* ed. John A. Garraty (Columbia, S.C., 1968) 55; Robert H. Wiebe, *The Search for Order, 1877–1920* (NY, 1967) esp.

25, 31; William Hope Harvey, *Coin's Financial School* (Chicago, 1894) preface, 130; and Alan Trachtenberg, *The Incorporation of America* (NY, 1982) 39, 211.

26. Simon N. Patten, *Over-nutrition and Its Social Consequences* (Philadelphia, 1897); Hunt, *Ellen Richards*, 233; Daniel M. Fox, *The Discovery of Abundance* (Ithaca, N.Y., 1967); and Daniel Horowitz, *The Morality of Spending: Attitudes Toward the Consumer Society in America, 1875–1940* (Baltimore, 1985) esp. 30–66.

27. The concern with overnutrition arose at the same time as a new disease was being identified among the well-to-do: kleptomania. Amidst the open splendors of the new department stores, women who could afford the merchandise were stealing it instead. Like overnutrition, kleptomania was considered a form of taking-without-needing. See Patricia O'Brien, "The kleptomania diagnosis," *JSH* 17 (1983) 65–78; William Leach, "Transformation in a culture of consumption: women and department stores, 1890–1925," *JAH* 71 (1984) 319–42; and William A. Hammond, "A problem for sociologists," *North Amer R* 135 (1882) 422–32.

28. Wilbur O. Atwater, "Pecuniary economy of food," *Century Mag* 35 (Jan 1888) 437, 442.

29. Wilbur O. Atwater, *Methods and Results of Investigations on the Chemistry and Economy of Food* (Washington, D.C., 1895); Charles E. Rosenberg, "Atwater, Wilbur Olin," *DSB* 1, 325–26; and Nelson, *Frederick W. Taylor*, 43, 60.

30. Cf. Naomi Aronson, "Social definitions of entitlement: food needs 1885–1920," *Media, Culture and Society* 4 (1982) 51–61; idem, "Nutrition as a social problem," *Social Problems* 29 (1982) 474–87.

31. See esp. Illinois Bureau of Labor Statistics, "Earnings, expenses and conditions of workingmen and their families," *Third Biennial Report* (Springfield, Ill., 1884), liberally excerpted in Garraty, ed., *Transformation of American Society*, 115–36.

32. Aronson, "Nutrition as a social problem," 482.

33. John L. Hess and Karen Hess, *The Taste of America* (NY, 1977) 56–61, 114, 125, 129, and Shapiro, *Perfection Salad*, ch. 8.

34. Charlotte Perkins Gilman, *The Home* (NY, 1903); Dolores Hayden, *The Grand Domestic Revolution: A History of Feminist Designs for American Homes, Neighborhoods and Cities* (Cambridge, Mass., 1981); Wright, *Moralism and the Modern Home* 158–60, 167, 294; and Handlin, *The American Home*, 388–404.

35. See e.g., Anna Merritt East, *Kitchenette Cookery* (Boston, 1917) with tips for small-quantity buying, 31.

36. Hunt, *Ellen Richards* 291 on inexorable law.

37. "Fat men and clams," *NYT* (Aug 15, 1879) 8:2; "Fat men dining by the sea," *NYDT* (Sept, 7, 1887) 2:1; "Fat men's club gives up," *NYDT* (Sept 11, 1903) 14:1; John Burke, *Duet in Diamonds: The Flamboyant Saga of Lillian Russell and Diamond Jim Brady* (NY, 1972) 126–27, and Lois Banner, *American Beauty* (NY, 1983) 135.

38. Robert D. Bowden, *Boies Penrose* rept. (Freeport, N.Y., 1971) 207–8; Rudolph Marx, *Health of the Presidents* (NY, 1960) 303 on Taft; *City Life, or the Boys of New York* (NY, 1889), board game in NY Historical Society collection; Mary N. Henderson, *Aristocracy of Health* (NY, 1906) 154; "Being fat is like having money in the bank," *NYT* (May 15, 1910) V, 11 on the suicide; and A. Johnson Dodge, "General or embalmers' anatomy," *Amer Undertaker* 1 (Dec 1900) 37. For the cartoons, see the Picture Collection, NY Public Library, 42d Street Branch, Obesity folders: *Hearth and Home* (May 24, 1873) 340; *Harper's Weekly* (Jan 24, 1874); Chester L. Garde, "Figures of speech," *Harper's Weekly* (March 6, 1909) and others.

39. "On growing fat," *Atlantic Monthly* 99 (March 1907) 430–31; *Yankee Notions* 1 (1852) 157, cartoon playing on ambiguities of "stout"; Brenda Ueland, *Me* (NY, 1939) 60 on "sod-packer"; and Burton Stevenson, *Home Book of Proverbs, Maxims and Familiar Phrases* (NY, 1961) 764–65 on Reed and Arbuckle. For the other words, see *OED* II, 399, 402; III, 715; VII, 1131; VIII, 1567; X, 1047–48; XI, 443; Laurence Urdang and Nancy La Roche, *Picturesque Expressions* (Detroit 1980) 57–58; Eric Partridge, *Dictionary of Slang and Unconventional English*, 7th ed. (NY, 1970) 446–47, 916; and Mitford M. Mathews, *Dictionary of Americanisms on Historical Principles* (Chicago, 1951) 916.

40. Shepard B. Clough, *A Century of American Life Insurance: A History of the Mutual Life Insurance Company of New York, 1843–1943* (NY, 1946) 77–78; Harold M. Frost, "History and philosophy of life insurance medicine," in *Life Insurance and Medicine*, eds. Harry E. Ungerleider and Richard S. Gubner (Springfield, Ill., 1958) 203–4; J. Adams Allen, *Medical Examinations for Life Insurance*, 2d ed. (Chicago, 1867) 56; "Excessive weight," *Med Record* 8 (1873) 584; Edward H. Sieveking, *The Medical Advisor in Life Insurance*, 2d ed. (Hartford, 1886) 38n; and Henry W. Coe, "Overweight," *Med Examiner* 5 (1895) 32. See also "Insurance and assurance," *Graham's Mag* 14 (1839) 265–68 for an account of an early insurance examination, with higher premiums for those of large girth.

41. William Cahn, *A Matter of Life and Death: The Connecticut Mutual Story* (NY, 1970) 146–47; Henry F. Pringle, *Life and Times of William Howard Taft* (NY, 1939) I, 3, 166–67 (quote), 286 (quote) and II, 1072; and Judith I. Anderson, *William Howard Taft* (NY, 1981)

quotes on 28, 29. For the older Big Man view, see Mark Sullivan, *Our Times. III. Pre-War America* (NY, 1930) 14–15 on Taft.

42. Noel F. Busch, *T.R.* (NY, 1963) 173–74; Sullivan, *Our Times. III. Pre-War America* 13 and *IV. War Begins* (NY, 1932) 300, 347; Dorothy P. Ryan, *Picture Postcards in the U.S. 1893–1918* (NY, 1982) 94, Taft as Possum; and Anderson, *Taft*, quote on 28.

43. Denis T. Lynch, *Grover Cleveland: A Man Four Square* (NY, 1932) 88; Siva, *A Man of Destiny* (Chicago, 1885) 11; *The Fat Knight* (n.p., 1896) Canto 1, lines 2–5; and Joseph Simms, *Physiognomy Illustrated*, 9th ed. (NY, 1889) 50.

44. Landauer, Green Box (Digestive, Box 3, Tonics and Bitters), file on Stomach Bitters, Mrs. President Cleveland portrayed on ad for A. P. Ordway, Boston, Sulphur Bitters; Leslie Dorsey and Janice Devine, *Fare Thee Well* (NY, 1964) 216; "Mr. Windom drops dead," *NYT* (Jan 30, 1891) 1:7–2:3; *Med Examiner* 5 (1895) 135 on banquet; T. J. Jackson Lears, *No Place of Grace* (NY, 1981) 12; and Harrietta O. Ward, *Sensible Etiquette of the Best Society*, 18th ed. (Philadelphia, 1878) 175, contrasted to Margaret W. Livingston, *Correct Social Usage*, 6th ed. (NY, 1906) II, 400–01, 404. See also Susan Williams, *Savory Suppers and Fashionable Feasts* (NY, 1985) and Harvey Green, *Fit for America* (NY, 1986) 160.

On cautions against overeating in middle age, see Mrs. E. G. Cook, "Sanitarian," *Demorest's Monthly Mag* 23 (1887) 716; Rachel B. Gleason, *Talks to My Patients*, 8th ed. (NY, 1887) 173; and Emma F. Angell Drake, *What a Woman of Forty-Five Ought to Know* (London, 1902) 61. On the proportion of older Americans, see David H. Fischer, *Growing Old in America* (NY, 1977) Table IV.

45. Lillian Russell, "Reminiscences," *Cosmopolitan* (May 1922) 92; Alan Dale (= Alfred Cohen), *Familiar Chats with Queens of the Stage* (NY, 1890) 87; George C. D. Odell, *Annals of the New York Stage* (NY, 1940) XII, 238, 355; Banner, *American Beauty*, ch. 7; and Dorsey and Devine, *Fare Thee Well*, 75.

46. René Edouard-Joseph, *Dictionnaire biographique des artistes contemporaines 1910–1930* (Paris, 1930) I, 178; Bouguereau paintings reproduced in *Famous Pictures Reproduced from Renowned Paintings by the World's Greatest Artists* (Chicago, 1902) 117, 140, 197, 243, 259, a collection of soft pornography; Susan C. Power, *The Ugly-girl Papers* (NY, 1875) 233, 226; Emma E. Walker, "Pretty girl papers," *LHJ* 22 (Jan 1905) 33; Daniel G. Brinton and George H. Napheys, *Laws of Health in Relation to the Human Form* (Springfield, Mass., 1871) 37; and Madame Qui Vive (= Helen F. Stevans Jameson), *The Woman Beautiful* (Chicago, 1901) 149.

47. Brinton and Napheys, *Laws of Health*, 9; Fischer, *Growing Old*, 83–85; "Ballad of Peter Smith," *Harper's Weekly* 1 (Oct 3, 1857) 628;

Frank Harris, *My Life and Loves*, ed. John F. Gallagher (NY, 1963) 160; and Sheila Jeffreys, "'Free from all uninvited touch of man': women's campaigns around sexuality, 1880–1914," *Women's Studies International Forum* 5 (1982) 639, 644.

48. Patrick Bade, *Femme Fatale* (NY, 1979); Martha Kingsbury, "The femme fatale and her sisters," in *Woman as Sex Object*, eds. Hess and Nochlin (NY, 1972) 182–205; Mario Praz, *The Romantic Agony*, trans. Angus Davidson (London, 1933) 258 for quote; Banner, *American Beauty*, 51–52; Ryan, *Picture Postcards*, 182–96; and Ann U. Abrams, "Frozen goddess: the image of woman in turn-of-the-century American art," in *Woman's Being, Woman's Place*, ed. Mary Kelley (Boston, 1979) 93–108.

49. Ryan, *Picture Postcards*, 195; Erik Nórgaard, *With Love To You: A History of the Erotic Postcard* (London, 1969) esp. 54–55; Ralph Stein, *The Pin Up* (Chicago, 1974); Mark Gabor, *The Pin-Up: A Modest History* (NY, 1972); William Culp Darrah and Richard Russack, *An Album of Stereographs* (Garden City, N.Y., 1977) esp. 12, 22, 36; Banner, *American Beauty*, chs. 7–8; Valerie Steele, *Fashion and Eroticism* (NY, 1985) ch. 6; and Jeanne M. Weimann, *The Fair Women* (Chicago, 1981) 475, reproduction of title page. The two images corresponded to a cultural ambivalence about abundance and self-control, an ambivalence elegantly dissected by Anita Clair Fellman and Michael Fellman, *Making Sense of Self: Medical Advice Literature in Late Nineteenth-Century America* (Philadelphia, 1981) esp. 137.

50. Alison Gernsheim, *Fashion and Reality 1840–1914* (London, 1963) 69–70, 77; Estelle A. Worrell, *American Costume 1840–1920* (Harrisburg, 1979) 91–94, 108–9, 130–32; Carol Wald, *Myth America: Picturing Women 1865–1945* (NY, 1975) 94–99; Anne Hollander, *Seeing Through Clothes* (NY, 1978) 152, 328, 332, 338–39, with the social impact of photography dated far too late; Gilbert Vail, *A History of Cosmetics in America* (NY, 1947) esp. 115; and Henry Blossom, *The Slim Princess*, musical comedy in three acts, music by Leslie Stuart and based on a novel by George Ade (1907), performed at the Globe Theatre on Jan 2, 1911, script at the NY Public Library, Theatre Collection, Lincoln Center of the Performing Arts.

51. "Being fat is like having money in the bank," *NYT* (May 15, 1910) V, 11.

52. Maria Parloa, *First Principles of Household Management and Cookery*, new ed. (Boston, 1888) 125; Mary Hinman Abel, *Practical Sanitary and Economic Cooking Adapted to Persons of Moderate and Small Means* (Rochester, N.Y., 1890) 67–69; and Sarah T. Rorer, "How to live on a thousand a year," *Table Talk* 4 (March 1889) 97.

53. Emma S. Weigley, *Sarah Tyson Rorer* (Philadelphia, 1977); Christine Frederick, *The New Housekeeping* (Garden City, N.Y., 1914) esp. ch. 16; Weimann, *Fair Women*, 459; Rorer, "How to live on a thousand a year," 97 for quote; and Schlesinger Library, Radcliffe College, Sarah Tyson Rorer Papers, 1929–1938, Dr. Dippell's eulogy.

54. Sarah Tyson Rorer, "The best foods for stout and thin women," *LHJ* 15 (July 1898) 23 (quote); idem, "Mrs. Rorer's cooking school," *LHJ* 18 (Nov 1901) 22; idem, *Mrs. Rorer's New Cook Book* (Philadelphia, 1902) 12; and Weigley, *Sarah Tyson Rorer*, 125–26, 140 (quote), 141, 147, 163 (quote).

55. Rorer, "Best foods," 23; idem, *New Cook Book*, 12; idem, "Mrs. Rorer's answers to questions," *LHJ* 16 (April 1899) 47 and 15 (Jan 1898) 31; and idem, "Food for fleshy people," *Household News* 3 (1895) 193. Cf. Shapiro, *Perfection Salad*, 17, 233.

56. See, e.g., *LHJ* 16 (Oct 1899) 48; *Household News* 4 (1896) 194; and Weigley, *Sarah Tyson Rorer*, 77.

57. American Medical Association (AMA), *Obesity Cure Fakes* (Chicago, 1914) 41–42; *Nostrums* II, 283–85; Warshaw, Collection 60, Box 51, Walker Pharmacal Co. "Too Much Fat Is Dangerous" (St. Louis, n.d.); Roland C. Curtin, "The heart and its danger in the treatment of obesity," *J of Balneology and Climatology* 12 (1908) 229–30 on phytolacca; James T. Whittaker, "On the use of arsenic in the treatment of obesity," *Cincinnati Lancet-Clinic* n.s. 1 (1878) 133–35; and Ernest F. Robinson, "Some experience with obesity treatment," *AJCM* 17 (1910) 392 on strychnine.

58. Samuel H. Adams, *The Great American Fraud* (NY, 1906) 144–46; *Nostrums* II, 676 (Biel); AMA, "*Obesity Cures*" (Chicago, 1929?) 9; Editorial, "Anti-fat remedies," *NYT* (Jan 7, 1906) 6:4–5 (quote); "Cult of slimness," *Living Age* 280 (Feb 28, 1914) 574; and Richard Hudnut, *On the Treatment of Obesity or Excess of Fat* (NY, 1896) 31, 33, 36. In George Burwell's *Obesity and the Cure* (Boston, 1892), twenty-five of the sixty testimonials were from men.

59. C. J. B. Williams, "Obesity," *Cyclopaedia of Practical Medicine*, ed. John Forbes et al. (Philadelphia, 1845) III, 410; Wooster Beach, *Family Physician* (Cincinnati, 1862) 467, 821; G. Hungerford, "A case in practice," *Chicago Med Times* 7 (1875) 145–47; A. W. Rogers, "Excessive deposit of fat over the abdomen," *New Jersey Med Soc Tr* (1876) 296; *National Druggist* 30 (1900) 395; and *Young Ladies J* 39 (1892) ad on 47.

60. "Corpulency and gluttony," *GJHL* 2 (1838) 293–94; "How to cure obesity," *Library of Health* 6 (1842) 152–54; and X.Y.Z., "How to get thin," *Harper's Bazaar* 41 (Sept 1907) 883.

61. Elmer V. McCollum, *A History of Nutrition* (Boston, 1957) 420, citing Beccari and Haller on gluten; William T. Cathell, "Overfatness," *Maryland Med J* 37 (1897) 163; A. W. Perry, "Nature and treatment of obesity, or corpulence of the middle-aged," *California St J of Med* 1 (1903) 357; Artemas Ward, *The Grocer's Encyclopedia* (NY, 1911) 246—these last three references giving variant proportions of fat and water in the body; Brinton and Napheys, *Laws of Health*, 43 on fluid bloat; Emma E. Walker, "The place of water in our diet," *Success Mag* (April 1906) in Walker Papers, Sophia Smith Collection, Smith College; James J. Walsh, "Some dangers of obesity cures," *Int Clinics* 24th ser., 4 (1914) 65–66 against restricting fluids; and Sarah T. Rorer, "Water fattening," *Household News* 2 (1894) 347. For a fine example of confusions about fluids, see William G. Sutherland, *On Corpulence and Thinness as Curable Conditions* (London, 1901) 8.

62. The milk cure was promoted in the late 17th century by Dr. Thomas Sydenham as an antidote to hysteria. *Works of Thomas Sydenham*, trans. R. G. Latham (London, 1850 [1685]) II, 105–6; Philippe Karell, "De la cure de lait," *Archives générales de médecine* ser 6, 8 (1866) 513–33, 694–704; George H. Rohé, "On corpulence, especially its treatment by a pure milk diet," *Maryland Med J* 20 (1889) 281–85; S. Weir Mitchell, *Fat and Blood* (Philadelphia, 1877) 27 and cf. 8th ed. (1902) 128–29, suggesting the use of skim milk for a reducing diet.

63. Walter Mendelson, "Physiological treatment of obesity," *Med Record* 37 (1890) 176–77, summary of the fuel-food/tissue-food theory, and Alice Worthington Winthrop, "Hygiene for the stout," *Harper's Bazaar* 33 (June 30, 1900) 565.

64. [William E. Aytoun], "Banting on corpulence," *Blackwood's Mag* 96 (Nov 1864) 607–17; J. S. Buist, "Mr. Banting's 'Excellent Adviser,' William Harvey, F.R.C.S. (1806–1876)," *Practitioner* 194 (1965) 415–20; Rodney Bennett-England, *As Young as You Look* (London, 1970) 76 on Wellington's coffin; William Banting, *Letter on Corpulence Addressed to the Public*, 3d ed. (London, 1864) and 5th ed., with Addendas and Remarks by Mr. Harvey, F.R.C.S. (London, 1865); William Harvey, *On Corpulence in Relation to Disease* (London, 1872); Power, *Ugly-girl Papers*, 175, 183; and *OED* I, 659. The contemporary physician John Harvey, often confused with William, also published a diet book, *Corpulence, Its Diminution and Cure*, 3d ed. (London, 1864), and he too referred to deafness being caused by fat pressing on the Eustachian tube, p. 18. Carol Guilford has conveniently reprinted the Banting 3d edition in her *The Diet Book* (NY, 1973) 163–200, arguing incorrectly that Banting's was the first high-fat low-carbohydrate diet.

65. Victor C. Vaughan, "Reduction of corpulency," *Physician and Sur-*

geon 1 (1879) 287; Alfred C. Croftan, "Dietetics of obesity," *JAMA* 47 (1906) 821; Mai Thomas, *Grannies' Remedies* (NY, 1967) 72–73; "Simple methods of flesh reduction," *Harper's Bazaar* 42 (July 1908) 704; and Lincoln, *Mrs. Lincoln's Boston Cook Book*, 432.

66. Clyde L. Cummer, "Dr. James H. Salisbury and the Salisbury diet," *Ohio St Archaeological and Historical Q* 59 (1950) 352–70; Richard J. Hooker, *Food and Drink in America* (Indianapolis, 1981) 246; James H. Salisbury, *The Relation of Alimentation and Disease*, 3d ed. (NY, 1895 [1888]) iii–v.

67. Cummer, "Dr. James H. Salisbury," and Salisbury, *Alimentation and Disease*, 18, 21, 145.

68. Salisbury, *Alimentation and Disease*, 97, 168, 172.

69. *Ibid.*, 97, 112; T. J. McGillicuddy, "Diet and regimen for the diminution of fat," *NY St Med Assoc Tr* 11 (1894) 308; James H. Robbins, "American dyspepsia," *BMSJ* 107 (1882) 133 (quote); and Crouch, *Dream of Wings*, 23. Cf. "Era of predigestion," *Atlantic Monthly* 104 (Nov 1909) 714.

70. William Towers-Smith, "Dietetic treatment of obesity," *Providence Med J* 10 (1891) 451; William Tibbles, *Dietetics or Food in Health and Disease* (Philadelphia, 1914?) 455; Isaac Burney Yeo, *Food in Health and Disease*, 2d ed. (Philadelphia, 1896?) 452.

71. Edward Hooker Dewey, *A New Era for Women* (Norwich, Conn., 1908 [1896]) 22, 40, 48, 114–15, 230–31, 311. On the popularity of Dewey's plan, see John J. Black, *Eating to Live*, 2d ed. (Philadelphia, 1907) 105.

72. Carl F. H. Immermann, "Corpulence," in *Cyclopaedia of the Practice of Medicine*, trans. E. B. Baxter, ed. Albert H. Buck, (NY, 1877) XVI, 686.

73. Charles Lowe, ed., *Bismarck's Table-Talk* (London, 1895) 276–79, reprinted in Louis L. Snyder, *The Blood and Iron Chancellor* (Princeton, N.J., 1967) 291-93; Isaac Burney Yeo, "The new cure for 'growing too fat,'" *Nineteenth Century* 24 (1888) 197; "Good news for fat folk," *NYDT* (April, 30, 1894) 4:5; Karl Ed. Rothschuh, "Ernst Schweninger," *Medizinhistorisches J* 19 (1984) 250–58; Jules Hoche, *Bismarck at Home*, trans. Thérèse Batbedat (London, 1899) 160–63, 177, though untrustworthy on Schweninger; Norman Rich and M. H. Fisher, eds., *The Holstein Papers. III. Correspondence 1861–1896* (Cambridge, 1961) 103 (letter of Feb 7, 1884); Werner Richter, *Bismarck*, trans. Brian Battershaw (NY, 1965) 263, 370; and Alan Palmer, *Bismarck* (London, 1976) 223–24, 229, 255.

74. Oscar Maas, *Die Schweninger-Kur*, 16th ed. (Berlin, 1895); Ernst Schweninger and F. Buzzi, *Die Fettsucht* (Vienna, 1894); Yeo, "New cure," 202; and Max J. Oertel, "Obesity," in *Twentieth Century Practice*, ed. Thomas L. Stedman (NY, 1895) II, 707.

75. Sinclair, I, 694–706, and II, 82–164; Walter Thom, *On Pedestrianism* (Aberdeen, 1813) 228–36, 243–45; Archibald MacLaren, *Training in Theory and Practice*, 2d ed. (London, 1874 [1866]); and Joshua Duke, *Banting in India*, 3d ed. (Calcutta, 1885) 20–26, with comments on usefulness of cocaine as a reducing agent, p. 55.

76. Jean François Dancel, *Traité théorique et pratique de l'obésité* (Paris, 1863) 149 on sex as exercise; J. L. H. Down, "On polysarcia and its treatment," *Clinical Lectures and Reports . . . London Hospital* 1 (1864) 99; Francis Smith Nash, "A plea for the New Woman and the bicycle," *AJOG* 33 (1896) 556–60; Heinrich Stern, "On the treatment of obesity," *JAMA* 38 (1902) 452; "Cult of slimness," *Living Age* 280 (Feb 28, 1914) 572 on the Kaiser; "New methods of flesh reduction," *Harper's Bazaar* 43 (Aug 1909) 810, on rolling on the floor; and Elizabeth Anstruther, *Complete Beauty Book* (NY, 1906) 164, the dash. On exercising machines, see Dick Sutphen, *The Mad Old Ads* (NY, 1966) 37–38, Health Jolting Chair; Patent 217,918, Marvin B. White, Exercising chair, July 29, 1879; Patent 232,022, Jesse H. Gifford and Charles H. Gifford, Combined portable health-exercising and gymnastic apparatus, Sept 7, 1880; Patent 243,309, Frank Saunders, Exercising or rowing machine, June 21, 1881; and Patent 281,097, William T. McGinnis, Electrical exercising apparatus, July 10, 1883.

77. Edwin Checkley, *A Natural Method of Physical Training* (Brooklyn, 1890) 90; Florence Bolton, *Exercises for Women* (NY, 1914) 119; Marie Montaigne et al., *How to Be Beautiful* (NY, 1913) 81–97; Emerson, *Physical Culture*, 47; John M. Taylor, "Obesity treated by systematic movements," *Int Med Mag* 10 (1901) 399–402; and Eduardo Fornias, "Obesity," *North Amer J of Homeopathy* 58 (1910) 76 (quote).

78. Walker, "Pretty girl papers," 33; Edward B. Warren and Mrs. Warren, "Answers to questions about health," *LHJ* 18 (1901) 44; G. Elliot Flint, "Dieting vs. exercise to reduce flesh," *Outing* 48 (1906) 408–11; Jørgen Peter Müller, *My System for Ladies*, new ed. (NY, 1911) 21, 67, 76, 81; and "Macfadden, Bernarr Adolphus,"*NCAB* XLV, 363–64.

79. Avery, *Dyspeptic's Monitor*, 138; Douglas Graham, *Practical Treatise on Massage* (NY, 1884); Thomas S. Dowse, *Lectures on Massage and Electricity* (NY, 1890) 147, 152; Maurice Steinberg, "Treatment of obesity by massage," *Maryland Med J* 35 (1896) 362–65; and G. H. Patchen, "Obesity," *Dietetic and Hygienic Gazette* 15 (1899) 195–99.

80. Margaret M. Lock, *East Asian Medicine in Urban Japan* (Berkeley, 1980) 54, 58, 179, and cf. 86–87 on meaning of abdomen in Japanese culture. Like the Turkish bath, massage in this era was not yet unavoidably linked with sex.

81. The Reducing-Machine Company, *Gardner Reducing Machine: The Easy Method* (Chicago, 1915?); Lindstrom, Smith Company, *Health and Beauty and How It Is Obtained Through Vibration* (Chicago, 1918) 51–62; Anna B. Both, *The Twentieth Century Method of Health Building and Weight Reducing* (Chicago, 1916?); "A machine that takes off fat," *Scientific Amer* 112 (1915) 366; and "Ring roller reducing machines," *Amer J of Electrotherapeutics and Radiology* 34 (1916) 52–53.

82. Cf. Cowan, *More Work for Mother*, esp. 172–78.

83. Madge E. Pickard and R. C. Buley, *The Midwest Pioneer* (Crawfordsville, Ind., 1945) 87; Burwell, *Obesity and the Cure*, 18; and Eric Jameson, *Natural History of Quackery* (Springfield, Ill., 1961) 136–37. On electricity as therapy, see Nicholas A. Cambridge, "Electrical apparatus used in medicine before 1900," *Royal Soc of Med Proc* 70 (1977) 635–41. Green, *Fit for America*, 168–79, 262–65.

84. Jean Alban Bergonié, "The cure of obesity by muscular action electrically provoked," *Archives of the Roentgen Ray and Allied Phenomena* 15 (Dec 1910) 255–56; Francis H. Humphris, "Electricity in the treatment of obesity," *BMJ* 2 (1912) 493–94; "Electric aid for the fat," *Literary Digest* 47 (July 26, 1913) 129; Heinrich F. Wolf, "General faradization (Bergonié) in the treatment of obesity," *Med Record* 87 (1915) 501; J. S. Kellett Smith, *The Cure of Obesity and Obese Heart* (London, 1916); and "A new obesity apparatus," *Modern Hospital* 7 (1916) 76.

85. Salisbury, *Alimentation and Disease*, 5–7.

86. Gail T. Parker, *Mind Cure in New England* (Hanover, N.H., 1973) esp. 20; Annie Payson Call, *Power Through Repose* (Boston, 1892); and Alice M. Long, *My Lady Beautiful*, rev. ed. (Chicago, 1908) 92.

87. Edward Stainbrook, "The use of electricity in psychiatric treatment during the nineteenth century," *BHM* 22 (1948) 168.

88. Call, *Power Through Repose*, 96, 122, 124, 93, and cf. her "Why fuss so much about what I eat?" *LHJ* 26 (Jan 1909) 22. Contrast T. J. Jackson Lears, "From salvation to self-realization: advertising and the therapeutic roots of the consumer culture, 1880–1930," in *The Culture of Consumption*, eds. Jackson and Richard W. Fox (NY, 1983) 12–17.

89. On tobacco, see "Corpulency," *A New and Complete Dictionary of Arts and Sciences* (London, 1754) I, 758; William Wadd, *Cursory Remarks on Corpulence*, 3d ed. (London, 1816) 20; and Immermann, "Corpulence," 712.

On soap, see F. Uzureau, "Comment on traitait l'obésité en Anjou au XVIIIe siècle," *Archives médicales d'Angers* 24 (1920) 77–80; Malcolm Flemyng, *A Discourse on the Nature, Causes, and Cure of Corpulency* (London, 1760) 19; Wadd, *Cursory Remarks*, 20–21, 24,

30; Sarah Josepha Hale, *New Household Receipt Book* (1853) cited in Hechtlinger, *Seasonal Hearth*, 35; W. H. Allchin, "Obesity," in *Dictionary of Medicine*, ed. Richard Quain, 7th ed. (NY, 1884) 1054; and *Nostrums* II, 684–85.

On vinegar, see John Arbuthnot, *Essay Concerning the Nature of Aliments* (Dublin, 1731) 90; Barnard Lynch, *A Guide to Health* (London, 1744) 244; Benjamin Waterhouse, *Cautions to Young Persons Concerning Health* (Cambridge, Mass., 1805) 20; *The Art of Beauty* (London, 1825) 80; and Professor De La Banta, *Advice to Ladies Concerning Beauty* (Chicago, 1878) 128.

On lemon juice and other acids, see "Obesity cures," *BMJ* 2 (1907) 25; Harvey Wiley and Anne Lewis Pierce, "Swindled getting slim," *GH* 58 (Jan 1914) 109–10; AMA, *Obesity Cure Fakes* (Chicago, 1914) 43–45; and *Nostrums* II, 679–80.

On creams and lotions, [John Dunton], *Ladies Dictionary* (London, 1694) 63; "Obesity cures," *BMJ* 2 (1907) 25; and *Nostrums* II, 677–79.

For Roman prescriptions, see esp. K. Guggenheim, "Soranus of Ephesus on obesity," *IJO* 1 (1977) 245–46, and Aulus Cornelius Celsus, *De Medicina*, trans. W. G. Spencer (Cambridge, Mass., 1948) I, 57–58.

90. AMA, *Obesity Cure Fakes*, 9 (quote), 12, 14, 31–40. For a recent modern example, consider the Silhouette Weight Loss Plan promoted by Health-Way Products, Milwaukee, in 1985: kelp (iodine, for which see Chapter V); soya lecithin (a "lipotrophic agent"); vitamin B-6 (a co-enzyme in fat metabolism; on vitamins see Chapter VII); cider vinegar—all in one "power-packed capsule."

91. E. S. McKee, "Obesity in its relation to menstruation and conception," *AJOG* 24 (1891) 301.

92. *Nostrums* II, 681.

93. Burwell, *Obesity and the Cure*, 6 (quote), and Jamieson B. Hurry, "Obesity and its vicious circles," *Practitioner* 99 (1917) 164–82.

94. N. E. Yorke-Davies, "Over-fatness," *Gentleman's Mag* n. s. 72 (1903) 571, and Pringle, *Life and Times of William Howard Taft*, I, 286.

CHAPTER FIVE
The Regulated Body

1. On Mollie Fancher, see *NYT* (Nov 25, 1878) 2:3 and (Dec 29, 1878) 12:3; and William H. Hammond, *Fasting Girls* (NY, 1879) 48 ff.

2. Petr Skrabanek, "Notes toward the history of anorexia nervosa," *Janus* 70 (1983) 109–28; Elizabeth A. Clark, "Ascetic renunciation and feminine advancement: a paradox of late ancient Christianity," *Anglican Theological R* 63 (1981) 240–57; Caroline W. Bynum,

"Women mystics and eucharistic devotion in the thirteenth century," *Women's Studies* 11 (1984) 179–214; Rudolph M. Bell, *Holy Anorexia* (Chicago, 1985;) William Wadd, *Comments on Corpulency* (London, 1829) 116; Percival B. Lord, *Popular Physiology*, 2d ed. (London, 1839) 106–10; Hammond, *Fasting Girls*; John Cule, *Wreath on the Crown: The Story of Sarah Jacob* (Llandyswl, 1967); and Eric N. Rogers, *Fasting* (Nashville, 1976) ch. 1. Prof. Joan J. Brumberg of Cornell is completing a book on the history of fasting girls.

3. "Moore, Ann," *DNB* XIII, 786–87; Hammond, *Fasting Girls*, 11.

4. Jane O'Hare-May, *Elizabethan Dietary of Health* (Lawrence, Kan., 1977) 124–26 on 17th-century Anglican fasting; Ronald A. Bosco, ed., *The Puritan Sermon in America, 1630–1750: Volume I. Sermons for Days of Fast, Prayer, and Humiliation and Execution Sermons* (Delmar, N.Y., 1978) introduction and, reproduced in Bosco, John Danforth, *The Vile Prophanations of Prosperity by the Degenerate Among the People of God* (Boston, 1704) 36; Robert Bolton, *A Three-Fold Treatise . . . or, Meditations Concerning the Word, the Sacrament of the Lord's Supper, and Fasting* (London, 1634) Part III, 22 (quote); Samuel Miller, "The duty, benefits and the proper method of religious fasting," *National Preacher* 5 (March 1831) 145–60; William A. Alcott, "How to keep fast," *Moral Reformer* 1 (1835) 127–28; and Protestant Episcopal Church in the United States, Diocese of New York, *Rules for Fasting* (Troy, N.Y., 1846).

5. "Dietetic charlatanry—new ethics of eating," *New-York R* 1 (Oct 1837) 349, and Jervis Robinson, "Starving the dyspepsia," *American Vegetarian and Health J* 1 (1851) 152–55.

6. L. S. F. Winslow, "Fasting and feeding; a detailed account of recorded instances of unusual abstinence from food . . . ," *Amer Psych J* n.s. 6 (1880) 258–64, 267, 273–74, and *NYT* (Nov. 25, 1878) 2:3.

7. Hammond, *Fasting Girls*, appendix. Young women in colonial New England who were either possessed or accused of witchcraft would frequently refuse to eat or be unable to eat. Cotton Mather noted, "It seems that long fasting is not only tolerable but strangely agreeable for such as have something more than ordinary to do with the invisible world." See John Putnam Demos, *Entertaining Satan* (Oxford, 1982) 164.

8. *NYT* (Dec 31, 1879) 2:5 and (July 5, 1880) 1:3; *NYDT* (Aug 9, 1880) 5: 1–3.

9. *NYDT* (Aug 9, 1880) 5:2–3; "Mrs. Tanner's revolt," *NYT* (Dec 29, 1882) 2:6; *NYT* (July 20, 1880) 2:3, (July 24, 1880) 2:6, and (Sept 10, 1880) 2:4; and Irving J. Eales, *Healthology* (London, 1913) 80.

10. *NYDT* (July 11, 1880) 6:4 quote, (Aug 9, 1880) 5:2 quote, and (Aug 8, 1880) 7:3; *NYT* (Dec 31, 1879) 2:5, (July 6, 1880) 8:3, and (Sept 10, 1880) 2:4; Winslow, "Fasting and feeding," 257; Eales, *Healtho-*

logy, 78, 80; and Frank Harris, *My Life and Loves*, ed. John F. Gallagher (NY, 1963) 96.

11. Based on a running series of reports in *NYT*; quotes from (July 4, 1880) 5:5 and (July 16, 1880) 8:1. See *NYDT* (Aug 8, 1880) on why Tanner abstained from water.

12. *NYT*, daily reports from July 11, 1880 on; *NYDT*, quotes from editorial, "The starvation comedy," (July 11, 1880) 6:3–4, and also (Aug 8, 1880) 7:2–5 and (Aug 13, 1880) 4:3.

13. *NYT* (Aug 7, 1880) 5:5, (Aug 8, 1880) 1:7–2:1, (Aug 9, 1880) 5:1, and (Aug 11, 1880) 2:3; *NYDT* (Aug 8, 1880) 7:2–5 with quote and (Sept 10, 1880) 8:4 quote; "Dr. Tanner's fast," *Kansas City R* 4 (1881) 285.

14. "Tanner, Henry S.," *Appleton's Cyclopaedia of American Biography*, rev. ed. (NY, 1900) VI, 32, and "Dr. Tanner passes," *Los Angeles Times* (Dec 29, 1918) I, 5:4.

15. *NYT* (Aug 29, 1886) 1:3, (Sept 13, 1886) 5:1, (Sept 19, 1886) 9:1, (Nov 8, 1886, 2:5, (Nov 28, 1886) 2:1, (Dec 16, 1886) 5:5, (Dec 23, 1886) 1:2, (Oct 21, 1888) 10:4 and (Dec 25, 1896) 3:2; *NYDT* (Sept 20, 1886) 4:3 and (Nov 6, 1890) 7:1 describing the elixir Succi used during his fasts as a compound of chloroform, morphine, ether and cannabis; "Succi, Giovanni," *Lessico universale Italiano* (Rome, 1979) XXII, 205; "Dieting and fasting not so new as we moderns think," *Mentor* 16 (April 1928) 57; and *NYDT* (Jan 24, 1883) 10:2 on Bunnell's Museum.

16. Paul Boyer, *Urban Masses and Moral Order in America, 1820–1920* (Cambridge, Mass., 1978) 127; Baker Business Library, Harvard University, Department of Archives and Manuscripts, Trade Card Collection, I, 33.

17. *NYT* (Aug 11, 1880) 2:3; Eales, *Healthology*, 120–21, 83–85 on Madison Square Garden; Robert B. Pearson, *Fasting and Man's Correct Diet* (Chicago, 1921) chart of forty-nine fasts, *NYDT* (Feb 11, 1900) III, 6:1, (July 23, 1902) 14:5, (March 15, 1903) 10:2 and (June 29, 1903) 12:5. See also *Chicago Record-Herald* (Jan 15, 1906) 1:6 and Helen Densmore, *How to Reduce Fat* (n.p., 1896) 7.

18. *NYT* (July 11, 1888) 5:3 and (July 13, 1888) 5:2.

19. *NYDT* (Nov 25, 1884) 2:1, (Feb 20, 1885) 1:4, (March 19, 1885) 5:2 and (April 12, 1885) 6:4, "The fasting girl problem"; Otoman Z. Hanish, *How to Fast Scientifically* (Chicago, 1912) 20–21 on Marie Davenport; *NYT* (March 31, 1910) 1:6 on a Cleveland girl fasting forty-five days; and Alfred Gradenwitz, "An apostle of hunger," *Technical World Mag* 13 (May 1910) 302–3. See John A. Sours, *Starving to Death in a Sea of Objects* (NY, 1980) ch. 3 for an historical survey of the anorexia diagnosis.

20. E. Sylvia Pankhurst, *The Suffragette* (London, 1911) 392, 431–35, 440–43, 482–86; Richard Pankhurst, *Sylvia Pankhurst Artist and*

Crusader (NY, 1979) 124, 156, 163–65; Doris Stevens, *Jailed for Freedom* (NY, 1920) ch. 10; and Dorothy P. Ryan, *Picture Postcards in the United States 1893–1918* (NY, 1982) 113 on suffragist slogan.

21. Stevens, *Jailed for Freedom*, 189–90, 201, 223.

22. Upton B. Sinclair, *The Fasting Cure* (Pasadena, Calif., 1923) quote on 25, and William Bloodworth, "From *The Jungle* to *The Fasting Cure*," *J of Amer Culture* 2 (1979) 444–453. Meanwhile, the marathon fasting went on; the most popular manual was by Edward E. Purinton, *The Philosophy of Fasting*, 2d ed. (Butler, N.J., 1915). The famous Sinn Fein hunger strikes began in September 1917. Gandhi's first political fast occurred in 1918.

23. Fletcher Correspondence, letter to James E. West, Jan 26, 1911, and letter to Russell Chittenden, Oct 15, 1909; Horace Fletcher, *Glutton or Epicure* (Chicago, 1899) 62; idem, *The New Glutton or Epicure* (NY, 1908) 81n; idem, *Fletcherism* (London, 1913?) 1–2; George H. Genzmer, "Fletcher, Horace," *DAB* III, 464–65; and James C. Whorton, "'Physiological Optimism': Horace Fletcher and hygienic ideology in Progressive America," *BHM* 55 (1981) 59–87; and Harvey Green, *Fit for America* (NY, 1986) ch. 11.

24. Fletcher Correspondence, letter to James E. West, Jan 26, 1911.

25. Fletcher, *New Glutton*, 274–75; idem, *Glutton or Epicure*, 27, 34, 36, and Whorton, "Horace Fletcher," 70n.

26. Fletcher, *Glutton or Epicure*, 34, 88, 118.

27. Robert Kingslake, "On dyspepsia," *Med Repository* 6 (1803) 106; William Kitchiner, *The Art of Invigorating and Prolonging Life* (London, 1822) 263; Sylvester Graham, *Treatise on Bread* (Boston, 1837) 17; Dio Lewis, *Our Digestion* (Philadelphia, 1872) 28; Arthur W. Brayley, *Bakers and Baking in Massachusetts* (Boston, 1909) 169; and Martin L. Holbrook, *Eating for Strength* (NY, 1888) 58.

28. Fletcher Correspondence, letter to John Harvey Kellogg, Nov 10, 1910, and letter to Mr. Erickson, Dec 21, 1910.

29. Fletcher, *New Glutton*, 73–75, 273, 325; Fletcher Correspondence, typescript letter to John Harvey Kellogg, Oct 31, 1909, and letter to same, Aug 6, 1910, and letter to Mary H. Waterman, Oct 31, 1909; Fletcher, *Fletcherism*, vii, on Rockefeller; A Mere Man (= F. W. Andrewes), "Women and food," *Harper's Bazaar* 43 (1909) 857; Sarah T. Rorer, "What nervous people should eat," *LHJ* 26 (Feb 1909) 40; Henry James, *Letters*, ed. Leon Edel (Cambridge, Mass., 1984) IV, 307, 374 (quote), 415 (quote); and Gilbert Seldes, *The Stammering Century* (NY, 1928) 370. See also Ronald M. Deutsch, *The Nuts Among the Berries*, rev. ed. (NY, 1967) 114–128 on Fletcher's popularity.

30. Fletcher Correspondence, letter to John Harvey Kellogg, Oct 31, 1909, and Fletcher, *New Glutton*, 325 (quote).

31. Fletcher, *Glutton or Epicure*, 16 (quote), 22, 30, 61, and Fletcher Correspondence, undated paper entitled "Department of Vital Economics," p. 4 on chauffeurs.

32. Fletcher, *Glutton or Epicure*, part II: *What Sense? or Economic Nutrition*, 69 (quote); idem, *The A.B.–Z. of Our Own Nutrition* (NY, 1903) 10–11 (quote); idem, *New Glutton*, 5, 142; and idem, *Fletcherism*, 104 (quote). Nina Tobier and Israel Steinberg, "Fletcherism," *NY St J of Med* 66 (1966) 2687–89, claim that Fletcher died of constipation.

33. Catharine E. Beecher, *Letters to the People on Health and Happiness* (NY, 1855) 73; H. C. Wood, "Cathartics," *Encyclopaedia Britannica*, 9th ed. (NY, 1886) Supp. I, 747; Rachel B. Gleason, *Talks to My Patients* (NY, 1871) 48; "Constipation and the corset," *Mind and Body* 5 (1896) 117; and David T. Courtwright, *Dark Paradise: Opiate Addiction in America before 1940* (Cambridge, Mass., 1982).

34. On obesity and constipation, see, e.g., H. S. Jones, "Some remarks on obesity," *Med Brief* 25 (1897) 1654.

35. Suellen M. Hoy, "'Municipal Housekeeping': the role of women in improving urban sanitation practices, 1880–1917," in *Pollution and Reform in American Cities, 1870–1930*, ed. Martin V. Melosi (Austin, Tex., 1980) 173–98; Marlene S. Wortman, "Domesticating the nineteenth-century American city," *Prospects* 3 (1977) 531–72; Gwendolyn Wright, "Sweet and clean: the domestic landscape in the Progressive Era," *Landscape* 20 (Oct 1975) 38–43; Carol Wald, *Myth America* (NY, 1975) 149 for Sapolio ad; Martin V. Melosi, *Garbage in the Cities* (College Station, Tex., 1981) 35, 110–11, 123–24 *et passim*; and Boyer, *Urban Masses*, 266–68.

36. Melosi, *Garbage in the Cities*, 42, 47–48, 161, 175–86, and George E. Waring, Jr., "The utilization of city garbage," *Cosmpolitan* 24 (Feb 1898) 405–12.

37. Fletcher Correspondence, letter to John Harvey Kellogg, Jan 2–4, 1912, f. 6v.

38. Melosi, *Garbage in the Cities*, 143–44; Stuart Galishoff, "Triumph and failure: the American response to the urban water supply problem, 1860–1923," in *Pollution and Reform*, 35–58; May N. Stone, "The plumbing paradox: American attitudes towards later nineteenth-century domestic sanitary arrangements," *Winterthur Portfolio* 14 (1979) 283–309; Joel A. Tarr et al., "Water and wastes: a retrospective assessment of wastewater technology in the United States, 1800–1932," *Technology and Culture* 25 (1984) 226–63; and Emma E. Walker, "The economy of the bathroom," *GH* (Aug 1906) 220–21.

39. Boyer, *Urban Masses*, 171 (quote), 200.

40. Christine Frederick, *Household Engineering* (Chicago, 1919) 486–87; W. Arbuthnot Lane, "The sewage system of the human body," *Amer Med* 29 (May 1923) 267; and Walter C. Alvarez, *Incurable Physician* (Englewood Cliffs, N.J., 1963) 57–58. The maxim "Disease is stench" underlay the popular dress and diet program of physician Gustav Jaeger and his Sanitary Woolen System; see his *Essays on Health Culture*, trans. and ed. Lewis R. S. Tomalin (London, 1887).

41. A. Lapthorn Smith, "What civilization is doing for the human female," *Southern Surgical and Gynecological Assoc Tr* 2 (1890) 354, and Charles J. Bouchard, *Lectures on Autointoxication*, trans. Thomas Oliver (Philadelphia, 1894) viii (quote), 93 (quote), 139, 177.

42. See Elmer V. McCollum, *A History of Nutrition* (Boston, 1957) ch. 12 for a good summary; also Gert H. Brieger, "Metchnikoff, Elie," *DSB* IX, 331–35. Bouchard did cite Sylvester Graham, who had had similar fears of fermentation and putrefaction in the intestines: *Lectures on Autointoxication*, 179.

43. Van Someren, "Was Luigi Cornaro right?" *BMJ* 2 (1901) 1082–84; Alcinous B. Jamison, *Intestinal Ills* (NY, 1901); *Therapeutic Med* 1 (1907) 86; John B. Huber, "Do we eat too much?" *Scientific Amer* 97 (Sept 7, 1907) 167; Emma E. Walker, "The prevention of colds," *Christian Advocate* (Dec 7, 1905); Ernest F. Robinson, "Some experience with obesity treatment," *AJCM* 17 (1910) 391; and Guillaume Guelpa, *Auto-intoxication and Disintoxication*, trans. F. S. Arnold (NY, 1914) esp. 29.

44. T. B. Layton, *Sir William Arbuthnot Lane, Bt.* (Edinburgh, 1956) esp. 88–91, 98–100; Harold Chapple, "The fundamental facts of chronic intestinal stasis," *Int J of Surgery* 27 (1914) 109–13; W. Arbuthnot Lane, "Civilization in relation to the abdominal viscera, with remarks on the corset," *Lancet* 2 (Nov 13, 1909) 1416–18; idem, *Blazing the Health Trail* (London, 1929) 31; and Logan Clendening, "A review of the subject of chronic intestinal stasis," *Interstate Med J* 22 (1915) 1191–1200. On the sudden popularity of appendectomies, see William F. Ross, *Medical Hygiene* (St. Louis, 1895) 22, and Special Collections, Bailey/Howe Library, Univ of Vermont, Vermont Homeopathic Medical Society Proceedings, 1898, E. E. Whitaker, "A plea for the appendix," 17–18.

45. T. J. Jackson Lears, *No Place of Grace* (NY, 1981) 116.

46. Monroe Lerner and Odin W. Anderson, *Health Progress in the United States, 1900–1960* (Chicago, 1963) 16.

47. Chittenden Papers, Box 2, Folder 35, p. 95 (quote); Russell H. Chittenden, *Physiological Economy in Nutrition* (NY, 1905) v, 8 (quote); Fletcher, *Fletcherism*, 12–14; and Whorton, "Horace Fletcher," 74–75.

48. Louis Berman, *Food and Character* (NY, 1932) 242–43 describing Voit; Fletcher Correspondence, letter to John Harvey Kellog, Jan 4, 1911, f. 2v, Wilbur O. Atwater, *Methods and Results of Investigations* (Washington, D.C., 1895) 213; Chittenden, *Physiological Economy*, 16–20; Chittenden Papers, Box 2, Folder 35, p. 98 on his own dieting; Chittenden, *Nutrition of Man* (NY, 1907) 272; and Whorton, "Horace Fletcher," 76–77.

49. Chittenden, *Physiological Economy*, 9, 12, 22–30, 466; Alexander Haig, *Uric Acid as a Factor in the Causation of Disease* (Philadelphia, 1892); C. Stanford Read, *Fads and Feeding* (London, 1908) 94–104; James C. Whorton, *Crusaders for Fitness* (Princeton, N.J., 1982) 239–40, 247, 255; James G. Kiernan, "Inter-complications of neurasthenia," *JAMA* 29 (1897) 582; and Josephine Goldmark, *Fatigue and Efficiency* (NY, 1912) 13.

50. Chittenden, *Physiological Economy*, 12, 16, 21, 473 (quote); idem, *Nutrition of Man*, 197; Chittenden Papers, Box 2, Folder 35, p. 107; and William S. Nicholl, "An experiment with Fletcherism," *J of Amer Osteopathic Assoc* 10 (1911) 438–41.

51. James Crichton-Browne, *Parcimony in Nutrition* (London, 1909) opposing Chittenden, 17 ff.; Harvey Cushing, *Life of Sir William Osler* (London, 1940) II, 85, mocking Chittenden; Francis G. Benedict, *A Study of Prolonged Fasting* (Washington, D.C., 1915); idem, "Food conservation by reduction of rations," *Nature* 101 (July 4, 1918) 355–57; and Eales, *Healthology*, 211–20.

52. Edward Glas, "Bio-science between experiment and ideology," *Studies in the History and Philosophy of Science* 14 (1983) 39–57; Frederic L. Holmes, *Claude Bernard and Animal Chemistry* (Cambridge, Mass., 1974); Joseph Larner, "The discovery of glycogen and glycogen today," in *Claude Bernard and Experimental Medicine*, eds. F. Grande and M. B. Visscher (Cambridge, Mass., 1967) 137–39; Jacques Martinie, *Notes sur l'histoire de l'obésité* (Paris, 1934) 46–48; Frederic L. Holmes, "Voit, Carl von," *DSB* XIV, 63–67; and E. Heinrich Kisch, "Obesity and its cure," *Post-Graduate* 25 (1910) 708.

53. Wilhelm Ebstein, *Corpulence and Its Treatment on Physiological Principles*, trans. and adapted by Emil W. Hoeber (NY, 1884) 18.

54. K. E. Rothschuh, "Rubner, Max," *DSB* XI, 585–86, and Atwater, *Methods and Results*, 15.

55. Chittenden, *Nutrition of Man*, 163.

56. Irving Fisher, "A new method for indicating food values," *Amer J of Physiology* 15 (1906) 417–32; Chittenden, *Nutrition of Man*, 283; Irving N. Fisher, *My Father, Irving Fisher* (NY, 1956) esp. 41, 49, 124 (quote), 215 (quote); and Whorton, "Horace Fletcher," 79–83.

57. Henry James, *Letters*, IV, 547 (quote), 596; *NYT* (May 1, 1912) 1:3;

Los Angeles Examiner (April 30, 1912) Want Ad section, p. 1, and (May 2, 1912) 2.

58. Everett Mendelsohn, *Heat and Life: Development of the Theory of Animal Heat* (Cambridge, Mass., 1964) esp. ch. 6; Thomas M. Carpenter, "Historical development of metabolism studies," *JADA* 25 (1949) 837–41; Graham Lusk, "A history of metabolism," in *Milestones in Nutrition*, eds. S. A. Goldblith and M. Joslyn (Westport, Conn., 1964) 19–94; Frederic L. Holmes, "Carl Voit and the quantitative tradition in biology," in *Transformation and Tradition in the Sciences*, ed. E. Mendelsohn (NY, 1984) 455–70; and Atwater, *Methods and Results*, ch. 7 and 157 on women. For a critique of Atwater's assumptions about women and children, see Laura Shapiro, *Perfection Salad* (NY, 1986) 166–67.

59. Leonard Landois defined "luxus consumption" but dismissed it as a theory in his *Manual of Human Physiology*, trans. from 4th German ed. (Philadelphia, 1885) I, part iv, 477. George M. Gould, *Illustrated Dictionary of Medicine, Biology and Allied Sciences*, 4th ed. (Philadelphia, 1899) I, 710, credited the introduction of the term to Friedrich H. Bidder and Carl Schmidt, *Verdauungssäfte und der Stoffwechsel* (Leipzig, 1852). The usual reference for the application of the term to human metabolism is R. O. Neumann in 1902; see William Bennett and Joel Gurin, *The Dieter's Dilemma* (NY, 1982) 79–82.

60. These paragraphs and the accompanying table are based on Carl F. H. Immermann, "Corpulence," in *Cyclopaedia of the Practice of Medicine*, trans. E. B. Baxter, (NY, 1877) XVI, 603–736; W. H. Allchin, "Dietetic treatment of obesity," *Practitioner* 76 (1906) 514–26; T. Harold Sunde, "Obesity," *Southern California Practitioner* 21 (1906) 408–11; James M. Anders, "Obesity" in *Modern Medicine*, eds. William Osler and Thomas McCrae (Philadelphia, 1907) I, 845–63; Kisch, "Obesity and its cure," 707–22; O. Rozenraad, "Lecture on obesity and certain changes of metabolism," *Lancet* 2 (1910) 1873–75; Joseph Di Rocco et al., "The treatment of obesity," *NY Med J* 93 (1911) 376–78, 423–27, 473–76; and J. Madison Taylor, "Reduction cures for overweight," *Med Times* (NY) 45 (1917) 217–20. For comparison, see the trifold scheme of Heinrich Stern, "On the treatment of obesity," *JAMA* 38 (1902) 447–55, with a fine chart detailing the binary system begun by Immermann. Hilde Bruch, *The Importance of Overweight* (NY, 1957) 24–26, claims that Karl von Noorden's *Die Fettsucht*, 2d ed. (Vienna, 1910), was the first to use the terms endogenous and exogenous obesity; Allchin had used "extrinsic" and "intrinsic" in 1906.

61. Anders, "Obesity," stated that heredity was responsible for obesity in 60 percent of cases for *both* plethoric and anemic types.

62. F. X. Dercum, "Three cases of a hitherto unclassified affection . . . Adiposis Dolorosa," *AJMS* n.s. 104 (1892) 521–35; Augustus A. Eshner, "Case of Adiposis Dolorosa," *JAMA* 31 (1898) 1156–60; F. X. Dercum, "Autopsy of a case of Adiposis Dolorosa," *JNMD* 27 (1900) 419–29; Frank Billings, "Adiposis Dolorosa—Dercum's Disease," *Illinois Med J* n.s. 5 (1903–4) 349–52; Michael G. Wohl and Nathan Pastor, "Adiposis dolorosa (Dercum's disease)," in *Cyclopaedia of Medicine*, ed. George M. Piersol (Philadelphia, 1950) I, 117–26.

63. F. X. Dercum, "Neurasthenia Essentialis and Neurasthenia Symptomatica," *JAMA* 30 (1898) 827–31.

64. McCollum, *History of Nutrition*, 106; Alfred H. Iason, *Thyroid Gland in Medical History* (NY, 1946) 77, 89; J. M. D. Olmsted, *François Magendie* (NY, 1944) 198; M. Donovan, "Fucus vesiculosus in obesity," *Dublin Med Press* 48 (1862) 638 on use in 1840s; John R. Wardell, "Remarks on obesity," *London Med Gazette* n.s. 8 (1849) 536; W. D. Briggs "Novel cure for obesity," *Nelson's Northern Lancet* 6 (1852) 43; Jonathan Pereira, *Elements of Materia Medica and Therapeutics*, ed. Joseph Carson, 3d Amer ed. (Philadelphia, 1852–54) II, 55; M. Duchesne-Duparc, "Sur les propriétés fondantes et résolutives du fucus vesicularius," *Compte rendus de l'Académie des Sciences (Paris)* 48 (1859) 1154; Richard Corson, *Fashions in Makeup* (NY, 1981) 123; Clarence Meyer, *American Folk Medicine* (NY, 1973) 265; Francis E. Anstie, "Corpulence," *Cornhill Mag* 7 (April 1863) 463; Joseph H. Wythe, *Physician's Dose and Symptom Book*, 13th ed. (Philadelphia, 1877) 80; Immermann, "Corpulence," 730; J. J. Mulheron, "Obesity," *New Preparations* (= *Therapeutic Gazette*) 3 (1879) 273, fucus as remedy of choice for "passive" obesity; Morrison, Plummer & Co., *Druggist's Ready Reference 1880* (Chicago, 1880) 31, with ad. opp. p. 32 vaunting fucus as new remedy; and "Obesity cures," *BMJ* 2 (1907) 209.

65. Iason, *Thyroid Gland*; Henry D. Jump, "Use and abuse of the thyroid in obesity," *Pennsylvania Med J* 16 (1912) 28–30; D. M. Lyon and D. M. Dunlop, "Treatment of obesity," *Q J of Med* ser. 2, 1 (1932) 337 on early use of thyroid extract; and N. E. Yorke-Davies, "Thyroid tablets in obesity," *BMJ* 2 (1894) 42–43. Thyroxine itself was isolated in 1915 by Edward C. Kendall.

66. Leonard Williams, "Some further aspects of obesity," *Practitioner* 86 (1911) 548.

67. Francis W. Crowninshield, *Manners for the Metropolis* (NY, 1909) 48.

68. Leon de Saravel, *Concerning the Beauty of a Woman* (Paris, 1910) 2 (quote); Stern, "On the treatment of obesity," 453; *Nostrums* I, 458–59, 203–15; British Medical Assoc, *More Secret Remedies* (London,

1912) 112–13; and James Harvey Young, *Medical Messiahs* (Princeton, N.J., 1967) 122–27, 211–16 on Marmola.

69. On the dangers of thyroid treatments and the need for supervision, see esp. Alfred Stengel, "Obesity," *Progressive Med* 2 (1899) 350; Stern, "On the treatment of obesity," 452; and Jump, "Use and abuse of the thyroid in obesity," 29–30.

70. Richard N. Smith, *An Uncommon Man: The Triumph of Herbert Hoover* (NY, 1984) 79–80 (quote), 82, 84; David Burner, *Herbert Hoover* (NY, 1979) 96–113; Fletcher Correspondence, letter to John Harvey Kellogg, July 13, 1915; and Mark Sullivan, *Our Times, V. Over Here* (NY, 1933) 408–22.

71. Maxey R. Dickson, *The Food Front in World War I* (Washington, D.C., 1944) 43, 60, 63–66, 73, 75, 121, and Irving Fisher, *Life Extension: A Talk at Vassar College* (Poughkeepsie, N.Y., 1917) 20.

72. Dickson, *Food Front*, 60, 64, 111; Naomi Aronson, "Social definitions of entitlement: food needs 1885–1920," *Media, Culture and Society* 4 (1982) 58; Charlotte H. Ormond, *The Abingdon War-Food Book* (NY, 1918); Richard Barry, "Less sugar means good-bye to your surplus fat," *NYT Mag* (Nov 4, 1917) 2; Alice Bradley, "Revising your cook book," *WHC* 45 (Feb 1918) 33; Belle Jessie Wood-Comstock, *The Home Dietitian*, 2d ed. (Washington, D.C., 1922) 201–3, 274; and William D. Halliburton, ed., *Physiology and National Needs* (London, 1919) 13, 21.

73. [Eugene L. Fisk], *Food, Fuel for the Human Engine . . . based on the Diet Squad Experiment* (NY, 1917); Francis G. Benedict, "Food conservation by reduction of rations," *Nature* 101 (July 4, 1918) 355–57; Benedict et al., *Human Vitality and Efficiency Under Prolonged Restricted Diet* (Washington, D.C., 1919); HEBE ad in *WHC* 45 (May 1918) 83; and Smith, *An Uncommon Man*, 86.

74. Graham Lusk, "Economy in diet," *Proc of the National Conference of Social Work* (Chicago, 1917) 231, 240; Barry, "Less sugar"; Benedict, "Food conservation," 357; and "War, the character builder," *WHC* 45 (Feb. 1918) 2.

75. Luella E. Axtell, "Misconceptions concerning obesity and its treatment," *Med Standard* 42 (1919) 18; idem, "An analysis of obesity with outline of treatment," *Wisconsin Med J* 14 (1915) 52; idem, "Obligation of the physician in regard to obesity," *Woman's Med J* 26 (1916) 36–38; idem, *Grow Thin on Good Food* (NY, 1931) 3, 7; and F. McKelvey Bell, "The 'why' of obesity," *NY Med J* 99 (1914) 733. For biographical data on Axtell, I have used Ellis B. Usher, *Wisconsin: Its Story and Biography 1848–1913* (Chicago, 1914) VIII, 2385–86; Wisconsin State Historical Society (Madison), Board of Medical Examiners, Series 1606, Applications for Licenses, 1897–1907, A-

Col, *sive* Axtell, Application #882, License #861; and *Marinette City Directory* (Marinette, Wisc., 1921), this last kindly provided me by George S. Robbins, manager of the Marinette Area Chamber of Commerce.

76. John Higham, *Strangers in the Land: Patterns of American Nativism, 1860–1925*, 2d ed. (NY, 1965) 63, 118, 124–25, and ch. 9; Franz Boas, *Changes in Bodily Form of Descendants of Immigrants* (Washington, D.C., 1910) esp. 6; Thomas S. Dowse, *Lectures on Massage and Electricity* (NY, 1890) 160 on Jews, as also William E. Preble, "Obesity and malnutrition," *BMSJ* 172 (May 20, 1915) 741, and James M. Anders and H. Leon Jameson, "Adiposity and other etiological factors in diabetes mellitus," *AAPT* 40 (1925) 236–37; and Frederick, *Household Engineering*, 156 on absorption.

77. Warren Webster, "Auto-intoxication more deadly than warfare," *Every Week* (Feb 9, 1918) 23, ad disguised as article.

78. Mark Sullivan, *Our Times: IV. The War Begins* (NY, 1932) 18; Alice S. Cutler, "Corsets versus backache and fatigue," *BMSJ* 175 (1916) 168–69; Amelia Summerville, *Why Be Fat?* (NY, 1916) 28–29; Grace M. Gould, "The indispensable corset," *WHC* 45 (March 1918) 54; and Arthur W. Pearce, *The Future Out of the Past: An Illustrated History of the Warner Brothers Company* (Bridgeport, Conn., 1964) 26–29.

79. War Department, *Hearings before the Committee on Military Affairs, House of Representatives, 66th Congress 1st Session, on H.R. 4096* (Washington, D.C., 1919) 7; and Cocroft ad, *WHC* 47 (April 1920) 143. For biographical data, see University of Wisconsin (Madison) archives, Susie Cocroft academic record 1886–87 (furnished courtesy of Herbert D. Evert, Asst. Registrar); *Amer School Board J*, edited by Cocroft Jan–June, 1892 (= vol. 4); A. C. Beckwith, *History of Walworth County*, Wisconsin (n.p., 1912) 698–99; "Cocroft, Susanna," *Woman's Who's Who of America*, ed. John W. Leonard (NY, 1914) 189; "Cocroft, Susanna," *Clark J. Herringshaw's City Blue-Book of Biography. Chicagoans of 1920* (Chicago, 1919); and Albert N. Marquis, ed., *The Book of Chicagoans* (Chicago, 1917) 142.

80. Cocroft ad, *Amer Med* 22 (1916) p. 37 of ad pages; Susanna Cocroft, *Self-Sufficiency—Mental Poise*, 2d ed. (Chicago, 1912) esp. 17; idem, *The Woman Worth While* (NY, 1916) 1 (quote), 21–22 (quote), 43 (quote); idem, *Poise and Symmetry of Figure: Obesity, Leanness—Their Causes and Effects*, 3d ed. (Chicago, 1914) esp. 23, 25, 27, 30, 37, 49 (quote); and idem, *What to Eat and When*, 4th ed. (NY, 1916) vii on preparedness.

81. War Department, *Hearings*.

82. Cocroft ad, *WHC* 47 (April 1920) 143.

CHAPTER SIX:
The Measured Body

1. Arthur MacDonald, *Abnormal Woman* (Washington, D.C., 1895) 3, 61–62.

2. *Ibid.*, 172, and James B. Gilbert, "Anthropometrics in the U.S. Bureau of Education: the case of Arthur MacDonald's 'Laboratory,'" *History of Educ Q* 17 (1977) 169–85.

3. MacDonald, *Abnormal Woman*, 39–40.

4. *Ibid.*, quotes on 67, 108.

5. "Psychometry in Brooklyn," *NYT* (Dec 29, 1878) 12:3, and Madge E. Pickard and R. Carlyle Buley, *The Midwest Pioneer* (Crawfordsville, Ind., 1945) 227–28, 234.

6. See, e.g., Violet McNeal, *Four White Horses and a Brass Band* (Garden City, N.Y., 1947).

7. There is now a science devoted to this. Ray Birdwhistell, *Kinesics and Context* (Philadelphia, 1970).

8. Edwin G. Boring, *Sensation and Perception in the History of Experimental Psychology* (NY, 1942) 34–45; Julian Jaynes, "Fechner, Gustav Theodor," *DSB* IV, 556–59; "Modern experimental psychology— its methods and apparatus," *Scientific Amer* 97 (Sept 7, 1907) 164–66; and Stephen Jay Gould, *The Mismeasure of Man* (NY, 1981) 122–43 on Lombroso.

9. The same principles also underlay the new science of graphology or handwriting analysis, which was immediately and often applied to criminology. See Emilie de Vars, *Histoire de la graphologie* (Paris, 1874); Jean Hippolyte Michon, *La méthode pratique de graphologie* (Paris, 1878); and Jules Crépieux-Jamin, *L'écriture et le caractère*, 4th ed. (Paris, 1896).

10. Carl Georg Lange and William James, *The Emotions* (Baltimore, 1922), comprising essays published in 1885 (Lange) and in 1884 and 1893 (James); see also Magda B. Arnold, *Emotion and Personality* (NY, 1960) II, 3–8, for Walter B. Cannon's critique of the James-Lange theory.

11. Luigi Belloni, "Riva-Rocci, Scipione," *DSB* VII, 354b, and Audrey B. Davis, *Medicine and Its Technology* (Westport, Conn., 1981) 125, 129–30.

12. Matthew N. Chappell, "Blood pressure changes in deception," *Archives of Psych* 105 (1929); Leonarde Keeler, "A method for detecting deception," *Amer J of Police Science* 1 (1930) 38–51; and John Augustus Larson with George W. Haney and Leonarde Keeler, *Lying and Its Detection* (Montclair, N.J., 1969 [1932]) esp. ch. 11, and xx for quote, from Paul Schilder.

13. J. E. D. Esquirol, *Mental Maladies*, trans. E. K. Hunt (Philadelphia, 1845) 389; Thomas King Chambers, "On corpulence," *Lancet* 2 (1850) 441; "Thirty-Seventh Meeting of the Association of German Naturalists and Physicians, 1862," *J of Mental Science* 9 (1864) 242–45; Cesare Lombroso and A. Laurent, "Du poids du corps chez les aliénés," *Annales médico-psychologiques* 4th ser., 9 (1867) 217–24; "Bodily weight in mental disease. Marburg dissertation 1872," *J of Mental Science* 18 (1872) 614; A. R. Turnbull, "Psychological retrospect," *ibid.* 23 (1877) 303–4; "English retrospect," *ibid.* 31 (1885) 122–23; and K. Planansky, "Changes in weight in patients receiving a tranquilizing drug," *Psychiatric Q* 32 (1958) 296–301 for a literature review.

14. Caesar Lombroso and William Ferrero, *The Female Offender* (NY, 1899) 48; August Drähms, *The Criminal* (NY, 1900) with introduction by Lombroso, and see 116; Israel Castellanos, *El peso corporal en los delincuentes de Cuba* (Havana, 1935) with literature review, 69–74; Earnest A. Hooton, *Crime and the Man* (Cambridge, 1939) 87, 93; and Arthur E. Fink, *Causes of Crime: Biological Theories in the United States, 1800–1915* (Philadelphia, 1938) chs. 5–6, esp. 127, 131 (on Kellor).

15. Haley Fiske, "Fifty years of life insurance," *Med Insurance* 41 (1926) 384.

16. Viviana A.R. Zelizer, *Morals and Markets: Development of Life Insurance in the United States* (NY, 1979) 6, 40, 45–56, 59, 92n, 106–7, 123, 126, 134.

17. Edwin J. Faulkner, *Health Insurance* (NY, 1960) 512–35, 564; Jerome L. Schwartz, "Early history of prepaid medical care plans," *BHM* 38 (1965) 452–53, 457, 471–72; Metropolitan Life Insurance Company, *An Epoch in Life Insurance*, 2d ed. (NY, 1924) 211, 237; and Louis I. Dublin, *A Family of Thirty Million: The Story of the Metropolitan Life Insurance Company* (NY, 1943) 89–90, 192–206, 441.

18. Angela Nugent, "Fit for work: the introduction of physical examinations in industry," *BHM* 57 (1983) 578–95; Harry A. Nelson, "Pre-employment examination," *Industrial Med* 9 (Sept 1940) 451–52; Davis, *Medicine and Its Technology*, 221; Dublin, *Family of Thirty Million*, 406–7; and James A. Tobey, "A layman's view of health examinations," *BMSJ* 191 (Nov 6, 1924) 875–78.

19. Nugent, "Fit for work," 588–89; Davis, *Medicine and Its Technology*, 192–93; Harold M. Frost, "History and philosophy of life insurance medicine," in *Life Insurance and Medicine*, eds. Ungerleider and Gubner (Springfield, Ill., 1958) 203–4, 216–17; Marquis James, *The Metropolitan Life* (NY, 1947) 270, 327; and C. C. Bombaugh, "Medical examination in life insurance," *Insurance Monitor* 30 (1882) 200–201 (quote).

20. Nina W. Putnam, "Reductio ad absurdum," *SEP* 194 (Dec 31, 1921) 62.

21. G. A. Heron, "Bearing of obesity on health," *Dietetic and Hygienic Gazette* 15 (1899) 219; George R. Shepherd, "Relation of build to longevity," *Med Examiner* 9 (1899) 209–16; and Oscar H. Rogers, "Build as a factor influencing longevity," *Assoc of Life Insurance Med Directors Proc* 12 (1901) 280.

22. Actuarial Society of America and the Association of Life Insurance Medical Directors, *Medico-actuarial Mortality Investigations* (NY, 1912–14) II, 9–14, 18, 34 See F. Parkes Weber, *Disease in Relation to Obesity* (London, 1916) for other data.

23. See the review by Herbert H. Marks, "Body weight: facts from life insurance records," in Josef Brożek, ed., *Body Measurements for Human Nutrition* (Detroit, 1956) 107–21.

24. John K. Gore, "Should life [insurance] companies discriminate against women?" *Papers and Tr of the Actuarial Soc of Amer* 6 (1900) 380–88, and Shepherd, "Relation of build to longevity," 212–13. See also the critique in William Bennett and Joel Gurin, *The Dieter's Dilemma* (NY, 1982) 125–29.

25. On aging and weight-gain, see esp. Henry W. Coe, "Overweight," *Med Examiner* 5 (1895) 30–32; "Influence of over-weight and underweight on vitality," *Amer Insurance Digest* 56 (1908) 385; Dudley A. Sargent, "Are you too fat, or too thin?" *Amer Mag* 92 (Nov 1921) 13; K. H. Beall, "Parasitism of fat," *Southern Med J* 17 (1924) 323, comment by Dr. Seale Harris; W. R. P. Emerson and Frank A. Manny, "Underweight and overweight in relation to vitality," *JAMA* 92 (1929) 457; and Rollo H. Britten, "Physical impairment and weight," *Public Health Reports* 48,31 (1933) 926–44.

    On percentage overweight deemed excessive, see esp. *Med Examiner* 5 (1895) 109 (15 %); John M. Keating, *How to Examine for Life Insurance*, 3d ed. (Philadelphia, 1898) 24 (20 %); William E. Preble, "Obesity: observations on one thousand cases," *BMSJ* 188 (1923) 617–21 (10 lbs); and Henry Gauss, "Obesity," *Colorado Med* 24,3 (1927) 88–96 (15 %, with a graduated table on excess mortality).

26. On Dublin, see his *After Eighty Years* (Gainesville, Fla., 1966) 192–94, and Bennet and Gurin, *Dieter's Dilemma*, 130–38. On the term "ideal weight," see Frederick J. Stare, "Ideal intake of calories and specific nutrients," *AJPH* 37 (1947) 519n.

27. Luella E. Axtell, "Obligation of the physician in regard to obesity," *Woman's Med J* 26 (1916) 36; Frank McCoy, *The Fast Way to Health* (Los Angeles, 1923) 150; Claes J. Enebuske, "Place of physical training in a rational education," in *Physical Training*, ed. Isabel C. Barrows (Boston, 1890) 39; Helen G. Buttrick, *Principles of Clothing Se-*

lection (NY, 1926) 70; Milo Hastings, *Reducing and How!* (NY, 1930) 9–11, 14; and Woods Hutchinson, "Defense of fat men," *SEP* 196 (June 7, 1924) 8.

28. *APER* 18 (1913) 295–303; Edward M. Hartwell, "Physical training in American colleges and universities," *U.S. Bureau of Education Circulars of Information* No. 5 for 1885 (Washington, D.C., 1886) 36; Milicent L. Hathaway and Elsie Foard, "Heights and weights of adults in the United States," *Home Economics Research Reports* No. 10 (Washington, D.C., 1960) 3–4, 20, 30; "Point of view: Dr. Sargent's average American," *Scribner's* 14 (1893) 130; "The ideal girl," *Med Examiner* 5 (1895) 63; Howard V. Meredith, "Stature and weight of private school children in two successive decades," *AJPA* 28 (March 1941) 4–5, 8–11, quoting Dudley Sargent in 1908, who believed that college students were an inch taller and 4–8 lbs heavier than a generation before; and David L. Wilkinson, "Some remarks concerning education and the results of the examination of over two thousand young college women," *Med Assoc of the St of Alabama Tr* (1903) 168–76. Weights were usually for nude men, clothed women.

29. Benjamin A. Gould, *Investigations in the Military and Anthropological Statistics of American Soldiers* (NY, 1869) ch. 11; T. B. Macaulay, "Weight and longevity," *Amer Statistical Soc Publications* 2 (1891) 287–96; Hathaway and Foard, "Heights and weights," 81–82; U.S. War Department, *Defects Found in Drafted Men* (Washington, D.C., 1920) 62, 72, 95, 112, 203, 276, 304, 357–58; and Bernard D. Karpinos, "Height and weight of Selective Service registrants processed for military service during World War II," *Human Biology* 30 (1958) 292–321. Correcting for age, Karpinos calculated that World War II inductees were ⅔ inches taller and 10.7 lbs heavier than in World War I.

30. Howe Papers, Scrapbook, Part I, f. 5, clipping from the *Boston Journal* circa 1859, and f.6, from the *Boston Transcript; Insurance Monitor* 23 (1875) 92c; Hathaway and Foard, "Heights and weights," 20; Albert Damon, "Secular trends in height and weight within Old American families at Harvard, 1870–1965," *AJPA* 29 (1968) 45–50; and Jervis S. Wight, *The Weight and Size of the Body and Its Organs* (Brooklyn, 1881) 3.

31. Actuarial Society . . . , *Medico-actuarial Mortality Investigations* II, 14, suggests that insurance companies often refused ordinary term insurance to the significantly overweight; it is likely that weight was underestimated by applicants (and in 40 percent of the cases, weight was *only* estimated: I, 16). On tendencies in weight estimation, see Phyllis Pirie et al., "Distortion in self-reported height and weight data," *JADA* 78 (1981) 601–6; and Albert J. Stunkard and Janet

M. Albaum, "Accuracy of self-reported weights," *AJCN* 34 (1981) 1593–99.

32. Samuel H. Hurwitz, commenting on H. C. Shepardson and R. E. Allen, "Treatment of obstinate obesity," *California and Western Med* 26 (1927) 37 (quote); *NYT* (Feb 22, 1926) 3:6 and (Feb 23, 1926) 17:1. Morris Fishbein, ed., *Your Weight and How to Control It* (NY, 1927) prints the conference papers.

33. "Girth and death," *MLIC* 18 (1937) 2–5; "Ideal weights for women," *MLIC* 23 (Oct 1942) 6–8; "Ideal weights for men," *MLIC* 24 (1943) 6–8; Amy Porter, "Waistline by Uncle Sam," *Collier's* 111 (April 24, 1943) 64–65; "Overweight unpatriotic as well as unhealthy," *Science News Letter* 43 (Jan 16, 1943) 40; and "Anthropometric method," *New Yorker* 20 (Dec 30, 1944) 12–13. The lifeline-beltline slogan dated back to 1922: Herman N. Bundesen, *Dr. Bundesen's Diet Book* (Chicago, 1934) 22; Beall, "Parasitism of fat," 320; Metropolitan Life ad in *Hygeia* 15 (1937) 464; Weil Belt ad in *Esquire* (Aug 1937) 16; and Metropolitan Life ad in *Hygeia* 19 (1941) 816.

34. Ueland, "Fat or thin women," *SEP* 202 (May 10, 1930) 48, and idem, *Me* (NY, 1939) 59.

35. Edward Atkinson, "The American physique," *Science* 10 (Nov 11, 1887) 239–40; Harvey Levenstein, "The New England Kitchen and the origins of modern American eating habits," *Amer Q* (1980) 369–86; and Bruce Haley, *The Healthy Body and Victorian Culture* (Cambridge, Mass. 1978) 169.

36. Claudia B. Kidwell and Margaret C. Christman, *Suiting Everyone: The Democratization of Clothing in America* (Washington, D.C., 1974) 101–3, 107; Paul H. Nystrom, *Economics of Fashion* (NY, 1928) 453, 457, 463, 466; and Estelle A. Worrell, *American Costume 1840–1920* (Harrisburg, 1979).

37. Kidwell and Christman, *Suiting Everyone*, 106–9 (it was an engineer, Albert Malasin, whose measurements of women provided the sizings for his wife's business at Lane Bryant); Mary S. Woolman, *Clothing Choice Care Cost*, 3d ed. (Philadelphia, 1926) 6, 88, 90, 94, 128; Mark Sullivan, *Our Times. III. Pre-War America* (NY, 1930) 339–40; Diana de Marly, *The History of Haute Couture 1850–1950* (NY, 1980) 50, 101–3 and Nystrom, *Economics of Fashion*, 205, 213, 295 on mannequins; Lucy Christiana Sutherland, Lady Duff Gordon (Lucille), *Discretions and Indiscretions* (London, 1932) 67–75, 81 on dress parades; and Vern L. Bullough, "Female physiology, technology and women's liberation," in *Dynamos and Virgins Revisited*, ed. Martha M. Trescott (Metuchen, N.J., 1979) 236–51. A company that sold beauty and reducing aids was the one to put Tampax on the market in 1933: "Gertrude Nova 'obesity cure,' another dangerous nostrum of 'get-thin-quick' type," *JAMA* 104 (1935) 1441–42.

38. On weights, see Hathaway and Foard, "Heights and weights," 2. On optical illusions, see Mrs. Ralston, "Helpful suggestions for stout women," *LHJ* 22 (Jan 1905) 49 and 22 (May 1905) 68; Margaret Story, *How to Dress Well*, 2d ed. (NY, 1924) 155–61; Jane W. Wells, *Dress and Look Slender* (Philadelphia, 1925) esp. 16–36; and Woolman, *Clothing*, 128 (quote).

39. Gilbert Vail, *A History of Cosmetics in America* (NY, 1947) 106, and Stephen Kern, *Anatomy and Destiny* (Indianapolis, 1975) ch. 5.

40. Broadus Mitchell, "Patten, Simon," *DAB* VII, 298–300; Sudhir Kakar, *Frederick Taylor* (Cambridge, Mass., 1970) 26–27; Daniel Nelson, *Frederick W. Taylor and the Rise of Scientific Management* (Madison, 1980) 25–26; George M. Beard, *A Practical Treatise on Nervous Exhaustion*, ed. A. D. Rockwell, 5th ed. (NY, 1905) 40–43, 113; James H. Cassedy, *American Medicine and Statistical Thinking 1800–1860* (Cambridge, Mass., 1984) 39–40 (quote from 1828); W. A. Evans, *Dr. Evans' How to Keep Well* (NY, 1922) ch. 11; A. W. Calhoun, "Effects of student life upon the eyesight," *U.S. Bureau of Education Circulars of Information* No. 6 (Washington, D.C., 1881) 12–13; Wilkinson, "Some remarks concerning education," 170–72; and James Rorty and N. Philip Norman, *Tomorrow's Food*, 2d ed. (NY, 1956) 43 on World War I statistics. For the treatments, see Daniel Drake's review of *A Manual of Diseases of the Eye* by S. Littell, Jr., in *Western J of the Med and Physical Sciences* 2 (1837) 225–58, and Clarence Meyer, *American Folk Medicine* (NY, 1973) 109–14.

41. Edmund Morris, *The Rise of Theodore Roosevelt* (NY, 1979) 62, 620.

42. A. F. M. Willich, *Lectures on Diet and Regimen* (Boston, 1800) 299–301 on ready-made glasses; "Near-sightedness," *BMSJ* 55 (1857) 456; Hasket Derby, "Relations of the ophthalmoscope to legal medicine," *BMSJ* 66 (1862) 525–27; Adolf Zander, *The Ophthalmoscope*, trans. Robert B. Carter (London, 1864) esp. 200; Stanley J. Reiser, *Medicine and the Reign of Technology* (Cambridge, Mass., 1978) 47–49, 217, 223; and Davis, *Medicine and Its Techology*, 217.

43. "Ocular astigmatism: a historical sketch," *The Optician* 144 (Dec 7, 1962) 549–53; James E. Lebensohn, "Notes to 'Astigmatism,'" *Survey of Ophthalmology* 7 (1962) 177–83; James P. C. Southall, *Introduction to Physiological Optics* (London, 1937) 144–54; S. Weir Mitchell, *The Early History of Instrumental Precision in Medicine* (New Haven, 1892) 5; and W. A. Fisher, "What the general practitioner should know about diseases of the eye," *JAMA* 22 (1894) 150–52.

44. Evans, *How to Keep Well*, 116, 120–21; George M. Kober, "History of industrial hygiene and its effect on public health," in *A Half Century of Public Health*, ed. M. P. Ravenel (NY, 1921) 408; Bureau of

the Census, *Census of Manufactures* for 1905 (Part 1, General Tables, p. 14 Optical Goods), for 1927 (p. 1222) and for 1931 (p. 1129). I must thank Dr. Gil Iser for cautionary advice on this topic.

45. Edward T. Fairbanks, "The Fairbanks scale industry," in *The New England States*, ed. William T. Davis (Boston, 1897) III, 1559–64; George A. Owen, *A Treatise on Weighing Machines*, 2d ed. (London, 1928) 135; "History of weighing machines," *Scale J* 9 (Jan 10, 1923) 7, and Howe Papers, Box 1, folder 21.

46. Howe Papers, Scrapbook, Part I, *New York Herald Magazine* (May 1878) Grant on Howe scale, and Part II, *Charleston News & Courier* (Dec 15, 1880); Landauer, Measuring & Weighing, and Poster—Scales; and Warshaw, Scales, Howe Scale Company, Trade Cards.

47. Charles Roberts, *Manual of Anthropometry* (London, 1878) 32–33; Fairbanks Papers, *Catalog #234* (1891) 14. Physicians at the Massachusetts General Hospital and the New England Hospital for Women and Children, two of the more zealously scientific, record-keeping American hospitals, showed scant interest in precise weights or weight-changes of patients until the late 1880s. At the New England Hospital, weights were somewhat irregularly recorded from 1874; even when forms were introduced in 1886 with space for pulse, temperature, respiratory rate and weight, the weight—and only the weight—was often left blank. See records on deposit, Countway Medical Library Archives, Harvard University. The first doctor's scale was produced in 1865, shown me by Gerald "Red" Meade of the Antique Penny Scale Company.

48. Keating, *How to Examine for Life Insurance*, 24.

49. Meade interview, Feb 12, 1985. Meade estimates that a total of 175 companies at one time or another manufactured penny scales: Daniel R. Meade, "The scale King," *Loose Change* 5 (April 1982) 13, with an estimate (p. 14) of 750,000 penny scales manufactured by 1933. In Joseph Taylor, "The Farrs have been weighing in for over 50 years," *Joel Sater's Antiques and Auction News* 14 (Jan 1, 1983) 1, Ray Farr estimates 150 companies and 150,000 scales. On the City Hall scale, see Bundesen, *Dr. Bundesen's Diet Book*, 22.

50. Archibald M. Andrews, "Profits from pennies," *SEP* 203 (Nov 1, 1930) 10–11; "Weighing machines take up work of telling fortunes," *NYT* (Oct 7, 1928) Section X, 10:7; Ralph W. Smith, "What do you weigh to-day?" *Scientific Monthly* 35 (Dec 1932) 558; and Taft Museum, *The American Weigh* (Cincinnati, 1983) esp. 53.

51. W. W. Wagstaffe, "Ups and downs in our daily weight," *Knowlege* 22 (1899) 247–48; Andrews, "Profits from pennies," 90; Taylor, "The Farrs," with illustration of the 1904 scale; Ray Farr letter, Dec 31, 1984; and Meade interview.

52. Meade interview; Patent 1,774,622, Thomas W. B. Watling, Combi-

nation scale and fortune-telling machine, Sept 2, 1930; George V. N. Dearborn, "Get fat—and die," *Interstate Med J* 24 (1917) 156; Wells, *Dress and Look Slender*, 4 (quote); and Irvin S. Cobb, *Irvin Cobb at His Best* (Garden City, N.Y., 1929) 216 (quote).

53. "Penny scales make millions," *NYT* (July 10, 1927) VIII, 8:1; *Creative Art* (Sept 1928), clipping from Weight file, New York Public Library Picture Collection; Andrews, "Profits from pennies," 11; Mills Novelty Co., *A Big Little Penny* (Chicago, 1932?) 4, 7, 9, 12, 17 (quote) and Rockola Manufacturing Corp., *Stepping Up with the New and Improved LoBoy Scale* (Chicago, 1937)—these two brochures at the Chicago Historical Society; "Height–weight–age tables for children," *JAMA* 101 (1933) 369 on Exposition profits; and Meade interview.

54. Andrews, "Profits from pennies," 11, and Smith, "What do you weigh to-day?" 557.

55. Wanda Moore, "Penny scales for thrift," *Bankers Mag* 122 (March 1931) 331–33; Dwight O'Hara, "Ruminations of an out-patient physician," *BMSJ* 197 (1927) 265; Ken Rubin and Frank Rubin, *Drop Coin Here* (NY, 1979); and "Slot machine retailing literally arrives," *Advertising and Selling* 9 (Aug 24, 1927) 21.

56. Thomas Lawton, *Dr. Thomas Lawton's Automatic Waistline Reducer and Weight Control* (Brooklyn, 1923) 44–45; Lydia E. Pinkham Medicine Co., *How Phyllis Grew Thin* (Lynn, Mass., 1924?) 3, in the Lydia E. Pinkham Papers, Schlesinger Library, Radcliffe College, Box 121, folder 2447; Luella E. Axtell, *Grow Thin on Good Food* (NY, 1931) 30; Janet Lane, "You can't laugh it off," *Collier's* 97 (March 21, 1936) 43; and *Nostrums* II, 272.

57. Fairbanks Papers, *Catalog #329* (1901) 33, *Catalog #505* (1906) 297, *Catalog #512* (1908) 818; Howe Papers, *Catalog #45* (1917) 38; Standard Scale and Supply Co., *Catalog #A160* (Aug 1, 1912) 114, in Trade Catalogue collection, Beinecke Rare Book Library, Yale University (no bathroom scales appear in Standard Scale's 1904 or 1908 catalogs); and Standard Scale ad in *WHC* (June 1918) 83.

58. Earl Lifshey, *The Housewares Story* (Chicago, 1973) 216–18.

59. *Ibid*. 217–21, and interview with William J. Hutchinson, former Chief Executive Officer of the Continental Scale Company, Sept 17, 1984.

60. Lifshey, *Housewares Story*, 217–21, and Hutchinson interview.

61. "Jacobs, Aaron Jacob," *NCAB* XLV, 275; Lifshey, *Housewares Story*, 222–23; interview with Mack Rapp of the Detecto Scale Company, Oct 9, 1984; Warshaw, Scales, Box 2, Jacobs Bros., *Scales, Fixtures and Store Equipment* (Brooklyn, 1925?) 4; and Hanson Scale Co.,

Catalog (1927), photocopies supplied by Theresa Mercer of the Hanson Scale division of Sunbeam Corp.

62. Howe Papers, Scrapbook 1917–26: Fairbanks Health Scale brochure (1922), Detecto brochure (1922?), Howe brochure, *Health Wealth and Happiness* (1926); Howe Papers, *Catalog #47* (1919) 45; and Fairbanks Papers, *Catalog #67* (1918) 58–59.

63. Francis G. Benedict, "Rationale of weight reduction," *Scientific Monthly* 33 (1931) 266; Hutchinson interview; Hanson Scale Co., *The Book of Weight Control* (Chicago, 1934); Warshaw, Scales, Continental Scale Works, Health-O-Meter brochure (Chicago, 1920s) quote; and James M. Booher (medical director, Continental Scale Works), *Scientific Weight Control* (Chicago, 1925).

64. On streamlined low-profile scales, see Lifshey, *Housewares Story*, 221–23; Jacobs Bros., *Detecto Scales Catalog #237* (Brooklyn, 1937?) 25, provided by Mack Rapp; Borg ad, "An inventor's dream gave you weighing accuracy at home," *RD* 68 (April 1956) 181; and interview with Hyland B. Erickson, Chief Executive Officer of the Borg-Erickson Corp., Sept 18, 1984.

65. Jones Scale Works, *The Test* (Binghamton, N.Y., 1874) 2; Chicago Scale Co., catalogs for 1885(?), p. 22, and 1890(?), p. 13, on the Little Detective, both at the Chicago Historical Society; and interview with Bill Gould, Chief Executive Officer of the American Family Scale Co., Sept 19, 1984. On standardizing weights, see Boorstin, *The Democratic Experience*, 189–91.

66. F. S. Holbrook, *Manual of Inspection and Information for Weights and Measures Officials* (Washington, D.C., 1918) esp. 74; Malcolm W. Jensen and Ralph W. Smith, *The Examination of Weighing Equipment* (Washington, D.C., 1965) 52, 59; Isabel Bevier, "Story of scales," *Chautauquan* 30 (Jan 1900) 375–77; and Dorothy P. Ryan, *Picture Postcards in the United States 1893–1918* (NY, 1982) 21.

67. *GJHL* 1 (1837) 142; George M. Beard, *Eating and Drinking* (NY, 1871) 88; Martin L. Holbrook, *Eating for Health* (NY, 1888) 73; Heinrich Stern, "On the treatment of obesity," *JAMA* 38 (1902) 451; "Teach weight reduction," *NYT* (April 15, 1924) 11:2; and Elmer L. Sevringhaus, "Obesity: endocrine or dietary," *Wisconsin Med J* 25 (1926) 245.

68. On diabetes, see esp. Hugh C. Trowell, "Hypertension, obesity, diabetes mellitus and coronary heart disease," in *Western Diseases: Their Emergence and Prevention*, eds. Trowell and D. P. Burkitt (Cambridge, Mass, 1981) 14, 24–24. On its prevalence, see Charles W. Purdy, "Popular errors in living and their influence over the public health," *North Amer R* 164 (June 1897) 670, and Elliott P. Joslin, "Prevention of diabetes mellitus," *JAMA* 76 (1921) 79. On diets for

diabetics, see Joshua Duke, *Banting in India*, 3d ed. (Calcutta, 1885) 62, same diet as for the obese, and Karl von Noorden, "Treatment of obesity complicated by diseases of the circulatory organs," *Int Med Mag* 11 (1902) 463.

69. Louis W. Hill and Rena S. Eckman, *Starvation Treatment of Diabetes*, 2d ed. (Boston, 1916), and Elliott P. Joslin, "Fat and the diabetic," *NEJM* 209 (1933) 527.

70. John R. Brobeck, "Physiology of appetite," in *Overeating, Overweight and Obesity* (NY: National Vitamin Foundation, 1953) 102, and Joslin, "Prevention of diabetes," 81–83.

71. Joslin, "Fat and the diabetic," 527; Solomon Strouse and M. Dye, "Studies in the metabolism of obesity," *ARIM* 34 (1924) 272; and Horace Gray and Jean M. Stewart, "Quantitative diets vs. guesswork in the treatment of obesity and diabetes," *Scientific Monthly* 32 (Jan 1931) 48. On food scales, see Howe Papers, *Catalog #61* (1924) 122 for Chatillon Dietary Scales; Hanson Scale Co., *Catalog, 1927*, items 1440, 1460; Pelouze New Dietetic Scale ad in *JADA* 8 (1932) 201; Jacobs Bros., *Detecto Scales Catalog #237*, 23 on Detecto-Diet scale; and Hanson Scale Co., *Catalog #7. Supplement* (1941) 8, item 1450.

72. Joslin, "Prevention of diabetes," 82; idem, "Fat and the diabetic," 518–20; and L. H. Newburgh et al., "A new interpretation of diabetes mellitus in obese, middle-aged persons," *AAPT* 53 (1938) 245–57.

73. Emma S. Weigley, *Sarah Tyson Rorer* (Philadelphia, 1977) 84–85, 161, and B. W. Kunkel, "Calories and vitamines," *Scientific Monthly* 17 (Oct 1923) 361.

74. Gaertner, *Reducing Weight Comfortably* (Philadelphia, 1914) quote on 112; Thompson, *Eat and Grow Thin: The Mahdah Diets* (NY, 1914) 7, 13, 14; Joseph C. Furnas, *Great Times: An Informal Social History of the United States 1914–1929* (NY, 1974) 39; and *Who Was Who in America* I, 1234. For early medical use of the low-calorie diet, see Alfred C. Croftan, "Treatment of obesity," *Illinois Med J* 10 (1906) 280–81; "Adequate foods and hints on diet," *NYT* (Oct 24, 1909) 20:4; and Walter C. Alvarez, *Incurable Physician* (Englewood Cliffs, N.J., 1963) 52.

75. Rose, *Eat Your Way to Health* (NY, 1916) 30, and Herrick, *Lose Weight and Be Well* (NY, 1917) 88–89.

76. Furnas, *Great Times*, 39; Philip S. Marden, "Counting your calories," in his *Detours (Passable but Unsafe)* rept. (Freeport, N.Y., 1968 [1926]) 86–87; and Alice Payne Hackett and James H. Burke, *Eighty Years of Bestsellers, 1895–1975* (NY, 1977) 21–31.

77. "Excess weight her specialty," *Los Angeles Times* (May 13, 1923) II, 11:1; *Who Was Who in America*, I, 964; Thyra S. Winslow, *Winslow Weight Watcher* (NY, 1953) 121 on Peters; Lulu Hunt Peters, *Diet*

and Health, with Key to the Calories, 10th ed. (Chicago, 1921) 11, 12, 18, 96-97; Peters diet column, *Los Angeles Times* (April 25, 1922) II, 8:2 and (Jan 10, 1924) II, 7:2, "A disgrace to be fat."

78. Richard O. Cummings, *The American and His Food* (Chicago, 1940) 153-54; Dignam Papers, Package #1, 1923 ad; "Metropolitan's plan for reducing works," *NYT* (June 26, 1924) 38:3; Ella Mae Ives, comp., *The Home Dietitian*, 3d ed. (Philadelphia, 1928) 23-28; Irving Fisher and Eugene L. Fisk, *How to Live*, 18th ed. (NY, 1929) 37, 282-304; George C. Beach, "Obesity and its treatment," *Military Surgeon* 69 (1931) 485-86; Esther B. Tietz, "Pocket calorie index," *Hygeia* 14 (Jan 1936) 15; and Marden, *Detours*, 93.

79. Blythe, *Get Rid of That Fat* (NY, 1928) 22, 48, 54; Blake F. Donaldson, "Treatment of obesity," *MCNA* 8,1 (1924) 334; and Stern, "On the treatment of obesity," 450.

80. Henry J. Spencer, "Clinical observations concerning the obese," *MCNA* 12 (1928) 607; James M. Strang and Frank A. Evans, "Energy exchange in obesity," *J of Clinical Investigation* 6 (1926) 277-89; idem, "A departure from usual methods in treating obesity," *AJMS* 177 (1929) 339-48; idem, "Treatment of obesity with low caloric diets," *JAMA* 97 (1931) 1063-69; and Frank A. Evans, "Treatment of obesity with low-calory diets," *AAPT* 53 (1938) 352-55. For comparisons, see W. H. Allchin, "Dietetic treatment of obesity," *Practitioner* 76 (1906) 523, and Jack C. Drummond and Anne Wilbraham, *The Englishman's Food*, rev. ed. (London, 1958) 256, estimating Cornaro's diet at 800-1,100 calories.

81. Margaret Rossiter, "'Women's work' in science, 1880-1910," *Isis* 71 (1980) 384; Lois Banner, *American Beauty* (NY, 1983) 260-70; and Booher, *Scientific Weight Control*, symmetry table, 72.

82. Elizabeth Ewing, *Dress and Undress* (London, 1978) 115-51; Carl A. Naether, *Advertising to Women* (NY, 1928) esp. 141; Wells, *Dress and Look Slender*, 55-56; Betty Thornley, "Merrily we roll along: how to roll off the roll," *Collier's* 84 (Dec 7, 1929) 73 on invisible girdles; Caroline Bird, *Enterprising Women* (NY, 1976) 190-92 on the Maidenform bra; Carol Wald, *Myth America* (NY, 1975) 108, Kabo Corset ad, "The Live Model Corset"; Florence Courtenay, *Physical Beauty* (NY, 1922) 54, on corsets along natural lines; "The corset," *Fortune* 17 (March 1938) 95-99, 110, 113-14; and "Soft-spoken promotion widens market for 'ethical' products," *Sales Management* 50 (Jan 15, 1942) 28, 30, 32, on the "Transparent Woman," an anatomical display piece.

83. Nystrom, *Economics of Fashion*, 463, 467; Naether, *Advertising to Women*, 227-28, 327; Christine Frederick, *Selling Mrs. Consumer* (NY, 1929) 27; Gossard Corsets ad in *LHJ* 36 (Sept 1919) 50 on fitting

special body types; Dowager Corset ad in *LHJ* (Aug 1899) back cover; Scott Hip Form ad in *LHJ* 22 (April 1905) 60; and Flatter-U ad in *Corset and Underwear Review* (Aug 1922) referring to the *Kabo System of Healthful Reducing*, in Dignam Papers, Package #3, folder on National Advertising of Corsets.

84. Julius Preuss, *Biblical and Talmudic Medicine*, trans. and ed. Fred Rosner (NY, 1978 [1911]) 215; E. Jeanselme, "Comment on traitait les obèses à Byzance," *Bulletin de la société française d'histoire de la médecine* 20 (1926) 388–90; Frederick M. Grazer and Jerome R. Klingbeil, *Body Image: A Surgical Perspective* (St. Louis, 1980) 63–74; Henry W. Coe, "Overweight," *Med Examiner* 5 (1895) 32; "Trimmed fat man better," *NYT* (May 11, 1908) 4:5; "Under knife for obesity," *NYT* (Nov 15, 1911) 1:6; Max Thorek, "Possibilities in the reconstruction of the human form," *NY Med J* 116 (1922) 572–75; and Joseph Colt Bloodgood, "Possibilities and dangers of beauty operations, and the danger of excessive fat in surgery and disease," in *Your Weight and How to Control It*, ed. Morris Fishbein (NY, 1927) 51–66.

85. "Congressmen jocose in fat and lean debate," *NYT* (Feb 4, 1921) 2:5; Club SHRDLU history, p. 53, and typescript of the debate photocopied for me by Barbara Vandegrift, Archivist/Librarian of the National Press Club.

86. William M. Ballinger, "Treatment of obesity," *Southern Med J* 23 (1930) 1156.

87. On gum, see *JAMA* 87 (1926) 688–91, 1665–66. On cigarettes, see Luckies ads in *Literary Digest* 101 (April 13, 1929) 79, and *Forum* 81 (Jan 1929) li, 81 (Feb 1929) xlviii, and 81 (April 1929) xxxvii. See also National Better Business Bureau, *Bulletins* (Jan 25, 1930) and (Sept 1930); and Robert Sobel, *They Satisfy: The Cigarette in American Life* (NY, 1978) 100–102.

88. Rapp interview; Erickson interview.

89. *Nostrums* II, 676–77; AMA, *"Obesity Cures"* (Chicago, 1929?) 10–13; *JAMA* 87 (1926) 189–90, 88 (1927) 1920–21, 92 (1929) 2121 and 97 (1931) 122–23; and Vincent Tumminello, *Vincent Method of Bathtub Exercises* (New Orleans, 1939).

90. Charles Gaines, *Yours in Perfect Manhood, Charles Atlas* (NY, 1983); Battle Creek Health Builder ad in *Literary Digest* 95 (Oct 15, 1927) 73; and Philip B. Hawk, *Streamline for Health* (NY, 1935) 135 on Coolidge. Cf. Harvey Green, *Fit for America* (NY, 1986) ch. 8

91. Sylvia of Hollywood, *Hollywood Undressed* (NY, 1931) 11, 20, and Sylvia Ullback, *No More Alibis* (NY, 1936) quote on 15. College girls associated the vamp silhouette with dieting—and the vamp's power came from her silhouette; see the 1930 story by Mary Edna McChris-

tie, "Reductio ad absurdum," *Survey* 65 (Nov 1, 1930) 152–55, 192, in which the stout heroine, once slenderized, becomes "love-hungry, and filled with a sense of power." See also Paula Fass, *The Damned and the Beautiful: American Youth in the 1920s* (NY, 1978) 282, 458n.

92. Francis B. Floore, "Analysis of the Hollywood Eighteen Day Diet," *Hygeia* 9 (March 1931) 245–46; Lewis R. Wolberg, *Psychology of Eating* (NY, 1936) 128; James Harvey Young, *Medical Messiahs* (Princeton, N.J., 1967) 123 on Marmola and Tallmadge; Marmola ad in *Motion Picture* 38 (May 1929) 107; Fanny Hurst, *No Food with My Meals* (NY, 1935) 53; Llewellyn Louderback, *Fat Power* (NY, 1970) 108–9 on Hollywood deaths, as also Carl Malmberg, *Diet and Die* (NY, 1935) 16–18, and Y. Y. (= Robert Lynd), "Slimming," *New Statesman* 34 (April 5, 1930) 832; and "Wolheim, 'bad man' of movies, is dead," *NYT* (Feb 19, 1931) 25:1.

93. H. I. Phillips, "It is never too late to shrink," *Amer Mag* 100 (Dec 1925) 39, and Francis G. Benedict, "Rationale of weight reduction," *Scientific Monthly* 33 (Sept 1931) 264.

94. For the physical portrait of Kellogg, see Irving N. Fisher, *My Father, Irving Fisher* (NY, 1956) 108–9.

95. R. W. Schwarz, *John Harvey Kellogg, M.D.* (Nashville, 1970) and Horace B. Powell, *The Original Has This Signature—W. K. Kellogg* (Englewood Cliffs, N.J., 1956) provide most of the biographical in formation here.

96. Schwarz, *Kellogg*, 116–20, 209–14; Powell, *Kellogg*, 90–95; and Gerald Carson, *Cornflake Crusade* (NY, 1957) 4, 67, 117–22. Cf. Ronald M. Deutsch, *The Nuts Among the Berries*, rev. ed. (NY, 1967) 54–104.

97. Schwarz, *Kellogg*, 87; John Harvey Kellogg, *Home Handbook of Domestic Hygiene and Rational Medicine*, rev. ed. (Battle Creek, Mich., 1896) 276–80, 808 ff.; and idem, *Rational Hydrotherapy*, 2d ed. (Philadelphia, 1904) 1027.

98. Schwarz, *Kellogg*, 33–34, 76–77, 84–87, 98–99, 124–25; "Centennial exhibition sketches," *Health Reformer* 11 (1876) 237–38; Kellogg, *Home-Handbook*, Plates XXIII–XXVI; Albert W. Ferris, "Reduction of obesity," *Med Record* 89 (1916) 144; and Carson, *Cornflake Crusade*, 101, 108, 241.

99. Schwarz, *Kellogg*, 34; Carson, *Cornflake Crusade*, 106; James C. Whorton, *Crusaders for Fitness* (Princeton, N.J., 1982) 216, 221–23; Kellogg, *A Household Manual* (Battle Creek, Mich., 1877) 39, 43; idem, *Autointoxication or Intestinal Toxemia*, 2d ed. (Battle Creek, Mich., 1919) 5, 41, 43, 203–5; Donaldson, "Treatment of obesity," 333; Dignam Papers, Package #1, ad copy for Pillsbury's Health Bran

and Kellogg's All-Bran; and Mary I. Barber, ed., *History of the American Dietetic Association 1917–1959* (Philadelpha, 1959) 19, 40 (quote).

100. Schwarz, *Kellogg*, 46, 76, 87, 107; Carson, *Cornflake Crusade*, 137; Horace Fletcher, *New Glutton or Epicure* (NY, 1908) 58, 60, 67; idem, *Fletcherism* (London, 1913?) 35; and Fletcher Correspondence, letter to Kellogg, Nov 18, 1903, with his song, to the tune of "Montague Montrose."

101. Schwarz, *Kellogg*, 45, 125, 227–28; Horace Fletcher, *A.B.–Z. of Our Own Nutrition* (NY, 1903) xxxiv; Carson, *Cornflake Crusade*, 234; and Fisher, "A new method," 417.

102. Schwarz, *Kellogg*, 51, 76–77; Carson, *Cornflake Crusade*, 229; and Rorty and Norman, *Tomorrow's Food*, 123.

103. Schwarz, *Kellogg*, 79; Powell, *Kellogg*, 138.

CHAPTER SEVEN
Hearts of Darkness, Bodies of Woe

1. Simeon Shell, "Remarks on amblyopia from dinitrobenzol," *BMJ* 1 (1894) 449–54; W. C. Cutting et al., "Actions and uses of dinitrophenol," *JAMA* 101 (1933) 193–95; M. L. Tainter et al., "Use of dinitrophenol in nutritional disorders," *AJPH* 24 (1934) 1045–53; William E. Robertson, "Alpha dinitrophenol and its influence upon metabolism," *J of Laboratory and Clinical Med* 19 (1934) 1280–85; Carl Malmberg, *Diet and Die* (NY, 1935) 120, 130; E. R. Squibb & Sons, *Physicians' Reference Book*, 8th ed. (NY, Dec 1936) 149–50; Ruth de Forest Lamb, *American Chamber of Horrors* (NY, 1936) 94–97; A. S. Blumgarten, *Textbook of Materia Medica*, 7th ed. (NY, 1937) 658–59; "Weight controls," *JAMA* 111 (1938) 188–89; and Food Law Institute, *Federal Food, Drug and Cosmetic Law: Administrative Reports, 1907–1949* (Chicago, 1951) 819, 913, 929.

2. *New Republic* 75 (Aug 2, 1933) 300–301.

3. Philip B. Hawk, *Streamline for Health* (NY, 1935) 131, 152; Herman N. Bundesen, *Dr. Bundesen's Diet Book* (Chicago, 1934) 15; and Victor H. Lindlahr, *Eat—and Reduce* (NY, 1939) 98.

4. On New Deal economists and consumption, see esp. Daniel M. Fox, *The Discovery of Abundance: Simon N. Patten and the Transformation of Social Theory* (Ithaca, N.Y., 1967) 162–66.

5. Solomon Strouse and M. Dye, "Studies in the metabolism of obesity," *ARIM* 34 (1924) 267–81, 575–83 and 36 (1925) 397–417; Harry M. Jones, "Basal metabolic rate in simple and pathologic obesity," *J of Laboratory and Clinical Med* 11 (1926) 966; Eugene F. DuBois, *Ba-*

sal Metabolism, 2d ed. (London, 1927) 235–37; L. H. Newburgh and M. W. Johnston, "The nature of obesity," *J of Clinical Investigations* 8 (1930) 197–213; idem, "Endogenous obesity—a misconception," *JADA* 5 (1930) 275–85; Russell M. Wilder, "The treatment of obesity," *Int Clinics* 4 (1933) 17 (quote); and Frank A. Evans, "Treatment of obesity with low-calory diets," *AAPT* 53 (1938) 354.

6. Walter B. Cannon, *Mechanical Factors of Digestion* (London, 1911); Anton J. Carlson, *The Control of Hunger in Health and Disease* (Chicago, 1916); Jean Mayer and Donald W. Thomas, "Regulation of food intake and obesity," *Science* 156 (April 21, 1967) 328–37 for historical review, as also E. Stellar, "The CNS and appetite: historical introduction," *Appetite and Food Intake*, ed. Trevor Silverstone (Berlin, 1976) 15–20; and Samuel Lepkovsky, "The physiological basis of voluntary food intake (appetite?)," *Advances in Food Research* 1 (1948) 105–48.

7. Kendrick A. Clements, "Herbert Hoover and conservation, 1921–33," *AHR* 89 (1984) 67–88; David D. Lee, "The politics of less: the trials of Herbert Hoover and Jimmy Carter," *Presidential Studies Q* 13 (1983) 305–12; Lawrence Chenoweth, *The American Dream of Success* (North Scituate, Mass., 1974) 55, 59, 70 (quote), 71 (quote); and Caroline Bird, *The Invisible Scar* (NY, 1966) 24–30.

8. E. G. Boring and Amy Luce, "The psychological basis of appetite," *Amer J of Psych* 28 (1917) 443–53; Ivan P. Pavlov, *The Work of the Digestive Glands*, trans. W. H. Thompson, 2d English ed. (London, 1910) esp. 89–95; Alonzo E. Taylor, "The national overweight," *Scientific Monthly* 32 (1931) 395 on self-feeding; Clara M. Davis, "Self selection of diet by newly weaned infants," *AJDC* 36 (1928) 651–79, first in a series of studies; Hilda Weber, "Hunger and appetite," *J of Mental Science* 76 (1930) 724–63; Joseph C. Aub, "Treatment of obesity," *MCNA* 18 (1935) 1192–93; and "The wonders of diet," *Fortune* 13 (May 1936) 86.

9. Abraham Myerson, *The Nervous Housewife* (NY, 1920); Christine Frederick, *Selling Mrs. Consumer* (NY, 1929); Alice Kessler-Harris, *Out to Work* (NY, 1982) ch. 8; Dolores Hayden, *The Grand Domestic Revolution* (Cambridge, Mass., 1981) 274–75, 295; Estelle B. Freedman, "The New Woman: changing views of women in the 1920s," *JAH* 61 (1974/75) 373–93; and Kurt Lewin, "Forces behind food habits and methods of change," in *The Problem of Changing Food Habits* NAS-NRC Pub. No. 108 (Washington, D.C., 1943) 37 on women as gatekeepers.

10. Kessler-Harris, *Out to Work*, ch. 9; Barbara Ehrenreich and Deirdre English, *For Her Own Good* (Garden City, N.Y., 1978) 203–10; Lynn Y. Weiner, *From Working Girl to Working Mother: The Female Labor Force in the United States, 1820–1980* (Chapel Hill, N.C.,

1985) chs. 4–5; Maxine L. Margolis, *Mothers and Such* (Berkeley, Calif., 1984) 57–58, 130–47; Nancy Chodorow, *The Reproduction of Mothering* (Berkeley, Calif., 1978) 84–85, 99n, 185, 187, 212; David M. Levy, "Maternal overprotection," *Psychiatry* 1 (1938) 561–91, and his *Maternal Overprotection* (NY, 1943). Contrast Kim Chernin, *The Hungry Self* (NY, 1985).

11. Samuel Hochman, "Mental and psychological factors in obesity," *Med Record* 148 (1938) 108–11; George H. Reeve, "Psychological factors in obesity," *Amer J of Orthopsychiatry* 12 (1942) 674–79; Israel Bram, "Psychosomatic obesity, with comments on 924 cases," *Med Record* 157 (1944) 673–76; "Eating your heart out?" *Science Illustrated* 1 (Oct 1946) 40–41; Henry B. Richardson, "Obesity as a manifestation of neurosis," *MCNA* 30 (1946) 1187–1202; Herman Friedel, *You Can Be Thin! Slenderness Through Psychology* (NY, 1948) 2, 90–91; Walter W. Hamburger, "Emotional aspects of obesity," *MCNA* 35 (1951) 483–99; Alfred J. Cantor, *How to Lose Weight the Doctor's Way* (NY, 1959); George Krupp, "My mother made me fat: a Redbook symposium," *Redbook* 132 (Jan 1969) 52–54, 105; and Benjamin B. Wolman, ed., *Psychological Aspects of Obesity* (NY, 1982) esp. 88–103.

12. Thomas M. French, "Psychogenic factors in asthma," *Amer J of Psychiatry* 96 (1939) 87–101, and Neil T. McDermott and Stanley Cobb, "Psychiatric survey of fifty cases of bronchial asthma," *Psychosomatic Med* 1 (1939) 203–44.

13. Terence Du Quesne and Julian Reeves, *Handbook of Psychoactive Medicines* (London, 1982) 207–12; Charles O. Jackson, "Before the drug culture: barbiturate/amphetamine abuse in American society," *Clio Medica* 11 (1976) 47–58; M. H. Nathanson, "The central action of beta-aminopropylbenzene (Benzedrine)," *JAMA* 108 (1937) 529; Mark F. Lesses and Abraham Myerson, "Benzedrine sulfate as an aid in the treatment of obesity," *NEJM* 218 (1938) 119–24; and Gerhard Rosenthal and Harry A. Solomon, "Benzedrine sulfate in obesity," *Endocrinology* 26 (1940) 807–12.

14. Du Quesne and Reeves, *Handbook*, 210–11; Jackson, "Before the drug culture," 49; and Andrew C. Ivy and F. R. Goetzl, "α-Desoxyephedrine: a review," *War Med* 3 (1943) 60–77.

15. "Use of amphetamine sulfate in control of obesity," *JAMA* 123 (1943) 1117; "Benzedrine and dieting," *Newsweek* 30 (Sept 8, 1947) 48; Robert H. Williams et al., "Obesity and its treatment," *AIM* 29 (1948) 527; S. Charles Freed, "Psychic factors in the development and treatment of obesity," *JAMA* 133 (1947) 369–73; Edward H. Rynearson and Clifford F. Gastineau, *Obesity* (Springfield, Ill., 1949) 95 on cocktails; E. Philip Gelvin and Thomas H. McGavack, "Dexedrine and weight reduction," *NY St Med J* 49 (1949) 279–82 on ef-

fects wearing off; "Drugs for obesity," *BMJ* 2 (1963) 853–55; and Biphetamine ad in *Postgraduate Med* 38 (Sept 1965) A40–41.

16. Ads in *Postgraduate Med* 38 (Aug 1965) A40 for Biphetamine and (Sept 1965) A205 for Obedrin; and Wallace Laboratories promotional record for Appetrol in their Recorded Medical Library (1960?): "Every husband knows how irritable his wife can become while she is on a reducing regimen." Appetrol combined amphetamine and Miltown.

17. Chodorow, *Reproduction of Mothering*, 99n.

18. Bertram W. Sippy, "Gastric and duodenal ulcer," *JAMA* 64 (1915) 1626; John P. Street, "Skim milk as a human food," *Amer Food J* 11 (Sept 1916) 453–55; George A. Harrop, "Milk and banana diet," *JAMA* 102 (1934) 2003–5; Malmberg, *Diet and Die*, 101; Roberta Sainsbury and Margaret C. Smith, "Metabolic studies of human subjects on a skimmed milk and banana diet," *JHE* 29 (1937) 468–71; "Dr. Stoll's Diet-Aid," *JAMA* 100 (1933) 207–8; Norman Jolliffe, *Reduce and Stay Reduced* (NY, 1952) 149 on liquid formula; "Universal diet no. 1," *Newsweek* 44 (Sept 27, 1954) 91; D. C. Norman, "Fabulous formula," *LHJ* 73 (Dec 1956) 64–65, 155–59; Vincent P. Dole, "Publicity about a 'reducing diet,'" *JAMA* 161 (1956) 901; "Crazy about reducing," *Time* 68 (Aug 6, 1956) 32; Roy De Groot, *How I Reduced with the New Rockefeller Diet* (NY, 1956); Alvan R. Feinstein et al., "The use of a formula diet for weight reduction of obese outpatients," *AIM* 48 (1958) 330–43; and George W. Corner, *History of the Rockefeller Institute 1901–1953* (NY, 1964) 489–91. On Metrecal, see Peter Wyden, *The Overweight Society* (NY, 1965) ch. 3.

19. See C. J. Speas, "Liquid therapeutic diet," *J of Tennessee St Med Assoc* 43 (1950) 321–27.

20. "Another obesity cure," *Consumer Reports* 17 (July 1952) 347–48.

21. Horace W. Davenport, "Why the stomach does not digest itself," *Scientific Amer* 226 (Jan 1972) 87–93, and Gerald S. Lee, *Recreating Oneself* (Northampton, Mass., 1934) quotes on 52, 53.

22. Axel E. Gibson, *Facts and Fancies in Health Foods* (Los Angeles, 1921) 105 against mixtures; Bernard Bernard, *Correct and Corrective Eating* (Chicago, 1923) 11–12, 15, 19 concerning acids and starches; Rose Millen, *Light on Dietetics* (Boston, 1927) 15, 19; Sunolia V. Harter, *80/20 Cook Book and Food Manual* (Toledo, 1928) title page; and Henrietta Hayes, *Eat to Grow Young* (NY, 1934) 29, 37.

23. George H. Brinkler, *Foresight, Foundation of Fortunes* (NY, 1932) 433, and "Another Brinkler fraud order," *JAMA* 113 (1939) 1346–48.

24. William H. Hay, *Weight Control* (NY, 1935) esp. 14–17, 34, 41–43, 52–53, 72; Malmberg, *Diet and Die*, 65–74; Lewis E. Wolberg, "Hay food fantasy," *Hygeia* 16 (1938) 311–13, 372; Thomas J. Walsh,

Youth Again: Letters to an Overweight Friend (Chicago, 1933) on Ford; and Josephine Boyer and Katherine Cowdin, *Hay Dieting* (NY, 1934) 6.

25. Boyer and Cowdin, *Hay Dieting*, 5.

26. Victor G. Heiser, "We are what we eat," *Collier's* 98 (Oct 10, 1936) 18, 56–57; Weston A. Price, *Nutrition and Physical Degeneration* (Redlands, Calif., 1945 [1939]); Vilhjalmur Stefansson, *Not by Bread Alone* (NY, 1946), and for recent examples, Sally De Vore and Thelma White, *Dinner's Ready! An Invitation to Better Nutrition from Nine Healthier Cultures* (Pasadena, Calif., 1977); and William T. Jarvis, "Myth of the healthy savage," *Nutrition Today* 16 (March–April 1981) 14–23.

27. Hay, *Weight Control*, 11, 24.

28. Hawk, *Streamline for Health*, xix.

29. Hilde Bruch, *Importance of Overweight* (NY, 1957) 5–7, and Susan K. Deri, "A problem in obesity," in *Clinical Studies of Personality*, eds. Arthur Burton and Robert E. Harris (NY, 1955) 526.

30. On psychotherapy in conjunction with other therapies, see esp. Henry M. Ray, "The obese patient," *Amer J of Digestive Diseases* 14 (1947) 153–62.

31. Isador H. Coriat, "Sex and hunger," *Psychoanalytic R* 8 (1921) 375–81; Gustav Bychowski, "Neurotic obesity," *ibid.* 27 (1950) 301–19; Chodorow, *Reproduction of Mothering*, esp. 59, 63; and Elta Arnold, *Reduce Your Weight for Keeps* (n.p., 1949) 13, a quote seemingly taken out of context, but Arnold too accused the obese of "trying to eat your way to happiness," p. 8.

32. Frederick S. Perls, *Ego, Hunger and Aggression* (London, 1947) 192–99, and Perls et al., *Gestalt Therapy* (NY, 1951) 221–47.

33. Leonid Kotkin, *Eat, Think and Be Slender* (NY, 1954) 25.

34. Cyril Connolly, *The Unquiet Grave* (NY, 1945) quotation on p. 58. Jonathon Green, *Dictionary of Contemporary Quotations* (London, 1982) gives George Orwell's *Coming Up for Air* (1939) as the source for Connolly's maxim.

35. Ernest Kurtz, *Not-God: A History of Alcoholics Anonymous* (Center City, Minn., 1979); Mark E. Lender and James K. Martin, *Drinking in America* (NY, 1982) 182–90; and Bill (= William Wilson), *The A.A. Way of Life* (NY, 1967) quote on 90.

36. "Women in anti-fat contest," *NYT* (March 5, 1912) 1:3; Lulu Hunt Peters, *Diet and Health, with Key to the Calories*, 10th ed. (Chicago, 1921) 78–79; "Dr. Copeland starts fat-reducing contest," *NYT* (Oct 19, 1921) 33:2 and daily accounts through Nov 13, with quote (Oct 26, 1921) 36:3.

37. Linda Gordon, *Woman's Body, Woman's Right* (NY, 1976) 374–75; Robert M. Goldenson, *Encyclopedia of Human Behavior* (Garden City, N.Y., 1970) I, 77–79, 523–27; Franz G. Alexander and Sheldon T. Selesnick, *History of Psychiatry* (NY, 1966) 411–16; and S. R. Slavson, "Current trends in group psychotherapy," *Int J of Group Psychotherapy* 1 (1951) 7–15.

38. T. W. Adorno et al., *The Authoritarian Personality* (NY, 1950), and David Riesman, with Nathan Glazer and Reuel Denney, *The Lonely Crowd* (New Haven, 1950).

39. "Obesity is now no. 1 US nutritional problem," *Science News Letter* 62 (Dec 27, 1952) 408; and "Fat and unhappy," *Time* 59 (June 23, 1952) 64, Bortz quote.

40. B. G. Hauser, *Look Younger, Live Longer* (NY, 1950) 98–112; Cecile A. Hoover, "Food facts," *Service* 16 (April 1952) 13; Bernard Koten, *The Low-calory Cookbook* (NY, 1951) xii; Metropolitan Life Insurance Company, *A Report on the Group Approach for Weight Control* (NY, 1951); Joseph I. Goodman, *Diet and Live* (Chicago, 1966) 150 on group diets in Cleveland, 1950; Herrick Memorial Hospital, *A Study of Weight Reduction Using Group Methods* (Berkeley, Calif., 1953?); Marjorie Grant, "Group approach for weight control," *Group Psychotherapy* 4 (1951) 156–65; A. L. Chapman, "Weight control—simplified concept," *Public Health Report* 66 (1951) 725–31; "Obesity anonymous," *Newsweek* 37 (June 4, 1951) 84; Malcolm J. Ford, "Group approach to weight control," *AJPH* 43 (1953) 997–1000; L. J. Bowser et al., "Group therapy with individual clinic interviews," *JADA* 29 (1953) 1193–96; and "Plan for people who must lose weight," *GH* 138 (March 1954) 58–59, 230.

41. "TOPS takes off pounds," *Life* 30 (April 9, 1951) 137–38; W. W. Bauer, "The Editor cornered," *Today's Health* 31 (Oct 1953) 10; Thyra S. Winslow, *Winslow Weight Watcher* (NY, 1953) 312; "Obesity anonymous: TOPS," *Newsweek* 56 (Aug 1, 1960) 78; Esther S. Manz, *How to Take Off Pounds Sensibly* (Milwaukee, 1963); and Wyden, *Overweight Society*, 79–95.

42. Overeaters Anonymous, Inc., *Overeaters Anonymous* (Torrance, Calif., 1980) quotes on 5, 55; Wyden, *Overweight Society*, quote on 85; and interview with Rozanne S., Sept 5, 1984.

43. Jean Nidetch, *The Story of Weight Watchers* (NY, 1970) 104, 146, 148.

44. *Ibid.*, 147.

45. *Ibid.*, 137–39, 147. I have also used Natalie Allon, "Stigma of overweight in everyday life," in *Obesity in America*, ed. George A. Bray (Washington, D.C., 1975) 83–102; idem, "Group-dieting rituals," in *Deviant Life Styles*, ed. James M. Henslin (New Brunswick, N.J.,

1977) 101–14; idem, *Urban Life Styles* (Dubuque, 1979) ch. 2; Nora S. Kinzer, *Put Down and Ripped Off: The American Woman and the Beauty Cult* (NY, 1977) 31–55; and Marvin B. Sussman, "'The Calorie Collectors': a study of spontaneous group formation, collapse and reconstruction," *Social Forces* 34 (1956) 351–55.

46. Telephone interview with Jeff Salzman of Leo D. Bernstein & Sons, NY, Oct 9, 1984, on mannequins.

47. On secrecy, see, e.g., Jean Z. Owen, *It's More Fun to Be Thin* (Boston, 1939) 147; Annie W. Williams-Heller, *It's a Sin to Be Fat* (NY, 1947) 36, 163; and Alfred Toombs, "Quiet, I'm on a diet," *Atlantic* 188 (Sept 1951) 90–91.

48. Rozanne S. interview; Nidetch, *Story of Weight Watchers*, 57–59; and interview with Lois Lindauer, Nov 11, 1984.

49. Interview with Lynne Miller of Thin Forever! Inc., NY, Oct 18, 1984.

50. Elmer Wheeler, *Fat Boy's Book* (NY, 1950) quote on 160; idem, *Fat Boy's Downfall* (NY, 1952) 1, 141; "Diets for men," *Time* 57 (March 26, 1951) 63–64; and "Page-one fat boy," *Newsweek* 37 (March 26, 1951) 64.

51. Wheeler, *Fat Boy's Book*, slide rule at front, and *Fat Boy's Downfall*, thermometer at flyleaf, also 67, 114–16.

52. Wheeler, *Fat Boy's Book*, 3, 54, 134.

53. *Ibid.*, 57.

54. John Taylor, *The Olde, Olde, Very Olde Man* (London, 1635) quote on sig A4v.

55. William Harvey, "Anatomical examination of the body of Thomas Parr," in *Works*, trans. Robert Willis (London, 1847) 587–92, quote on 590.

56. William J. Ford, "Old Parr," *BHM* 24 (1950) 219–26, and William J. Thoms, *Human Longevity* (NY, 1979 [1873]) 85–94.

57. Harry L. Smith and Frederick A. Willius, "Adiposity of the heart," *ARIM* 52 (1933) 911.

58. Giovanni Maria Lancisi, *De Subitaneis Mortibus (On Sudden Deaths)* (1707), trans. Paul Dudley White and Alfred V. Boursy (NY, 1971) 133–39; John Baptist Morgagni, *The Seats and Causes of Disease* (1760), trans. Benjamin Alexander (NY, 1960) I, 802–3, 832–34; Dr. Wade, "Case of a preternatural fatness," *Med Observations and Inquiries* 3 (1767) 69–84, associating fat heart, obesity and reducing agents; John Fothergill, "Case of an angina pectoris," *ibid.* 5 (1779) 233–51, with "Farther account," 252–58; Smith and Willius, "Adiposity of the heart," 912; and Douglas Guthrie, "Evolution of cardiology," in *Science, Medicine and History*, ed. E. A. Underwood (NY, 1953) II, 511–14.

59. John Mason Good, *The Study of Medicine*, 4th Amer ed. (Philadelphia, 1825) IV, 201, citing Hunter; Lyman Spalding, "Change of a human body to a fatty substance, by submersion in water, after death," *Med Repository* 2d ser., 5 (1808) 325–36; and R. T. H. Laennec, *A Treatise on the Disease of the Chest* (1819), trans. John Forbes (NY, 1962) 284 ff.

60. William Wadd, *Cursory Remarks on Corpulence*, 3d ed. (London, 1816) 9–15; idem, *Comments on Corpulency* (London, 1829) 29; Good, *Study of Medicine*, IV, 201–2; Everard Home, "On the formation of fat in the intestines of living animals," *Philosophical Tr of the Royal Soc of London* (1813) 146; C. J. B. Williams, "Obesity," *Cyclopaedia of Practical Medicine*, ed. John Forbes et al. (Philadelphia, 1845) III, 405; and John R. Wardell, "Remarks on obesity," *London Med Gazette* n.s., 8 (1849) 535.

61. Evan Bedford, "The story of fatty heart: a disease of Victorian times," *British Heart J* 34 (1972) 23–28; Thomas King Chambers, "On corpulence," *Lancet* 2 (1850) 12, 350, 437; Alfred C. Croftan, "Treatment of obesity and its complications," *Illinois Med J* 10 (1906) 278, 283; Nellis B. Foster, "Treatment of hypertension," *JAMA* 79 (1922) 1089; William E. Preble, "Obesity," *BMSJ* 188 (1923) 618; Wingate Johnson, "The low-down on high blood pressure," *Hygeia* 10 (1932) 115 on miles of vessels; Don Marquis, "Eat, drink and be merry, for to-morrow ye diet," *Amer Mag* 92 (Oct 1921) 7–9; and K. H. Beall, "The parasitism of fat," *Southern Med J* 12 (1924) 322.

62. Louis I. Dublin et al., "Physical defects as revealed by periodic health examinations," *AJMS* 170 (1925) 583–85; Heart Counsel of Greater Cincinnati, *Life Conservation Studies* (Cincinnati, 1929–30); Actuarial Society of America, *Medical Impairment Study. Supplement* (NY, 1932) esp. 31; Louis I. Dublin and A. J. Lotka, *Length of Life* (NY, 1936) 204; J. E. Wood, Jr., and J. R. Cash, "Obesity and hypertension," *AIM* 13 (1939) 81–90; Actuarial Society of America and the Assoc of Life Insurance Medical Directors, *Blood Pressure Study 1939* (NY, 1940) esp. 19; "The heart and weight," *Newsweek* 43 (Jan 11, 1954) 78; Society of Actuaries, *Build and Blood Pressure Study* (Chicago, 1959–60).

63. Monroe Lerner and Odin W. Anderson, *Health Progress in the United States, 1900–1960* (Chicago, 1963) 16, 54–55.

64. Louis I. Dublin, "Overweight, America's no. 1 health problem," *Today's Health* 30 (Sept 1952) 18–21; Stanley J. Reiser, *Medicine and the Reign of Technology* (Cambridge, Mass., 1978) 65; "The wonders of diet," *Fortune* 13 (May 1936) 86; and Jacobs Bros., *Detecto Scales Catalog #237* (Brooklyn, 1937?) 24.

65. Heinrich Stern, "On the treatment of obesity," *JAMA* 38 (1902) 450, and F. McKelvey Bell, "The 'why' of obesity," *NY Med J* 99 (1914) 732 on the Dead Sea image.

66. On spontaneous combustion, see Wadd, *Cursory Remarks*, 59, and *Comments*, 23–24, 32; Henry T. Finck, *Romantic Love and Personal Beauty* (London, 1887) 382–83 on the body-fuse; and N. E. Yorke-Davies, "Over-fatness," *Gentleman's Mag* n.s. 72 (1903) 574, volcano image.

67. H. Gideon Wells, "Adipose tissue, a neglected subject," *JAMA* 114 (1940) 2177–78, and Friedrich Wasserman, "The concept of the 'fat organ,'" in *Fat as a Tissue*, eds. K. Rodahl and B. Issekutz (NY, 1964) 22–24.

68. E. T. Bell, "On the histogenesis of the adipose tissue of the ox," *Amer J of Anatomy* 9 (1909) 412–35, summary of debate and siding in favor of Toldt; Woods Hutchinson, "A defense of fat men," *SEP* 196 (June 7, 1924) 8; Smith and Willius, "Adiposity of the heart," 929; Wells, "Adipose tissue," 2179; H. E. Wertheimer, "Introduction—a perspective," *Handbook of Physiology. Section 5: Adipose Tissue* (Washington, D.C., 1965) 6–9; Paul S. Ross, "Obesity, cholesterol, arterial disease and hypertension," *Ohio St Med J* 47 (1951) 1109; and Better Homes and Gardens, *Diet Book* (Des Moines, 1955) 40 (quote).

69. William D. Reid, "Relation of obesity to heart disease," *Amer Heart J* 2 (1927) 311; Arthur M. Master and Enid T. Oppenheimer, "A study of obesity," *JAMA* 92 (1929) 1652–56; Smith and Willius, "Adiposity of the heart," 912–17; and Robert L. Levy et al., "Overweight: the prognostic significance in relation to hypertension and cardiovascular-renal diseases," *JAMA* 131 (1946) 951–53.

70. "Reductio ad absurdum," *JAMA* 117 (1941) 1556, and U.S. Senate, *Diet Pill Industry* (Washington, D.C., 1968) 23, 73, 125, 264 (Helen Bailey), 322, 348.

71. Elmer V. McCollum, *A History of Nutrition* (Boston, 1957) ch. 3; Emile Demange, "Obésité," *Dictionnaire encyclopédique des sciences médicales* (Paris, 1880) IV, 8–9; Elliott P. Joslin, "Fat and the diabetic," *NEJM* 209 (1933) 523–25; Maurice Bruger and Charles A. Poindexter, "Relation of the plasma cholesterol to obesity . . . ," *ARIM* 53 (1934) 423–34; Ross, "Obesity, cholesterol . . . ," 1113; Daniel C. Munro, *Slenderizing for New Beauty* (NY, 1953) 18; "Fat's the villain," *Newsweek* 44 (Sept 27, 1954) 90–91; Ancel Keys and Josef Brožek, "Body fat in adult man," *Physiological R* 33 (1953) 245–325; Ancel Keys, "Prediction and possible prevention of coronary diseases," *AJPH* 43 (1953) 1399–1407; Ancel Keys et al., "Effects of diet on blood lipids in men," *Clinical Chemistry* 1 (1955) 34–52; and George Christakis et al., "The Anti-coronary Club," *AJPH* 56 (1966) 299–314.

72. "The fat of the land," *Time* 77 (Jan 13, 1961) 49 (quote); Edward R. Pinckney and Cathey Pinckney, *The Cholesterol Controversy* (Los Angeles, 1973); and Edward C. Naber, "The cholesterol dilemma," *BioScience* 30 (1980) 571.

73. O. T. Williams, "Abnormal fat assimilation," *Bio-Chemical J* 2 (1907) 395; Maximilian Kern, "Status of physical therapy for obesity," *Archives of Physical Therapy* 9 (1928) 259–60; Norman Jolliffe, *Reduce and Stay Reduced* (NY, 1952); Wyden, *Overweight Society*, 149–152, 160–64; and Mohamed A. Antar et al., "Changes in retail market food supplies in the U.S. in the last seventy years in relation to the incidence of coronary heart disease," *AJCN* 14 (1964) 169–78. On February 4, 1980, the USDA and HEW released dietary guidelines suggesting that Americans avoid large amounts of saturated fat and cholesterol.

74. Keys and Brožek, "Body fat in adult man"; "Fat man's gravity," *Newsweek* 19 (March 30, 1942) 61–62; and A. R. Behnke, Jr., et al., "Specific gravity of healthy men," *JAMA* 118 (1942) 495–98.

75. See Alex F. Roche, "Anthropometric methods: new and old, what they tell us," *IJO* 8 (1984) 509–23.

76. J. M. Tanner, *A History of the Study of Human Growth* (Cambridge, 1981) 203; Ancel Keys, "Obesity measurement and the composition of the body," in *Overeating, Overweight and Obesity* (NY, 1953) 17–21; Carl C. Seltzer and Jean Mayer, "A simple criterion of obesity," *Postgraduate Med* 38 (Aug 1965) A101–106; Public Health Service, *Obesity and Public Health* (Washington, D.C., 1966) 12; and Sidney Abraham et al., *Obese and Overweight Adults in the United States* (Hyattsville, Md., 1983) 12–17.

77. Public Health Service, *Obesity*, 12–13.

78. James MacKenzie, *History of Health and the Art of Preserving It*, 2d ed. (Edinburgh, 1759) 224; William Nisbet, *A Practical Treatise on Diet* (London, 1801) 8–11; and "The Temperaments," *Amer Phrenological J* 1 (1839) 361–69. For a good historical review, see William B. Tucker and William A. Lessa, "Man: a constitutional study," *Q R of Biology* 15 (1940) 265–89, 411–53.

79. Ernst Kretschmer, *Physique and Character*, trans. W. J. H. Sprott, 2d ed., rev. (London, 1936) esp. 22–36, and Linford Rees, "Body build, personality, and neuroses in women," *J of Mental Science* 96 (1950) 426–34, following up Kretschmer. See also Anne Scott Beller, *Fat and Thin* (NY, 1977) ch. 5.

80. W. H. Sheldon and S. S. Stevens, *The Varieties of Temperament* (NY, 1942) 43, 255, 268.

81. J. Lawrence Angel, "Constitution in female obesity," *AJPA* ser. 2, 7 (1949) 459; Johanna T. Dwyer et al., "The social psychology of diet-

ing," *J of Health and Social Behavior* 11 (1970) 270; H. I. Douty et al., "Body characteristics in relation to life adjustment, body-image, and attitudes of college females," *PMS* 39 (1974) 499–521; and see literature review in Janet Polivy et al., "Causes and consequences of the current preference for thin female physiques," in *Physical Appearance, Stigma and Social Behavior*, eds. C. P. Herman et al. (Hillsdale, N.J., 1986).

82. Bruch, *Importance of Overweight*, 178–84, 195, 267–74, 288–89, 315, and B. Kotkov and M. Goodman, "The Draw-a-Person test of obese women," *J of Clinical Psych* 9 (1953) 362–64.

83. William Mortensen, *The Model: A Book on the Problems of Posing* (San Francisco, 1937) 16, 38, 114 and esp. 224; Liselotte Strelow, *Photogenic Portrait Management* (London, 1966) 58–59; and Ernest Havemann, "The wasteful, phony crash dieting craze," *Life* 46 (Jan 19, 1959) 103 on the effect of cameras on ideals of beauty. Cf. Liam Hudson, *Bodies of Knowledge* (London, 1982) 62, 107, 112.

84. Kretschmer, *Physique and Character*, 21; Sheldon, *Varieties of Temperament*, 39; Paul F. Secord and Sidney M. Jourard, "The appraisal of body-cathexis: body-cathexis and the self," *J of Consulting Psych* 17 (1953) 343–47; and idem, "Body cathexis and the ideal female figure," *J of Abnormal and Social Psych* 50 (1955) 243–46.

85. "Open letter to medical examiners: relation of build to mortality," *Med Insurance* 41 (1926) 382–83; Rollo H. Britten, "Physical impairment and weight," *Public Health Reports* 48, 31 (1933) 926, 931; Helen B. Pryor, *Width–Weight Tables* (Stanford, 1936); and Carl C. Seltzer and Jean Mayer, "Body build and obesity—who are the obese?" *JAMA* 189 (1964) 677–84.

86. Albert J. Stunkard et al., "The Night-Eating Syndrome," *Amer J of Med* 19 (1955) 78–86.

87. Chambers, "On corpulence," 440; Leonard Landois, *A Manual of Human Physiology*, from 4th German ed. (Philadelphia, 1885) IV, 488; James M. Anders, "Obesity" in *Modern Medicine*, eds. William Osler and Thomas McCrae (Philadelphia, 1907) I, 846; Charles B. Davenport, *Body Build and Its Inheritance* (Washington, D.C., 1923) 46–50, 97; C. H. Danforth, "Hereditary adiposity in mice," *J of Heredity* 18 (1927) 143–62; Henry J. Spencer, "Clinical observations concerning the obese," *MCNA* 12 (1928) 606; D. M. Dunlop and R. M. Murray Lyon, "A study of 523 cases of obesity," *Edinburgh Med J* 38 (1931) 566; and Ramsdell Gurney, "The hereditary factor in obesity," *ARIM* 57 (1936) 557–61.

88. See Frederick J. Simoons, *Eat Not This Flesh* (Madison, Wis., 1961); John Garcia, "Koalas, men, and other conditioned gastronomers," in *Food Aversion Learning*, eds. N. W. Milgram et al. (NY, 1977) 195–

218; Mary Douglas, "Food as an art form," *Studio* 188 (Sept 1974) 83–88; and Jack Goody, *Cooking, Cuisine and Class* (Cambridge, 1982).

89. Fielding H. Garrison, *An Introduction to the History of Medicine*, 4th ed. (Philadelphia, 1929) 49. On hunter-gatherers, see Beller, *Fat and Thin*, 70–73 and contrast C. M. Cassidy, "Nutrition and health for agriculturalists and hunter-gatherers," in *Nutritional Anthropology*, eds. N. W. Jerome et al. (Pleasantville, N.Y., 1980) 117–46.

90. Rose, "Weight reduction as an art," *Med R of Reviews* 34 (1928) 274; William M. Ballinger, "Treatment of obesity," *Southern Med J* 23 (1930) 1156; H. H. Fellows, "Studies of relatively normal obese individuals . . . ," *AJMS* 181 (1931) 301–12; Hugo R. Rony, *Obesity and Leanness* (Philadelphia, 1940) 266; T. S. Danowski and A. W. Winkler, "Obesity as a clinical problem," *AJMS* 208 (1944) 628; Albert J. Stunkard and Mavis McLaren-Hume, "The results of treatment for obesity," *ARIM* 102 (1959) 79–85; Public Health Service, *Obesity*, 56; and Kelly D. Brownell, "Obesity," *J of Consulting and Clinical Psych* 50 (1982) 820.

91. "Simple methods of flesh reduction," *Harper's Bazaar* 42 (July 1908) 702; B. B. Vincent Lyon, "The treatment of obesity," *Int Clinics* 26th ser., 3 (1916) 37 (quote); Ursula Parrott, "Nice people don't eat," *LHJ* 58 (March 1941) 58; Senate Subcommittee on Monopoly of the Select Committee on Small Business, *Advertising of Proprietary Medicines. Part 3.* (Washington, D.C., 1973) 1304; and Ellen S. Parham et al., "Weight control as portrayed in popular magazines," *J of Nutrition Educ* 14,4 (1982) 153–56 on beliefs in dieting success, and contrast Sandra Haber, "Effective treatment for obesity produces remission, not cure," *IJO* 4 (1980) 265–67.

92. Thyra S. Winslow, *Be Slim–Stay Slim* (NY, 1955) 205.

93. Reuben S. Clymer, *Dietetics* (Quakertown, Pa., 1917) 17 (quote); Charles H. Goudiss, *Eating Vitamines* (NY, 1922); G. Rosenfeld, "[Vitamins and treatment in obesity]," abstracted in *JAMA* 81 (1923) 174, vitamins against depression; Russell M. Wilder, "Treatment of obesity," *Int Clinics* 4 (1933) 13, vitamins in low-calorie diets; Karl M. Bowman and Herman Wortis, "Psychologic syndromes caused by nutritional deficiency," in *Role of Nutritional Deficiency in Nervous and Mental Disease* (Baltimore, 1943) 168–91; Ida Jean Kain, "Safe and sane reducing diets," *JADA* 17 (1941) 673; and Vita-Kaps ad in *What's New* (Feb 1943). On the appeal of vitamins, see A. J. Carlson, "Some obstacles in the path towards an optimum diet," *Science* 97 (1943) 414; "General Foods quiz shows women want more facts on nutrition," *Sales Management* (Feb 1, 1943) 26; and "The vitamin business," *Fortune* 31 (May 1945) 140. On the confusion of vitamins and calories, George H. Gallup, *The Gallup Poll* (NY, 1972)

I, 310, and Margaret Cussler and Mary L. de Give, *'Twixt the Cup and the Lip* (NY, 1952) 60. On vitamin fortification, see Lydia J. Roberts, "Beginnings of the Recommended Dietary Allowance," *JADA* 34 (1958) 903–8, and Russell M. Wilder and Robert R. Williams, *Enrichment of Flour and Bread* (Washington, D.C., 1944).

94. I. G. Macy and H. H. Williams, *Hidden Hunger* (Lancaster, Pa., 1945); Kellogg's ad in *JADA* 18 (1942) 353; and "Min-amin," *JAMA* 104 (1935) 335.

95. See Richard H. Follis, Jr., "Cellular pathology and the development of the deficiency disease concept," *BHM* 34 (1960) 291–317, and Charles E. Rosenberg, *No Other Gods* (Baltimore, 1976) 187.

96. Leo K. Campbell, "Obesity," *Industrial Med* 6 (1937) 613.

97. Ida Jean Kain, *Rx for Slimming* (Philadelphia, 1940), 3; Donald G. Cooley, *New Way to Eat and Get Slim* (NY, 1941) 2, 9; William Engel, *Sensible Dieting* (NY, 1939) 26–27; Blake Clark, "There's only one way to get thin," *Rotarian* 63 (Nov 1943) 58; Cyrus C. Sturgis, "Obesity," *Hawaii Med J* 7 (1948) 233; and Hazel M. Hauck, *How to Control Your Weight* (Ithaca, N.Y., 1942) II.

98. "Simple methods of flesh reduction," 704, and Brenda Ueland, "Fat or thin women," *SEP* 202 (May 10, 1930) 181.

99. Warshaw, Work Box P80, pamphlet by "Voice of Experience," *B. 4. Reducing—Part II.*

100. *OED* X, 1100 and XIII, 258; Eric Partridge, *Dictionary of Slang and Unconventional English*, 8th ed. (London, 1984) 1166; Celia Caroline Cole, "Streamline," *Delineator* 124 (March 1934) 16; Paul C. Bragg, *Personal Health Food Cook Book* (Burbank, Calif., 1935) 12; Franklin ad reproduced in Robert Atwan et al., *Edsels, Luckies, & Frigidaires* (NY, 1979) 166; and Renee Long, *Style Your Personality* (NY, 1939) 164 and cf. Sylvia of Hollywood, *Streamline Your Figure* (NY, 1939).

101. Carole Conover, *Cover Girls* (Englewood Cliffs, N.J., 1978); Clyde M. Dessner, *So You Want to Be a Model* (Chicago, 1943) 107; and Thyra S. Winslow, *Winslow Weight Watcher* (NY, 1953) 94–96.

102. Joe Bonomo, *How to Keep Physically Fit: A Health Manual for War Workers* (Deep River, Conn., 1943) 3, 6, 13 (quote), 24 (quote), 30; *Who Was Who in America* VII, 61. Bonomo's *Little Red Calorie Counter* later sold some twenty million copies. Edwin Bayrd, *The Thin Game* (NY, 1978) 57.

103. "Battle for Girdles," *Business Week* (June 19, 1943) 92, and Olga F. Ley, *It's Fun to Be Fit* (NY, 1942) 15.

104. Jantzen ad in *Life* 26 (June 13, 1949) 85; Thomas H. Etzold and John L. Gaddis, eds., *Containment* (NY, 1978) 87 and see 25–37; Melvyn P. Leffler, "The American conception of national security and the be-

ginnings of the Cold War, 1945–48," *AHR* 89 (1984) 346–81; Morris A. Bealle, *The Drug Story*, 3d ed. (Washington, D.C., 1949) 44–45; "President Eisenhower's calorie-count diet," *McCall's* 85 (Dec 1957) 98; Gallup, *Gallup Polls* II, 1463; and H. Harrison Clarke, "Contributions of physical education to physical fitness," in *An Introduction to Physical Education*, eds. H. S. Slusher and A. S. Lockhart, 2d ed. (Dubuque, Iowa, 1970) 145–56. In 1962 CBS-TV produced a documentary on "The Fat American," which also posed fatness within a Cold War frame.

105. Bonnie Prudden, "Keep Fit/Be Happy with Bonnie Prudden," Warner Bros. 1959 LP, WS 1358, album notes and quote from side one, cut two. Columbia Records that year produced "Reducing Off the Record"; two years before, Evelyn Loewendahl's "Reduce in Record Time" was issued by Crown Phonodiscs.

106. Jack LaLanne, *Food for Glamour* (Englewood Cliffs, N.J., 1961) 47; Huston Horn, "LaLanne a treat and a treatment," *Sports Illustrated* 13 (Dec 19, 1960) 28–31; Jim Scott, "Conscience of a million housewives," *TV Guide* 8 (Nov 12, 1960) 20–23; and Wyden, *Overweight Society*, 100–102, 119.

107. LaLanne, *Foods for Glamour*, quotes on 78, 117.

108. Jean Mayer and Frederick J. Stare, "Exercise and weight control: frequent misconceptions," *JADA* 29 (1953) 340–43; Ancel Keys, "Body composition and its change with age and diet," in *Weight Control*, eds. E. S. Eppright et al. (Ames, Iowa, 1955) 25; Anna-Marie Chirico and Albert J. Stunkard, "Physical activity and human obesity," *NEJM* 263 (1960) 935–40; Alton Blakeslee and Jeremiah Stamler, *Your Heart Has 9 Lives* (NY, 1963) 111–20; and LaLanne, *Foods for Glamour*, 119 (quote).

109. Vance Thompson, *Eat and Grow Thin* (NY, 1914) 22–23.

CHAPTER EIGHT
Thin Bodies, Fat Profits

1. G. [Baker], "The case of Mr. Thos. Wood," *Med Tr of the Royal College of Physicians in London* 2 (1772) 259–74, with "A sequel," 3 (1785) 309–18, quote on 266–67. A younger contemporary, William Stark (1740–70), "stout but not corpulent," put himself through a series of experimental diets, many precariously low in nutrients; he died of scurvy. Jack C. Drummond and Anne Wilbraham, *The Englishman's Food*, rev. ed. (London, 1958) 459–61.

2. Borg scale ad in *House Furnishing R* 108 (May 1948) 69; Borg scale ad in *Life* (May 22, 1950) 58; Zemco, Inc., brochure, "Datatrim: a new concept in computerized weight management" (San Ramon,

Calif., 1983); and Healthtronic brochure for X-Pounder 2000, marketed as Sunbeam Motivator (Lauderhill, Fla., 1984?) 2.

3. Thomas Short, *A Discourse Concerning the Causes and Effects of Corpulency* (London, 1727); Malcolm Flemyng, *A Discourse on the Nature, Causes and Cure of Corpulency* (London, 1760); Emile Demange, "Obésité," *Dictionnaire encyclopédique des sciences médicales* (Paris, 1880) XIV, 35–38, listing many dissertations; John Dunton, *Ladies Dictionary* (London, 1694) 62; Jean D'Alembert, "Obésité," *Encyclopédie* (Neufchastel, 1765) XI, 300–301; Hilary Whelan, *Obesity, A Bibliography 1964–1973* (London, 1974); Anne Smith, *Obesity: A Bibliography 1974–1979* (London, 1980); David M. Garner et al., "Cultural expectations of thinness in women," *Psych Reports* 47 (1980) 489; W. Stewart Agras and Betty G. Kirkley, "Bulimia: theories of etiology," in *Handbook of Eating Disorders*, eds. K. D. Brownell and J. P. Foreyt (NY, 1986), on frequency of dieting articles; and Ellen S. Parham et al., "Weight control as portrayed in popular magazines," *J of Nutrition Educ* 14,4 (1982) 153.

4. On breads, see *Nostrums* II, 670–71; Thyra S. Winslow, *Winslow Weight Watcher* (NY, 1953) 226; and "Continental wants okay for weight-loss claims," *AA* 47 (Aug 2, 1976) 1. On meats, M. M. Hamdy, "Soybean proteins in prudent-diet foods," *Amer Oil Chemists' Soc J* 54 (Feb 1977) 87A–89A, and Oscar Mayer ad in *Restaurant Business* 83 (May 1, 1984) 46–47. On milk and dairy products, "Insurance ads pave the way for dietary and 'health' foods," *Business Week* (Dec 6, 1952) 46; "Battle of the bulge," *Time* 62 (Aug 10, 1953) 80–81; Genevieve Smith, "35,000,000 overweights tip scales toward low-calorie foods," *Printers' Ink* 250 (Feb 11, 1955) 27; "McCall's Diet of the Month," *McCall's* (June 1970) 42; Herbert Seal, "How to succeed with dietary dairy foods," *Amer Dairy R* 37 (Aug 1975) 8–9; and "Moo juice is sales, not slang, for low-fat milk," *ibid.* 40 (July 1978) 68. On beverages, John J. Riley, *A History of the American Soft Drink Industry* (Washington, D.C., 1958); "What gives the light to light beer?" *FE* 50 (Sept 1978) 101–5; and Laura C. Jacobs, "Enologists develop light wine technology," *FPD* 15 (Aug 1981) 14–15, 18. On new foods, "125 'light' foods," *FE* 54 (Oct 1982) 94–95, and Mary Johnson, "Shoppers say 'yes' to less," *Progressive Grocer* (May 1984) 191–92.

5. A.I.B. ad in *JADA* 15 (1939) 717. The American Meat Institute, the Wheat Flour Institute, and the National Dairy Council have been the most active trade associations trying to link their interests to those of dieters, since dieters have tended to abandon whole milk, bread and fatty meats on the slightest provocation.

6. On changes in restaurant menus, I have benefited from a conversation with Joan Bakos, editor of *Restaurant Business*, Oct 19, 1984.

See also Rona Gindin, "Lo-cal burgers poise D'Lites for heavy expansion," *Restaurant Business* (Sept 1, 1983) 110; Christine Van Lenten, "Serving up health: nutrition in today's restaurant," *National Restaurant Assoc News* (Aug 1983) 11–14; and "Light touch," *Forbes* 131 (Sept 12, 1983) 134–35. On lo-cal frozen dinners, Mike Pehanich, "Heavyweights battle in 'light' entree category," *Processed Prepared Foods* 152 (Sept 1983) 15.

7. Excelsior Fitness Equipment Co. ad in *WW* (Feb 1983); Robert Sherrill, "Before you believe those exercise and diet ads . . . ," *Today's Health* 49 (Aug 1971) 35, 70; and Nike ad in *Rolling Stone* 409 (Nov 24, 1983).

8. Eleanor Harris, "Reducing at $500 a week," *Look* 22 (April 29, 1958) 35–38; Peter Wyden, *The Overweight Society* (NY, 1965) 122–30; Kitty Kelley, *Glamour Spas* (NY, 1976) quote on 161; and Emily Wilkens, *Secrets from the Super Spas* (NY, 1976) 78–81, 104–16.

9. American Society of Bariatric Physicians pamphlets, "What is the Obesity Foundation?" (Englewood, Colo., 1984?), "Standards of bariatric practice" (adopted 1974, revised 1982) and "History" (updated Jan 29, 1982); "Bariatrician," *Melloni's Illustrated Medical Dictionary* (Baltimore, 1979), a disparaging entry; and interview with Dr. James M. Ferguson, member of the ASBP, Sept 10, 1984.

10. "Machines attack the solid flesh," *Life* 9 (Nov 4, 1940) 54–55 on Mac-Levy; "MacLevy 'slenderizing' racket," *JAMA* 116 (1941) 1083; "Re making your measurements," *Vogue* 129 (Jan 15, 1957) 56–57 on Stauffer in particular; Robert O'Brien, "Secret of Slenderella," *Collier's* 138 (Dec 21, 1956) 40–42; Walter Goodman, "Shake to size: slimming by Slenderella," *Nation* 182 (March 3, 1956) 176–78; and "Lean times for Slenderella," *AA* 30 (Aug 3, 1959) 3, 80.

11. "Lean times for Slenderella," 3; "Tannyed and fit," *Time* 77 (Feb 10, 1961) 76; and "The Tanny tumble," *Newsweek* 62 (Dec 23, 1963) 60.

12. Letter from Marlene Johnson, Manager, Consumer Public Relations, The Pillsbury Company, Nov 28, 1984, concerning consumer use of the toll free number; interview with Lois Lindauer, International Director of Diet Workshop, Inc., Nov 5, 1984; Diet Center ad in *Brookline Chronicle* (Sept 27, 1984) 11; Nutritional Management ad in *Boston Globe Mag* (April 22, 1984) 53; interview with Lynne Miller, founder of Thin Forever! Inc., Oct 18, 1984; Gloria Marshall and Schick ads in *Los Angeles Times* (Jan 16, 1984) Part V, 4, 6; mailer from YMCA, Encinitas, Calif., Jan 1985; and Forever Thin brochure from Scripps Clinic and Research Foundation, La Jolla, Calif., 1984.

13. To follow the rising profits, see Russell Chappell, "Big bulge in profits," *Newsweek* 48 (July 23, 1956) 61–63; Norman Bussel, "Sales

grow fat on low-cal foods," *Progressive Grocer* 45 (Nov 1966) 162–86; "How to cash in on the low-cal revolution," *ibid.* 48 (March 1969) Supplement, 180–202; D. H. Engstrom, "Present and future markets of dietetic foods," *FPD* 11 (Feb 1977) 50, 54; "Food giants see the 'light,'" *Business Week* (June 1, 1981) 112–14; "Diet foods may represent $41 billion market by 1990," *Grocery Communications* (Sept–Oct 1984) 32; Stratford P. Sherman, "America's new abstinence," *Fortune* 111 (March 18, 1985) 20–23; and Eric Gelman et al., "Calories and cash," *Newsweek* (Aug 26, 1985) 54–55.

14. "Anti-obesity market products," *Grocery Communications* (Jan 1978) 16–17; "Off the fat of the land," *Financial World* 150 (Jan 1, 1981) 25–26; "Reducing aids on a media binge," *Market and Media Decisions* 16 (Sept 1981) 76–78; "Diet aids," *Drug Topics* 125 (July 3, 1981) 83; and "35th Annual Report on Consumer Spending," *ibid.* 126 (July 4, 1983) esp. 3, 70, 72.

15. "Remaking your measurements," 57, 111; Sherrill, "Before you believe," 35–36, 70; "Body building," *Fortune* 35 (Oct 1947) 94–101; Goodman, "Shake to size," 176; O'Brien, "Secret of Slenderella," 42; and "Lean times for Slenderella," 3.

16. "Weight Watchers success story," *Mag of Wall Street* 128 (July 3, 1971) 22–23; Robert J. Cole, "Weight Watchers, noted successful loser, expecting rich fare from Heinz," *NYT* (May 6, 1978) 29, 33; Susan Antilla, "Living off the fat of the land," *Dun's Business Month* 118 (Oct 1981) 73–74 on Nutri/System; Carnation Company, *Every Pound of the Weigh* (May–June 1984); and ad in *Los Angeles Times* (Jan 16, 1984) V, 2.

17. A. A. Wittenberg, "Recent conceptions of obesity," *J of the Michigan St Med Soc* 32 (1933) 500; Thomas C. Desmond, "Fat men can't win," *Science Illustrated* 4 (June 1949) 47; Senate Select Committee on Nutrition and Human Needs, *Nutrition and Diseases. Part I. Obesity and Fad Diets* (Washington, D.C., 1973) v on percentage overweight; Wyden, *Overweight Society*, 1–2 on the 79 million; H. Woodward, "Executive paunch," *Sales Management* 91 (July 5, 1963) 66 on those over thirty; and John W. Farquhar, *The American Way of Life Need Not Be Hazardous to Your Health* (NY, 1978) 143, claiming 80–90 percent overweight. For data on actual changes in weight, see Jean Roberts, "Weight by height and age of adults," *Vital and Health Statistics*, series 11, no. 14 (1966).

18. Johanna T. Dwyer and Jean Mayer, "Potential dieters: who are they?" *JADA* 56 (1970) 511; George H. Gallup, *The Gallup Poll 1935–1971* (NY, 1972) II, 984–85, 1352; idem, *The Gallup Poll: Public Opinion 1972–1977* (Wilmington, 1978) I, 170–71; Joseph W. Newman, *Motivation Research and Marketing Management* (Boston, 1957) 320–42, Young & Rubicam survey in 1955 contrasting beliefs

about being overweight with actual overweight, p. 327; Jane E. Ful-
larton, "Obesity: a new social policy perspective," *IJO* 2 (1978) 170;
Karen Anderegg, "Are we fatness crazy?" *Vogue* 172 (March 1982)
428; and L. M. Boyd, "Grab-Bag," *San Francisco Chronicle* (Jan 17,
1981) 33. See, most recently, a *Glamour* survey reported by Carol
Sternhill, "We'll always be fat, but fat can be fit," *Ms.* (May 1985)
66.

19. Dwyer and Mayer, "Potential dieters," 511; Gallup, *Gallup Poll
1972–1977*, I, 171; John Krueger, "America's nutritional habits: who's
dieting and why," *Processed Prepared Food* (July 1978) 88; C. I.
Beck, "Reduced calorie foods—once we create them, do they help?"
FPD 12 (March 1978) 72. A 1980–81 menu census study—in which
people are less likely to claim to be doing what they think they should
be doing—discovered that 20 percent of men and 38 percent of
women were following weight-loss or weight-maintenance diets.
Market Research Corporation of America, *Menu Census Dieters
Study, July 1980–June 1981*, summary kindly provided by Peter
Arato of Lever Brothers; and "Dieting: the losing game," *Time* 129
(Jan 20, 1986) 54.

20. Vance Packard, *The Pyramid Climbers* (NY, 1962) 99–100; Richard
F. Shepard, "Etiquette of the executive lunch," *Esquire* 60 (Nov
1963) 142; Thomas R. Brooks, "Dollars in figures," *Duns R and Modern Industry* 85 (April 1965) quote on 62; *Modern Materials Handling* 24 (Sept 1969) 92, with article, "Weight Watchers and the
heavy executive" in subsection, *Executive Life*; Robert Half, "Fatter
execs get slimmer paychecks," *Industry Week* 180 (Jan 14, 1974) 21,
24; *Computer World* (May 14, 1971) cited in Marvin Grosswirth, *Fat
Pride* (NY, 1971) 158–59; Walter McQuade, "Why are they running,
stretching, starving?" *Fortune* 82 (Aug 1970) 132–35; "Joe, when are
you going to lose some weight?" *Industry Week* 174 (Aug 21, 1972)
45–47; "The new Rx for better health," *Business Week* (Jan 5, 1974)
69–74; "Trimming the fat from overweight executives," *ibid.* (March
29, 1976) quote on 94; Sylvia Auerbach, "Obesity: an obstacle to
managerial success," *Computer Decisions* 14 (1982) 166–68; and
Timken ad in *Iron Age* (Jan 2, 1984) 26.

21. Peter M. Silverberg, "Stop being an overweight engineer," *Chemical
Engineering* 85 (Aug 28, 1978) 117–18; Ten High ad in *Collier's* 109
(Feb 7, 1942) inside back cover; E. P. Luongo, "'Fat cats' in laborers'
ranks," *Science Digest* 32 (Aug 1952) 49; Wayne W. Massey, "Ex-
athletes gain more weight," *ibid.* 37 (May 1955) inside cover; Peter
Wyden and Barbara Wyden, *Growing Up Straight* (NY, 1968) 47–49
and cf. David A. Sleet, "Physique and social image," *PMS* 28 (1969)
295–99; and Wyden, *Overweight Society*, 119. It was no coincidence
that the weighing-in ceremonies for boxers would become in the

1960s the central points of athletic drama and assertion of manhood; see esp. George Plimpton, *Shadow Box* (NY, 1977) 99–100. By 1969, weight-watching had reached the most stalwart of manhood magazines: "After 25, watch your weight!" *True* 50 (Aug 1969) 18.

Treatment of obesity with human chorionic gonadotropin, a growth hormone excreted in the urine during pregnancy, began in the early 1950s for fat women in particular, but it has grown more popular with men as fears of impotence have been associated with male obesity. See esp. James H. Hutton, "The overweight problem," *Industrial Med* 34 (Aug 1965) 623–27, and George A. Bray and Frank L. Greenway, "Phamacological approaches to treating the obese patient," *Clinics in Endocrinology and Metabolism* 5 (1976) 471–75.

22. On the stereotyping, see George D. Maddox et al., "Overweight as social deviance and disability," *J of Health and Social Behavior* 9 (1968) 287–98, and "TV stars stay fat to succeed," *Jet* 55 (Dec 21, 1978) 28–31. For diet columns and articles, see "Health hints: weight control," *The Crisis* 57 (March 1950) 190–94; Cecile Hoover Edwards, "Food facts," *Service* 16 (April 1952) 13, 22, and 17 (Sept 1952) 20–21, (Nov 1952) 13, (Dec 1952) 14; Gallup, *Gallup Poll 1972–1977*, I, 170; "Hints on keeping slim from famous personalities," *Ebony* 30 (Nov 1974) 76–80; "Slimming! Dianne Johnson, the woman who won the war against fat," *Essence* 4 (Jan 1974) 56–57; Stan Pantovic, "How to lose weight and like it," *Sepia* 24 (Nov 1975) 60–64; and Harmon Perry, "Maynard Jackson tells how he lost 110 pounds," *Jet* 52 (April 7, 1977) 52–53.

23. "How to stay slim after losing weight," *Ebony* 31 (Sept 1976) 87–88; Naomi Sims, *All About Health and Beauty for the Black Woman* (Garden City, N.Y., 1976) 159 (quote); Shawn D. Lewis, "Are we overdoing the diet thing?" *Ebony* 33 (Feb 1978) 43–44 and quote on 48; Lalita Kaul et al., "Management of obesity in black females in a community model clinic," *National Med Assoc J* 71 (Jan 1979) 81–83; R. L. Gamble, "The calorie dilemma," *Essence* 1 (Feb 1971) 56–57 on soul food; Charles L. Sanders, "Barry White," *Jet* 15 (May 8, 1980) 22–25; Norge W. Jerome, "Diet and acculturation: the case of Black-American in-migrants," in *Nutritional Anthropology*, eds. Jerome et al. (Pleasantville, N.Y., 1980) 275–325; and Herbert Temple, "Did your mother make you fat?" *Ebony* 32 (May 1977) 59–60. Cf. Elijah Muhammad, *How to Eat to Live* (Chicago, 1967) 43–48, and Dick Gregory's new Slim-Safe Bahamian Diet.

24. Emily B. Massara, "¡Que Gordita! A Study of Weight Among Women in a Puerto Rican Community," Ph.D. thesis, Bryn Mawr, 1979, esp. 93, 128, 145n, 156, 160–61, 191, 193, 206.

25. David H. Fischer, *Growing Old in America* (NY, 1977) 222; "Lose

weight the 'Satchmo way,'" *Ebony* 11 (April 1956) 35–37; Prudden, *How to Keep Slender and Fit After Thirty*, new ed. (NY, 1969 [1961]) back cover; Irwin M. Stillman and Samm S. Baker, *The Doctor's Quick Weight Loss Diet* (NY, 1967) 229; Barbara Edelstein, *The Woman Doctor's Diet for Women* (NY, 1977) 31; and Nathan Pritikin, *Pritikin Program for Diet and Exercise* (NY, 1979) 90–116. The first height–weight tables for older Americans appeared in 1960: Arthur M. Master et al., "Tables of average weight and height of Americans aged 65 to 94 years," *JAMA* 172 (Feb 13, 1960) 658–67. The first diet book devoted to older Americans was perhaps Charles N. Aronson, *Regimen for Weight Control in Retired Couples* (Arcade, NY, 1973). On the health attitudes and practices of older people, see National Analysts, Inc., *A Study of Health Practices and Opinions: Final Report* (Philadelphia, 1972) xii–xiii *et passim*, and cf. Roberta E. Cozens, "Obesity in the aged: not just a case of overeating," *Nursing Clinics of North Amer* 17 (June 1982) 227–32.

26. E. M. Geraghty, "Watch your diet: article for those whose weight is normal," *Hygeia* 15 (Jan 1937) 32–36; "Overeating shortens life," *U.S. News and World Report* 38 (Jan 7, 1955) 50–54, interview with Stare; Hilde Bruch, *The Importance of Overweight* (NY, 1957) ch. 14; and Gulielma F. Alsop, *Hold Your Weight Losses* (NY, 1953) quote on 137; Chris Chase, *The Great American Waistline* (NY, 1981) 46 on Julia Child. On dieting in the military, see "A general thins his ranks," *Life* 41 (Sept 10, 1956) 87–88; Albert J. Stunkard, *The Pain of Obesity* (Palo Alto, Calif., 1976) 138–41; Wyden, *Overweight Society*, 307; and Anne Hoiberg et al., "Correlates of obesity," *J of Clinical Psych* 36 (1980) 983–90. Keeton quote is from her "Facts and figures," *Viva* 5 (July 1978) 8.

27. Katherine S. Z. Mitchell, *The Deuce of Reducing* (NY, 1937) 108–11; Helen Terkelsen, "But you can't insult your hostess, can you?" *Amer Home* 27 (March 1942) 36–37; Thyra S. Winslow, *Be Slim—Stay Slim* (NY, 1955) ch. 19; Louis Stern, *After Reducing, What?* (NY, 1955) 54; Harry Botsford, "The crazy calorie chase and how to avoid it," *Amer Mercury* 81 (Nov 1955) 11; and Harvey Chipkin, "A do's and don'ts guide to fitness etiquette," *Woman's Day Super Special* (May 1985) 24, 26.

28. "CDS History" statement provided by Beth Hvass, Consumer Products Division, Sandoz Nutrition Corp., now owners of Chicago Dietetic Supply; interview with Steven Bernard, son of Jules and present executive of the company, Sept 21, 1984; clippings and fact sheet, "Who Is Tillie Lewis" provided by Alilea Haywood Martin, personal secretary to Tillie Lewis from 1959, in letter of Dec 17, 1984; "Tillie's unpunctured romance," *Time* 58 (Nov 19, 1951) 103–5; "Tillie of the Valley," *RD* 61 (Aug 1952) 101–4; "Tillie Lewis: most famous woman

in food," *Good Packaging* 36 (Dec 1975) 6–8; and Caroline Bird, *Enterprising Women* (NY, 1976) 199–203.

29. Wyden, *Overweight Society*, ch. 3; "Battle of the bulge," *Financial World* 114 (Nov 30, 1960) 4–5; Lawrence Bernard, "Calorie-metered food sales . . . ," *AA* 31 (Dec 5, 1960) 104–6, with account of an earlier reducing formula marketed by Life Products International since 1954 (Wey-rite); "Potential radio-television gold mine: Metrecal is first of food concentrates buying tv," *Broadcasting* 59 (Dec 12, 1960) 36; "A booming new industry watches Metrecal," *Sponsor* 15 (Jan 9, 1961) 27–30, 47 (quotes); "Metrecal's semi-institutional approach," *Broadcasting* 60 (Jan 9, 1961) 30–31 (quote from Central Park commercial); David C. Stewart, "Daring innovation can be both soul- and sales- satisfying," *ibid.* 60 (Feb 6, 1961) 22; and "Here's how Metrecal did it," *Sponsor* 16 (July 9, 1962) 30–31, 48–49.

30. "Overweight seize on meal-in-a-glass diet," *Business Week* (Oct 22, 1960) 26–28; Bernard, "Calorie-metered food sales"; Richard F. Janssen, "Diet drinks," *Wall Street J* 157 (Jan 10, 1961) 1, 18; "Pet Milk sets 'Sego' debut in NY area," *Editor and Publisher* 95 (Sept 22, 1962) 46; "Tying up a market by tying in fashion," *Printers' Ink* 287 (May 8, 1964) 39–41; "Heavyweights in radio audience," *Broadcasting* 67 (Aug 3, 1964) 26; "The race is to the smart," *Forbes* 94 (Oct 1, 1964) 24; "Sego offers lure of slim figure for summer slimming," *AA* 36 (April 12, 1965) 55; "Join Metrecal for lunch bunch, says initial Ogilvy drive," *AA* 36 (March 1, 1965) 2; Jean McAlister, "Fat market," *Sales Management* 96 (April 1, 1966) 46–50; Herbert P. Sarett, "Use of formula diets," in *Conference on Nutrition in Space and Related Waste Problems* (Washington, D.C., 1964) 353–62; and Wyden, *Overweight Society*, 51–52.

31. "Duffy-Mott tackles a weighty problem," *Food Business* 10 (Feb 1962) 26–29; Wyden, *Overweight Society*, 69, 71; "The General Mills way to reduce," *Business Week* (Sept 23, 1972) 82; "CDS History" statement; Bernard interview; "How to cash in on the low-cal revolution," 182; Peter Jauquet, "Diet food sales increase nearly 50%," *Supermarket Business* 10 (Oct 1979) 22; R. D. Rauch, "Diet aids capture more attention as volume surges," *ibid.* 35 (April 1980) 1; idem, "Health and dietetic foods outgrow fad image with more shelf space among regular groceries," *ibid.* 35 (June 1980) 21; and "Fat market for thin foods," *Market and Media Decisions* 15 (April 1980) 72–73, quote on 73.

32. Albert J. Stunkard, "The obese: background and programs," in *U.S. Nutrition Policies in the Seventies*, ed. Jean Mayer (San Francisco, 1973) 29; Irwin M. Rosenstock et al., "Public knowledge, opinion and action concerning three public health issues," *J of Health and Human Behavior* 7 (1966) 91–98; Edwin Bayrd, *The Thin Game*

(NY, 1978) 30; interview with Tom K. Mura, Senior Consultant, Communications, Blue Cross and Blue Shield Assoc, Sept 19, 1984, who also provided me with a copy of their N. W. Ayer commercial, production date June 9, 1977; and "When God created man" ad, about 1975.

33. Summary of consulting group report on "Dieting and the Diet Food Business" for Lever Brothers, Oct 1982, kindly furnished by Peter Arato and Geraldine Russo; Craig Norback, ed., *Complete Book of American Surveys* (NY, 1980) 212, reprinting a 1978 Harris poll; "Diet market facts," *Food Distributors Mag* (Sept–Oct 1983) 14; and Janet Neiman, "Execs watch for Weight Watchers move," *AA* 53 (Jan 18, 1982) 14 on Nestlé.

34. The Pantene Company exploited the flood of promotions for thinness and lightness by advertising its thickening shampoo with the banner headline, "There's one part of you which should definitely not be thin." *Cosmopolitan* (May 1977) 209.

35. "How to cash in on the low-cal revolution," 184; "Low-cals are booming all over the market," *Progressive Grocer* 49,2 (Sept 1970) 169; "Putting the light in 'lite,'" *Prepared Foods* (July 1984) 112; ad in *WW* (March 1984) 27; Gallup, *Gallup Poll 1937–71*, III, 1743; idem, *Gallup Poll 1972–77*, 1200–1201; Jean Rosenblatt and Sandra Stencel, "Weight control: a national obsession," *Editorial Research Reports* 2 (Nov 10, 1982) 867 on exercising; W. Nelson Francis and Henry Kučera, *Frequency Analysis of English Usage* (Boston, 1982); Ellen T. Crowley, ed., *Trade Names Dictionary* (Detroit, 1979); and Kevin J. Hannigan, "It's a new and coming market . . . reduced calorie foods," *FE* 51 (May 1979) 114–16.

36. See esp. Ann A. Hertzler and Helen L. Anderson, "Food guides in the U.S.: an historical review," *JADA* 64 (1974) 19–28, and Henry C. Sherman, *Nutritional Improvement of Life* (NY, 1950) 131. There were also a Basic 8 and Basic 12. Cf. I. Leitch, "Evolution of dietary standards," *Nutrition Abstracts and R* 11 (1942) 502–21.

37. "The vulgar and common error about 'light food,'" *GJHL* 3 (May 11, 1839) 166; Margaret T. Cussler and Mary L. de Give, *'Twixt the Cup and the Lip* (NY, 1952) 36, 158; and Lowell Edmunds, "Ancient Roman and modern American food: a comparative sketch of two semiological systems," *Comparative Civilizations R* 5 (Fall 1980) 52–69.

38. Letitia Brewster and Michael F. Jacobson, *The Changing American Diet* (Washington, D.C., 1978) 4–5, 39; Richard Prescott, *Charts on U.S. Food Consumption* USDA Economics Research Service Staff Report No. AGES821124 (Washington, D.C., 1983) 13–16, 19; National Restaurant Assoc, *Current Issues Report* (Aug 1983) 5; Alexis Bespaloff, "White wine has fewer calories than red. Right? Wrong," *Food*

and Wine 7 (May 1984) 44–45; Slimtech ad in *Natural Foods Merchandiser* 6 (Oct 1984) 25; and Knox ad in *Cosmopolitan* 149 (Sept 1960) 135.

39. Brewster and Jacobson, *Changing American Diet*, 4–5, 22, 59; Prescott, *Charts*, 21–22; Otto F. Hunziker, *The Butter Industry*, 3d ed. (La Grange, Ill., 1940) 569; Martha F. Trulson, "The American diet—past and present," *AJCN* 7 (1959) 93–94; and Nucoa ad in *JADA* 18,9 (1942) 5. For a critique of methods of calculating the actual percentage of fat in the diet, see David L. Call and Ann M. Sanchez, "Trends in fat disappearance in the U.S. 1909–65," *J of Nutrition* supp. 1, part 2, 93 (Oct 1967) 1–28.

40. Lincoln, *Boston Cook Book*, 430; Laura Shapiro, *Perfection Salad* (NY, 1986) 204–205; John L. Hess and Karen Hess, *The taste of America* (NY, 1977) 59–61; Henry C. Sherman, *Food Products* (NY, 1917) 440–44; Vilhjalmur Stefansson, *Not by Bread Alone* (NY, 1946) 118–19 on rations; Ralph Bolton, "The hypoglycemia-aggression hypothesis," *Current Anthropology* 25 (Feb 1984) 1–54; William F. Dufty, *Sugar Blues* (Radnor, Pa., 1975); Prescott, *Charts*, 20, 28–30, 41; National Restaurant Assoc, *Current Issues Report* (Aug 1983) 5; Charles I. Beck, "Application potential for aspartame," is Basant K. Dwivedi, ed., *Low Calorie and Special Dietary Foods* (West Palm Beach, 1978) 61 on change in consumer habits; J. Daniel Palm, *Diet Away Your Stress, Tension and Anxiety: The Fructose Diet Book* (NY, 1976); and Sally DeVore and Thelma White, *Dinner's Ready!* (Pasadena, 1977) 240 quote. Cf. Sidney W. Mintz, *Sweetness and Power* (NY, 1985) and Rosalind Coward, *Female Desire* (London, 1984) ch. 8.

On candy as a reducing aid, see *Beauty and Hygiene* (NY, 1897) 40, Spanish bonbon fat reducer; *Nostrums* II, 684, Morlene; Roland Marchand, *Advertising the American Dream* (Berkeley, Calif., 1985) 98–99; Wyden, *Overweight Society*, 246–47 on Ayds, as also Bayrd, *Thin Game*, 82–84; George E. Anderson and Paul C. Eschweiler, "Diet control," *Med Times* 63 (1935) 108; "Fool-the-eye diet," *Look* 17 (May 19, 1953) 120–21; Gerold Nelson, "Candy that makes you thin," *Coronet* 37 (April 1955) 29–31; "Old style copy brings Ayds back after slump," *AA* 37 (Sept 12, 1966) 3; and Sonja Eiteljorg, *A Sweet Way to Diet* (NY, 1968).

41. W. A. Evans, *How to Keep Well* (NY, 1922) 635 on salt; "Hypertension—salt poisoning?" *Lancet* (1978) 1136–37; Food Marketing Institute, *Trends: Consumer Attitudes and the Supermarket* (Washington, D.C., 1984) 40, kindly provided by Susan Borra, Manager, Consumer Information, FMI; Martin Lederman, *The Slim Gourmet* (NY, 1955) quotes on 19, 24; Ernest Dichter, *Handbook of Consumer Motivations* (NY, 1964) 39; and Schiffman, interviewed on "All Things Considered," National Public Radio, March 7, 1985.

On flavor and taste cues, see Stanley Schacter, "Obesity and eating," *Science* 161 (1968) 751–56 and his "Don't sell habit breakers short," *Psych Today* (Aug 1982) 31; Lynn Spitzer and Judith Rodin, "Human eating behavior," *Appetite* 2 (1981) 293–329; and F. M. Toates, "Control of ingestive behavior by internal and external stimuli," *ibid.*, 35–50. For insightful analysis of American patterns of flavoring, see Octavio Paz, "Eroticism and gastrosophy," *Daedalus* 101,4 (1972) 67–85.

42. On cooking and food transformation, see Claude Levi-Strauss, "The culinary triangle," *Partisan R* 33 (1966) 586–95; Adrienne Lehrer, "Cooking vocabularies and the culinary triangle of Levi-Strauss," *Anthropological Linguistics* 14 (1972) 155–71; and Mary Douglas, *In the Active Voice* (London, 1982) ch. 9. On consumption of processed and prepared foods, see Prescott, *Charts*, 30–38, and Brewster and Jacobson, *Changing American Diet*, 28, 30.

On grazing, see Christine Frederick, *Selling Mrs. Consumer* (NY, 1929) 115–17—the first notice of the phenomenon, perhaps; "Eat often with McCall's new diet for men and women," *McCall's* 81 (April 1954) 36–37; Annemarie F. Crocetti and Helen A. Guthrie, "Food consumption patterns and nutritional quality of U.S. diets," *Food Technology* 35 (Sept 1981) 47; and Claude Fischler, "Gastro-nomie et gastro-anomie," *Communications* 31 (1979) 189–210. On fiber, see esp. Franklin C. Bing, "Dietary fiber—a historical perspective," *JADA* 69 (Nov 1976) 498–505. Also see ads for Diet Master in *RD* 68 (April 1956) 223, and Osterizer in *WW* (Feb 1968) 11.

43. Roland Barthes, "Toward a psychosociology of contemporary food consumption," in *Food and Drink in History*, eds. Robert Forster and Orest Ranum, trans. Elborg Forster and Patricia M. Ranum (Baltimore, 1979) 166–73; Richard J. Hooker, *Food and Drink in America* (Indianapolis, 1981) 357; Mary Bralove, "Most people have no taste: it's been lost in the process," *Wall Street J* (April 30, 1974) 1, 41; John A. Amoore, "Synthetic flavors," *Chemical Senses and Flavor* 2 (1976) 27–38; and Robert M. Hadsell, "Food processing: search for growth," in *The Feeding Web*, ed. Joan D. Gussow (Palo Alto, Calif., 1978) 137. I have taken into consideration the methodological warnings of Carol Laderman, "Food ideology and eating behavior: contributions from Malay studies," *Social Science and Med* 19 (1984) 547–59.

44. Gallup, *Gallup Poll 1935–71*, I, 488.

45. For the Butter Rebellion and adulteration, see Emma S. Weigley, "Food in the days of the Declaration of Independence," *JADA* 45 (1964) 39, and Drummond and Wilbraham, *Englishman's Food*, 41, 239, 296. On margarine I have used Matej K. Schwitzer, *Margarine and Other Food Fats* (London, 1956); Christian Guy, *La vie quoti-*

dienne de la société gourmande en France au XIXe siècle (Paris, 1971) 52–55; J. van Alphen, "Hippolyte Mège Mouriès," in *Margarine: An Economic, Social and Scientific History 1869–1969*, ed. J. H. van Stuyvenberg (Toronto, 1969) 5–8; James Harvey Young, "'This greasy counterfeit': butter versus oleomargarine in the U.S. Congress, 1886," *BHM* 53 (1979) 392–414; Richard A. Ball and J. Robert Lilly, "The menace of margarine: the rise and fall of a social problem," *Social Problems* 29 (1982) 488–98; William R. Pabst, *Butter and Oleo Margarine: An Analysis of Competing Commodities* (NY, 1937); K. F. Mattil, "The visible fats in our diet," *Food Technology* 13 (Jan 1959) 46–49; Katharine Snodgrass, *Margarine as a Butter Substitute* (Stanford, Calif., 1930); Gallup, *Gallup Poll 1935–71* II, 795, 814, 1141; and Siert F. Riepma, *The Story of Margarine* (Washington, D.C., 1970) with updates and revisions kindly furnished by Mr. Riepma and the National Assoc of Margarine Manufacturers.

46. Soon there may be, as chemists develop sucrose polyesters: Helmut L. Merten, "Low calorie lipids," *J of Agricultural and Food Chemistry* 18 (1970) 1002–4; Kevin J. Hannigan, "Fat replacer cuts calories in fatty foods," *FE* 53 (Sept 1981) 105; and Mae Rudolph, "New agent bats for fat," *Amer Health* 1 (March–April 1982) 87.

47. Chris Lecos, "The sweet and sour history of saccharine, cyclamate, aspartame," *FDA Consumer* 15,7 (1981) 8–11, quote on 8; Mary B. McCann et al., "Non-calorie sweeteners and weight reduction," *JADA* 32 (1956) 327–30; Karl M. Beck, "Practical requirements for the use of synthetic sweeteners," in Dwivedi, *Low Calorie and Special Dietary Foods*, 61–114; and "Consumers who like sugar-free products are on the rise," *FPD* 13 (May 1979) 28.

48. Telephone interview with Marvin Eisenstadt, Oct 18, 1984.

49. Eisenstadt interview; Wayne L. Pines, "The cyclamate story," *FDA Consumer* 8,10 (Dec 1974–Jan 1975) 19–20, 25–27; and Lecos, "Sweet and sour history."

50. Catherine Gonthier-Fishman, "Food additive regulation: the issue of saccharin," in *Controversial Nutrition Policy Issues*, eds. G. R. Solimano and S. A. Lederman (Springfield, Il., 1983) 209–23; Murray D. Sayer, "Artificial sweeteners—their impact on the food laws," *Food Drug Cosmetic Law J* 21 (1966) 111–23; Lecos, "Sweet and sour history"; Eisenstadt interview; Calorie Control Council pamphlet, *Epidemiology* (Atlanta, 1983); and *Congressional Record* (Feb 20, 1985) S1598–99.

51. Robert H. Mazur, "Discovery of aspartame," in Lewis D. Stegink and L. L. Filer, Jr., eds., *Aspartame: Physiology and Chemistry* (NY, 1984) 2–3, a copy kindly furnished by Annette Ripper, formerly of G. D. Searle & Co., who was also the one to credit the General Foods lawyer in an interview, Sept 21, 1984.

52. Stegink and Filer, *Aspartame*, articles by Inglett and section on metabolism, 29–199, 509–54; "Gumballs," 1984 ad created by Ogilvy & Mather for G. D. Searle; and "Aspartame is here," *General Foods News* (Feb–March 1983) 12–14.

53. "Business Times," National Public Radio, Jan 18, 1985, on profit figures, and "Aspartame—too good to be true?" *FE* 56,3 (1984) 16–18, 20.

54. "Polydextrose, a new ingredient for reduced-calorie foods," *FE* 53 (June 1981) 140–41, 143, and "Polydextrose," *Food Processing* 45 (April 1984) 29–30.

55. Louise Fenner, "That lite stuff," *FDA Consumer* (June 1982) reviews the labeling regulations. For legal and technical confusions, see H. L. Hensel, "Dietary version of a standardized food—is it an imitation?" *Food Drug Cosmetic Law J* 13 (March 1958) 172–77; E. J. Bigwood, "What is a dietetic food?" *ibid.* 37 (Jan 1972) 13–18; Stephen H. McNamara, "When does a food become a drug?" *ibid.* 37 (1982) 222–31; and "1980: decade of nutrition guidelines, fortification guidelines, and nutritional labeling," *Food Processing* 41 (April 1980) 30–35.

56. Cf. Mary Douglas, *In the Active Voice* 101–10, and Jack Goody, *Cooking, Cuisine and Class* (Cambridge, 1982) 154–90.

CHAPTER NINE
Baby Fat

1. Edmund S. Morgan, *The Gentle Puritan: A Life of Ezra Stiles, 1727–1795* (New Haven, 1962) 126; George F. Dow, ed., *Holyoke Diaries, 1709–1856* (Salem, Mass., 1911) 3, 17, 18, 23, 26, 29; Patricia C. Cohen, *A Calculating People: The Spread of Numeracy in Early America* (Chicago, 1982) 4 (quote), 111, 134; and "Journal of an infant," *Library of Health* 5 (1841) 108–10. For the Holyoke reference I thank Laurel Ulrich, who has also drawn my attention to a set of weighings recorded by Benjamin Vaughan, 1796, in the Samuel Vaughan Journal, photocopy at Hubbard Free Library, Hallowell, Me.

2. Francis Stone, letter to Lucy Stone, June 6, 1847, in Gerda Lerner, ed., *The Female Experience* (Indianapolis, 1977) 86; Carlo Ginzburg, *The Night Battles*, trans. John Tedeschi and Anne Tedeschi (Baltimore, 1983) 27, 148, 150, 162; Karl Knortz, *Amerikanischer Aberglaube der Gegenwart* (Leipzig, 1913) 9; Edwin M. Fogel, *Beliefs and Superstitions of the Pennsylvania Germans* (Philadelphia, 1915) #142; David Macrae, *Americans at Home*, rev. ed. (Glasgow, 1875 [1860]) 29.

3. Mr. and Mrs. Chetwood Smith, *Rogers Groups* (Boston, 1924) 41, 84; David H. Wallace, *John Rogers* (Middletown, Conn., 1967) xiii, 241, 301, 304; and Allan Nevins, *Emergence of Modern America 1865–1878* (NY, 1927) 206, unattributed anecdote.

4. Ethel Lynn, "Weighing the baby," *Hill's Manual* (Chicago, 1887) 508, reprinted in Clifton J. Farness, ed., *The Genteel Female* (NY, 1931) 231; Maud Skinner and Otis Skinner, *One Man in His Time: The Adventures of H. Watkins* (Philadelphia, 1938) 192; Theodore Stanton and Harriot S. Blanch, eds., *Elizabeth Cady Stanton* (NY, 1922) II, 44, letter of Oct 22, 1852; and Schlesinger Library, Radcliffe College, Lydia E. Pinkham Medical Company Records, Medical Notebooks 1878–1888 (M79 v.1), Dec 19, 1882, p. 80.

5. Jonathan Swift, *A Modest Proposal* (Dublin, 1729) in *Prose Works* (London, 1925) VII, 210; Hermann Boerhaave, *Academical Lectures on the Theory of Physic* (London, 1742) III, 390n; Thomas E. Cone, "De pondere infantum recens natorum. The history of weighing the newborn infant," *Pediatrics* 28 (1961) 490–98; Richard E. Scammon, "The literature on the growth and physical development of the fetus, infant, and child," *Anatomical Record* 35 (1927) 241–67; Wilton M. Krogman, "Growth of man," *Tabulae Biologicae* 20 (1941) 63; Howard V. Meredith et al., "Early seriatim research on human somatic growth," *Growth* 45 (1981) 151–67; and J. M. Tanner, *A History of the Study of Human Growth* (Cambridge, 1981) ch. 11.

6. Edward Meeker, "The improving health of the United States, 1850–1915," *Explorations in Entrepreneurial History* 2d ser., 9 (1972) 353–74.

7. Robert H. Bremner, ed., *Children and Youth in America: A Documentary History. Vol. II, 1866–1932. Parts 7–8* (Cambridge, Mass., 1971) 965–67; Nancy Weiss, "Save the Children: A History of the Children's Bureau, 1903–18," Ph.D. thesis, UCLA, 1974, esp. 10–13, 187–93; and Isaac F. Abt, ed., *Abt-Garrison History of Pediatrics* (Philadelphia, 1965) 150–68.

8. Stanford E. Chaillé, "Infants, their chronological progress," *New Orleans Med and Surgical J* n.s. 14 (1886–87) 910, cited by James Allen Young, "Height, weight, and health: anthropometric study of human growth in 19th-century American medicine," *BHM* 53 (1979) 233; Kathleen W. Jones, "Sentiment and science: the late 19th-century pediatrician as mother's advisor," *JSH* 17 (1983) 79–86; and Thomas E. Cone, Jr., *History of American Pediatrics* (Boston, 1979) 101, 151.

9. Jones, "Sentiment and science," 82–84.

10. See Edward Shorter, *Making of the Modern Family* (NY, 1975) 175–90; Randolph Trumbach, *Rise of the Egalitarian Family* (NY, 1978)

197–208; and George D. Sussman, *Selling Mothers' Milk: The Wet-Nursing Business in France, 1715–1914* (Urbana, Ill., 1982).

11. Ian G. Wickes, "A history of infant feeding. Parts I–V," *ADC* 28 (1953) 151–58, 232–40, 332–40, 416–22, 495–502.

12. *Ibid.*, 421; Smith, *Treatise*, 59 and Appendix A, extracts from C. H. F. Routh's *Treatise on Infant Feeding*, and 716–17 on Liebig's Soup; and Abraham Jacobi, *Infant Diet* (NY, 1873) 29.

13. John Ruhräh, comp., *Pediatrics of the Past* (NY, 1925) reviews many of these manuals.

14. Wickes, "History of infant feeding," 335, and Cone, *American Pediatrics*, 135–36.

15. Disney H. D. Cran, "Breast feeding: Dr. Variot's teaching," *Lancet* 2 (1913) 1659–60; and Wickes, "History of infant feeding," 339–40, 501.

16. Cone, *American Pediatrics*, 136–39; John L. Morse, "Recollections and reflections on forty-five years of artificial infant feeding," *JP* 7 (Sept 1935) 303–7. In the 1890s, Seibert's Bottles were marked for size and weight of the infant.

17. Manfred J. Waserman, "Henry L. Coit and the certified milk movement," *BHM* 46 (1972) 359–90; Bremner, *Children and Youth in America*, 812, 867–74; and Norman Shaftel, "History of the purification of milk in New York," *NY St J of Med* 58 (1958) 911–28.

18. Ira V. Hiscock, "Development of neighborhood health services in the U.S.," *Milbank Memorial Fund Q Bulletin* 13 (1935) 30–51; Patricia M. Melvin, "Milk to motherhood: the New York Milk Committee and the beginning of well-child programs," *Mid-America* 65 (1983) 111–34; Isaac A. Abt, *Baby Doctor* (NY, 1944) 128–33; George Rosen, "The first neighborhood health center movement," *AJPH* 61 (1971) 1620–35; Paul Starr, *Social Transformation of American Medicine* (NY, 1982) 192; Bird T. Baldwin, "Physical growth of children from birth to maturity," *Univ of Iowa Studies in Child Welfare* 1 (1921) 36; and Sheila M. Rothman, "Women's clinics or doctors' offices: the Sheppard–Towner Act and the promotion of preventive health care," in *Social History and Social Policy*, eds. David J. Rothman and Stanton Wheeler (NY, 1981) 75–202.

19. Fairbanks Papers, *Catalog #512* (1908) 817; Howe Papers, *Catalog #61* (1924) 57, 60, and *Catalog #48* (1920) 46.

20. Eugene Wood, "The new baby," *Amer Mag* 64 (1907) 486, and Smith College (Northampton, Mass.), Margaret Long Papers 1893–1929, folder 14, letter of May 20, 1913, from Mendenhall, quoted with permission from Thomas Mendenhall.

21. Phineas T. Barnum, *Struggles and Triumphs*, new ed. (Buffalo, 1878) 56, 65–66; Jane Mulligan, "Madonna and Child in American Cul-

ture, 1830–1916," Ph.D. thesis, UCLA, 1976, ch. 8; Agnes Ditson, "Human stock show," *JAMA* 61 (1913) 111–13; Anna S. Richardson, "News of Better Babies contests," *WHC* 41 (Jan 1914) 35, 46, and also (Feb 1914) 48–49, (March 1914) 19–20, 69, (April 1914) 46–47, (July 1914) 9; Frederick S. Crum, "Anthropometric statistics of children—ages six to forty-eight months," *Amer Statistical Assoc Tr* 15 (1916) 332–36; "Better Babies Bureau," *WHC* 45 (Jan 1918) 46 and (Feb 1918) 28; and Children's Bureau, *April and May Weighing and Measuring Test* Pub. No. 38 (Washington, D.C., 1918).

22. Joyce Antler and Daniel M. Fox, "The movement toward a safe maternity: physician accountability in New York City, 1915–1940," *BHM* 50 (1976) 569–95, and Fred L. Adair, "Maternal, fetal and neonatal morbidity and mortality," *AJOG* 29 (1935) 384–94.

23. C. Henry Davis, "Weight in pregnancy: its value as a routine test," *AJOG* 6 (1923) 575–81; Calvin R. Hannah, "Weight during pregnancy," *Texas St J of Med* 19 (1923) 224–26; idem, "Weight during pregnancy," *AJOG* 9 (1925) 854–63; and William Kerwin, "Weight estimates during pregnancy and puerperium," *AJOG* 11 (1926) 473–77.

24. See Myron Winick, "Food and the fetus," *Natural History* 90 (Jan 1981) 76–81, and Judith E. Brown, *Nutrition for Your Pregnancy* (Minneapolis, 1983) 34.

25. See F. E. Hytten and A. M. Thomson, "Maternal physiological adjustments," *Maternal Nutrition and the Course of Human Pregnancy* (Washington, D.C., 1970) 41–73; Gail S. Brewer, *What Every Pregnant Woman Should Know* (NY, 1977) 11–14, 18–19; and Annette Gormican et al., "Relationships of maternal weight gain, prepregnancy weight and infant birthweight," *JADA* 77 (1980) 662–67.

26. For a worst-case scenario, see J. William Finch, "The overweight obstetric patient with special reference to the use of dexedrine sulfate," *J of Oklahoma St Med Assoc* 40 (1947) 119–22; cf. Dawn C. Norman, ed., "I dieted during my second pregnancy . . . and what a difference!" *LHJ* 70 (Nov 1953) 166–71.

27. Richard W. Wertz and Dorothy C. Wertz, *Lying-In: A History of Childbirth in America* (NY, 1977) 168; and Rima D. Apple, "'To Be Used Only Under the Direction of a Physician': commercial infant feeding and medical practice, 1870–1940," *BHM* 54 (1980) 402–17.

28. James A. Greene, "Clinical study of the etiology of obesity," *AIM* 12 (1939) 1798, and Ann Williams-Heller, "Control your weight after the baby comes," *PM* 20 (June 1945) 44–45. Cf. Lillian C. Robbins, "Parental recall of child-rearing practices," *J of Abnormal and Social Psych* 66 (1963) 261–70, on more accurate memories of birth weights than of any other feature of childrearing.

29. T. A. Emmett, *Principles and Practice of Gynaecology* (Philadelphia, 1879) cited in Tanner, *Human Growth*, 190.

30. Young, "Height, weight and health"; Henry P. Bowditch, "Growth of children" (1879) in his *Papers on Anthropometry* (Boston, 1894) 65–116; W. Townsend Porter, "On the application to individual school children of the mean values derived from anthropological measurements," *Amer Statistical Assoc* 3 (1893) 576–87; idem, "Physical basis of precocity and dullness," *Academy of Science of St. Louis Tr* 6 (1895) 161–81; Tanner, *Human Growth*, 234–53 on Boas; Arthur MacDonald, *Experimental Study of Children* (Washington, D.C., 1899); Frederick Burk, "Growth of children in height and weight," *Amer J of Psych* 9 (1898) 253–326; and Agnes Wayman, "What to measure in physical education," *Research Q* 1,2 (1930) 97–110.

31. Porter, "On the application," 586; Luther H. Gulick and Leonard P. Ayres, *Medical Inspection of Schools*, rev. ed. (NY, 1913) esp. physical record cards on 54–57; Bremner, *Children and Youth in America*, 826, 952; Lucy Wood Collier, "A pair of scales in every school," *LHJ* 36 (Sept 1919) 125; "Wisconsin to have a demonstration band of Food Scouts," *Crusader* 10,1 (1919) 3–5; Hyman Krakower, "Anthropometry," *Research Q* 8,4 (1937) 85–95, historical survey; Tanner, *Human Growth*, 299–344; Elizabeth Irwin, "What the child's weight tells," *Delineator* 97 (Dec 1920) 29; and Fairbanks Papers, *Catalog #1100-C* (1925) 70–71.

32. "Significance of weight as an index to health," *Elementary School J* 31 (Sept 1930) 11–12; "Height–weight–age tables for children," *JAMA* 101 (1933) 369–70; and Vernette S. Vickers and Harold C. Stuart, "Anthropometry in the pediatrician's office," *JP* 22 (1943) 155–69.

33. Taylor's article appeared on March 15, 1922. Mrs. Grant's rebuttal came on May 10 (pp. 67–68) with Taylor's comment, "More enlightenment wanted," 68–69, and Holt's answer, June 7, 1922, pp. 248–49.

34. Borden S. Veeder, "The overweight child," *JAMA* 83 (1924) 486–89; Bird T. Baldwin, "Use and abuse of weight–height–age tables," *JAMA* 92 (1924) 1–4; Norman K. Nixon, "Obesity in children," *JP* 4 (1934) 295–306; and Adelaide R. Ross, "Case studies of overweight children," *Hygeia* 15 (1937) 456–57, 474, 476. The first popular article may have been R. P. Emerson, "Over-weight child," *WHC* 47 (April 1920) 31.

35. Quote from the Peters comments after paper by Veeder, "Overweight child," 489, and see her "The fat child—No. 1," *Los Angeles Times* (Feb 5, 1924) II, 6:7; McHale, *Comparative Psychology*, 78; Thomas D. Wood, "The overweight child," in *Your Weight and How to Control It*, ed. Morris Fishbein (NY, 1927) 136; and Rachel Bevington and Ruth Hall, "Dieting," *Hygeia* 9 (Aug 1931) 656–57.

36. Jean Piaget, *Six Psychological Studies*, trans. Anita Tenzer, ed. David Elkind (NY, 1967) 43–46; Frank B. Murray and Paul E. Johnson, "Relevant and some irrelevant factors in the child's concept of weight," *J of Educ Psych* 67 (1975) 705–11; Adelaide Ross, "Is the overweight child getting a square deal?" *Hygeia* 15 (1937) 360–61; and Frank H. Richardson, "What are you going to do with your underweight child?" *GH* 90 (Jan 1930) 34–35, 142, 144.

37. Clara E. Sears, *Some American Primitives* (Port Washington, N.Y., 1968) 31–50, illustrations 62–76, on Prior; Currier & Ives prints on display at the Margaret Woodbury Strong Museum (Rochester, N.Y.) in 1984 exhibit, "A Century of Childhood 1820–1920"; Dorothy P. Ryan, *Picture Postcards in the U.S. 1893–1918* (NY, 1982) 74, 196–205; Maurice Horn, ed., *World Encyclopedia of Comics* (NY, 1976) esp. 223 on Drayton; Constance E. King, *Dolls and Dolls' Houses* (London, 1977) 22–26, 66–101, 114–16; Joseph J. Schroeder, Jr., *The Wonderful World of Toys, Games and Dolls 1860–1930* (Chicago, 1971) 195 on kewpies, 240 on 1930 "Kidiline" thin dolls; and Margaret B. McDowell, "The children's feature," *Midwest Q* 19 (Autumn 1977) 36–50, esp. on Bogart.

38. Veeder, "Overweight child," 488.

39. Bremner, *Children and Youth in America*, 1089; Caroline Bird, *The Invisible Scar* (NY, 1966) 27; Carroll E. Palmer, "Children and the Depression," *School and Society* 42 (1935) 318–19; Georg Wolff, "A study on the trend of weight in white school children from 1933 to 1936," *Child Development* 11 (1940) 159–79, with follow-up articles 12 (1941) 183–206 and 13 (1942) 65–77; Howard V. Meredith, "Stature and weight of private school children in two successive decades," *AJPA* 28 (1941) 32, 34; John B. Youmans et al., "Surveys of the nutrition . . . in a rural population in middle Tennessee. Part 2," *AJPH* 33 (1943) 58–72; Richard O. Cummings, *The American and His Food* (Chicago, 1940) 180–87, 216; Calla Van Syckle, "Some pictures of food consumption in the U.S. Part II. 1860–1941," *JADA* 21 (1945) 691; Esther F. Phipard, "How good is our national diet?" *Annals of the Amer Academy of Political and Social Science* 225 (Jan 1943) 67–69; and George H. Gallup, *Gallup Poll 1935–71* (NY, 1972) I, 395, question of July 25, 1943, "Have you lost weight or gained weight since food rationing began?" See also Mayhew Derryberry, "Reliability of medical judgments of malnutrition," *Public Health Reports* 53 (1938) 263–68.

40. Veeder, "Overweight child," 488; Baldwin, "Physical growth of children," 143; McHale, *Comparative Psychology*, 13–18; Ellen Grindell, ed., "If your child is overweight. As told by a mother to Ellen Grindell," *Hygeia* 12 (1934) 1015–16; Mildred H. Bryan, "Don't let your child get fat!" *Hygeia* 15 (1937) 801–3.

41. Bremner, *Children and Youth in America*, 1040–57, 947–49, quote on 1051, and J. C. McCullers and J. M. Love, "The scientific study of the child," in *Issues and Ideas in America*, eds. Benjamin J. Taylor and Thomas J. White (Norman, Okla., 1976) 189–216.

42. Bremner, *Children and Youth in America*, 1054; Dom Cavallo, "From perfection to habit: moral training in the American kindergarten, 1860–1920," *History of Educ Q* 16 (1976) 147–61; and Fanny E. Lawrence, "Rhythm in the nursery school," *Amer Childhood* 13 (Nov 1927) 31–32.

43. Alice Guppy, *Children's Clothes, 1939–1970* (Poole, 1978) 1–2, 8–9; Montgomery Ward & Co., *Catalog #97* (Chicago, 1922) esp. 232; Hillel Schwartz, "The zipper and the child," *Notebooks in Cultural Analysis, Vol. II* eds. Norman F. Cantor and Nathalia King (Durham, N.C., 1985) 1–28. Ruth O'Brien and Meyer A. Girschick in 1939 determined that weight was the best single measure to use for sizing children's clothes: *Children's Body Measurements for Sizing Garments and Patterns* (Washington, D.C., 1939) 4.

44. Harry F. Dowling, *Fighting Infection* (Cambridge, Mass., 1977) 203–19; Monroe Lerner and Odin W. Anderson, *Health Progress in the U.S., 1900–1960* (Chicago, 1963) 151–60; and Victor Cohn, *Sister Kenny* (Minneapolis, 1975) quotes on 79, 126.

45. Emile Demange, "Obésité," *Dictionnaire encyclopédique des sciences médicales* (Paris, 1880) XIV, 10; William R. P. Emerson, *Nutrition and Growth in Children* (NY, 1926) 158; Dowling, *Fighting Infection*, 210; Editorial, "Infantile paralysis," *Hygeia* 19 (1941) 777; Gallup, *Gallup Poll 1935–71*, II, 845–46; and Benjamin P. Sandler, *Diet Prevents Polio* (n.p., 1951) quote on 54.

46. Cohn, *Sister Kenny*, 137.

47. Ross, "Case studies," 474.

48. Beatrice Black, "Give the fat child a chance," *PM* 16 (Oct 1941) 34, 93–95.

49. Hilde Bruch, *The Importance of Overweight* (NY, 1957) 5–6, 20, 23; H. Gardiner-Hill and J. Forest Smith, "Pituitary obesity in adolescence," *Q J of Med* 18 (1924/25) 309–26; Leonard Williams, "Some further aspects of obesity," *Practitioner* 86 (1911) 548; William Engelbach, "Juvenile adiposity," *Annals of Clinical Med* 3 (1924) 198–208; Norman Jolliffe, *Reduce and Stay Reduced* (NY, 1952) 229, quoting Froehlich; L. Napoleon Boston, "Juvenile adiposity," *Amer Physician* 31 (1926) 77–81; and Gavin Fulton, "Evaluation of reducing diets," *Kentucky Med J* 34 (1936) 519.

50. Bruch, *Importance of Overweight*, 6–9; Hilde Bruch and Grace Touraine, "Obesity in childhood: family frame of obese children," *Psychosomatic Med* 2 (1940) 141–206; and Hilde Bruch, "Obesity in

childhood: III. Physiologic and psychologic aspects of the food intake of obese children," *AJDC* 59 (1940) 739–81. Cf. I. P. Bronstein et al., "Obesity in childhood: psychologic studies," *AJDC* 63 (1942) 239. There were certain quite rare conditions (Laurence-Moon-Bardet-Biehl Syndrome, Prader-Willi Syndrome and Morgagni-Stewart-Morel Syndrome) in which childhood fatness seemed to be genetically transmitted and was sometimes associated with endocrine or pituitary disorders.

51. Two articles by same author in same journal twenty years apart: J. H. Kenyon, "Is your child too thin?" *GH* 82 (April 1926) 102, and "Don't let your child get fat," *GH* 121 (Oct 1945) 62; J. Sanford Kruglick, "Overstuffed babies," *PM* 15 (Feb 1940) 28; Morse, "Recollection," 324; C. Anderson Aldrich and Mary M. Aldrich, *Feeding Our Old Fashioned Children* (NY, 1941) v, 75; Celia B. Stendler, "Sixty years of child training practices," *JP* 36 (1950) 122–34; Clark E. Vincent, "Trends in infant care ideas," *Child Development* 22 (1951) 199–210; Michael Gordon, "Infant care revisited," *J of Marriage and the Family* 30 (1968) 578–83; Jay Mechling, "Advice to historians on advice to mothers," *JSH* 9 (1975) 44–63; and Gladys D. Shultz, "Forget that clean-plate bogey!" *Better Homes and Gardens* 21 (Sept 1942) 46.

   For early American studies of anorexia, see John M. Berkman, "Functional anorexia," *MCNA* 23 (1939) 901–12, discussing 117 cases diagnosed at the Mayo Clinic, 1917–30; John V. Waller et al., "Anorexia nervosa and psychosomatic entity," *Psychosomatic Med* 2 (1940) 3–16, stressing family dynamics; and Jules H. Masserman, "An analysis of a neurotic character with psychodynamisms of vomiting and anorexia nervosa," *Psychoanalytic Q* 10 (1941) 211–42, with fifty-six references.

52. On "good" food as medicine, see Helen Woodward, *It's an Art* (NY, 1938) 141, 150–51; for Mead's insights, see her "Dietary patterns and food habits," *JADA* 19 (1943) 1–5 and cf. William S. Langford, "The psychological aspects of feeding in early childhood," *JADA* 17 (1941) 208–16. Mothers had *more* feeding problems with their children if they had studied home economics, reported Winona L. Morgan, *The Family Meets Depression* (Minneapolis, 1939) 30–32.

53. For psychological tacks, see Marion J. Barnes, "Some reasons why obese children find dieting difficult," *Smith College Studies in Social Work* 11 (1941) 342–75, exemplary of transition between endocrine and psychotherapy; Israel Bram, "The fat youngster," *Archives of Pediatrics* 60 (1943) 239–49; and Herman N. Bundesen, "Overweight in children," *LHJ* 60 (July 1943) 115–16. The first report on the use of amphetamines with specifically obese children seems to have been Ralph H. Kunstadter, "Experience with benzedrine sulfate in the treatment of obesity," *JP* 17 (1940) 490–501.

54. "Slimming fare: Barnard girls lose weight through new diet," *Literary Digest* 123 (April 10, 1937) 35–36, and Regina J. Woody, "Reducing the adolescent," *Hygeia* 19 (1941) 476–82.

55. F. W. Schultz, "What to do about the fat child at puberty," *JP* 19 (1941) 376–81; Lulu G. Graves, "Should the teens diet?" *PM* 15 (April 1940) 76; and Woody, "Reducing the adolescent," 477.

56. Mary L. Johnson et al., "Prevalence and incidence of obesity in a cross-section of elementary and secondary school children," *AJCN* 4 (1956) 231–38; Ruth L. Huenemann et al., "A longitudinal study . . . in a teen-age population," *AJCN* 18 (May 1966) 325–38; Hermann H. Remmers and D. H. Radler, *The American Teenager* (Indianapolis, 1957) 63; R. W. Deisher and C. A. Mills, "The adolescent looks at his health and medical care," *AJPH* 53 (1963) 1929; Johanna T. Dwyer et al., "Adolescent dieters: who are they?" *AJCN* 20 (1967) 1047; Alexander Frazier and Lorenzo K. Lisonbee, "Adolescent concerns with physique," *School R* 58 (1950) 397–405; Luther Emmett Holt, Jr., "The obese child," *GH* 141 (Nov 1955) 304; and James F. Adams, "Adolescents' identification of personal and national problems," *Adolescence* 1 (1966) 240–50.

57. Benjamin Spock, *Common Sense Book of Baby and Child Care*, new ed. (NY, 1957) 433–34; Harold C. Stuart, "Obesity in childhood," *Q R of Pediatrics* 10 (1955) 131–45; Albert A. Schaal, "Overweight in young children," *GH* 148 (April 1959) 30–31; Marguerite Rittenhouse and Ruth Kamerman, "Overweight child," *Cosmopolitan* 149 (July 1960) 74; Edward T. Wilkes, "Chubby children need your help," *Today's Health* 40 (May 1962) 39; and "Teen-age gluttons," *Newsweek* 55 (March 14, 1960) 88.

58. A. G. Mullins, "Prognosis in juvenile obesity," *ADC* 33 (1958) 307–14; Sidney Abraham and Marie Nordsieck, "Relationship of excess weight in children and adults," *Public Health Report* 75 (1960) 263–73; June K. Lloyd et al., "Childhood obesity," *BMJ* 2 (1961) 145–48; and Patria Asher, "Fat babies and fat children" *ADC* 41 (1966) 672–73; *GH* 157 (Oct 1963) 195. The figure became 85 percent in John E. Allen et al., *Practical Points in Pediatrics*, 2d ed. (Flushing, N.Y., 1977) 244; it became 90 percent in Pasquale J. Accardo, ed., *Failure to Thrive in Infancy and Early Childhood* (Baltimore, 1982) 308. Restated by Stunkard, the odds against an obese child's becoming a normal-weight adult were more than 4 to 1, and if there were no weight reduction in adolescence, the odds were 28 to 1. Albert J. Stunkard, *The Pain of Obesity* (Palo Alto, Calif., 1976).

59. Tanner, *Human Growth*, 297–98; Peter Laslett, *Family Life and Illicit Love in Earlier Generations* (Cambridge, 1977) 214–32; Rose E. Frisch and Roger Revelle, "Height and weight at menarche and a hypothesis of critical body weights and adolescent events," *Science* 169

(July 24, 1970) 397–99; James Trussell, "Statistical flaws in evidence for the Frisch hypothesis that fatness triggers menarche," *Human Biology* 52 (1980) 711–20; and Stanley M. Garn and Joan A. Haskell, "Fat and growth during childhood," *Science* 130 (Dec 18, 1959) 1711–12. European and American children who are fat seem to be proportionately fatter than obese children in previous generations. Growing concern with obesity in children may therefore be due in part to a more remarkable obesity in the same percentage of the population. See Peter V. V. Hamill et al., *Height and Weight of Children: United States* Public Health Service Pub. No. 1000, series 11, #104 (Rockville, Md., 1970) esp. 16; M. Börjeson, "Prevention of obesity in childhood," in *Obesity in Childhood*, eds. E. Cacciari et al. (London, 1978) 239; and Wilton M. Krogman, *Child Growth* (Ann Arbor, Mich., 1972) 38–41.

60. Beryl Tucker, "They're better dressed today," *PM* 26 (Oct 1951) 144 and Chubbette ad, *PM* 15 (Feb 1940) 80; Geneen Roth, *Feeding the Hungry Heart* (Indianapolis, 1982) 112 on wearing Chubbettes; E-Z underwear ad in *PM* 28 (April 1953) 26, labeled by weight as well as size; and R. Duffy Lewis and Dorothy Stote, *How to Build an Infant's, Children's and Sub-Teens Business* (NY, 1956) 25, 32–34. On classroom weighing, see Judy Blume's novel, *Blubber* (NY, 1974) 77–79.

61. For the new tables, see Susan P. Souther et al., "A comparison of indices used in judging the physical fitness of school children," *AJPH* 29 (1939) 434–38; Norman C. Wetzel, "Physical fitness . . . ," *JAMA* 116 (1941) 1187–95; Howard V. Meredith, "Stature and weight of children in the U.S.," *AJDC* 62 (1941) 909–32; Harold C. Stuart and Howard V. Meredith, "Use of body measurements in the school health program, Parts I, II," *AJPH* 36 (1946) 1365–86; J. D. Ratcliff, "Wetzel grid tells how children grow," *Science Illustrated* 2 (Oct 1947) 66–70; and J. M. Tanner, "Standards from birth to maturity for height, weight, height velocity, and weight velocity: British children, 1965," *ADC* 41 (1966) 454–71, 613–35.

62. James Trager, *The . . . Bellybook* (NY, 1972) 452 on ads; White House Conference on Food, Nutrition and Health, *Final Report* (Washington, D.C., 1976) 49; A. B. Silverstein and H. A. Robinson, "Representation of physique in children's figure drawings," *J of Consulting Psych* 25 (1961) 146–48; J. Robert Staffieri, "A study of social stereotyping of body image in children," *J of Personality and Social Psych* 7 (1967) 101–4; Albert J. Stunkard and Myer Mendelson, "Obesity and the body image, II," 1443–47; Richard M. Lerner and Elizabeth Gellert, "Body build identification, preference and aversion in children," *Developmental Psych* 1 (1969) 456–62; Shelia R. Caskey, "Your responsibility toward the fat child," *School and Community* 57

(Feb 1971) 12–13; Susan C. Wooley et al., "Theoretical, practical, and social issues in behavioral treatments of obesity," *J of Applied Behavior Analysis* 12 (1979) 18; and "On a diet," *Boston Globe* (Feb 5, 1983) 2 on Campbell Kids.

63. Graves, "Should teens diet?" 76; Fred W. Norris, "Girth control," *Hygeia* 19 (1941) 780; and Alice Lake, "Tell me doctor: When should my child diet?" *LHJ* 83 (Feb 1966) 42.

64. Jerome L. Knittle and Jules Hirsch, "Effect of early nutrition on the development of rat epididymal fat pads," *J of Clinical Investigation* 47 (1968) 2091–98; idem, "Cellularity of obese and nonobese human adipose tissue," *Federation Proc* 29 (1970) 1516–21; and Jerome L. Knittle, "Obesity in childhood: a problem in adipose tissue cellular development," *JP* 81 (1972) 1049.

65. Lester David, "The fat child can be helped," *GH* 154 (Feb 1962) 53, quoting Garn; G. L. Whitelaw, "Prevalence and prognosis of obesity in infancy," in Cacciari, ed. *Obesity in Childhood*, 128; Lawrence D. Robinson, "The obese child," *Essence* 3 (Sept 1972) 15; Robert W. Mack and Mary Ellen Kleinhenz, "Growth, caloric intake and activity levels in early infancy," *Human Biology* 46 (1974) 345–54, first eight weeks as critical; and Daniel W. Schiff, "The case for routine visits," in *Controversies in Child Health*, eds. Daniel H. Smith and Robert A. Hoekelman (NY, 1981) 194.

00. Felix P. Heald and Mushtaq Ahmad Khan, "Obesity in childhood and adolescence," in *Endocrine and Genetic Diseases of Childhood and Adolescence*, ed. Lytt I. Gardner, 2d ed. (Philadelphia, 1975) 1152–53; June K. Lloyd, "The young child: obesity" in *Human Nutrition. Vol. 2: Nutrition and Growth*, eds. D. B. Jelliffe, and E. F. P. Jelliffe (NY, 1979) 233; Judith E. Singer et al., "Relation of weight gain during pregnancy to birth weight . . . ," *Obstetrics and Gynecology* 31 (1968) 417–23; "Influence of intrauterine nutritional status on the development of obesity in later life," *Nutrition R* 35 (May 1977) 100–102, first and second trimesters as critical; Abby A. Belson, "Obesity and the unborn child," *WW* 6 (Jan 1974) 20–22, 49; "Compound controls weight in pregnant," *Amer Druggist* 165 (Jan 24, 1972) 43; Seymour Isenberg, *Keep Your Kids Thin* (NY, 1982) 31–38, and cf. Clara J. McLaughlin, *Black Parents Handbook* (NY, 1976) 33.

67. See John T. Noonan, Jr., *A Private Choice: Abortion in America in the Seventies* (NY, 1979); Bernard N. Nathanson, *Aborting America* (Garden City, N.Y., 1979); and Kristin Luker, *Abortion and the Politics of Motherhood* (Berkeley, Calif., 1984).

68. I have benefited here from conversations with the psychologist Dori Winchell and with William N. Davis, executive director of the Center for the Study of Anorexia and Bulimia in New York City. On ano-

rexia, see esp. Marlene Boskind-Lodahl, "Cinderella's stepsisters: a feminist perspective on anorexia nervosa and bulimia," *Signs* 2 (1976) 342–56; Marilyn Lawrence, "Anorexia nervosa—the control paradox," *Women's Studies Int Q* 2 (1979) 93–101; Vicki Druss and Mary Sue Henifin, "Why are so many anorexics women?" in *Women Look at Biology Looking at Women*, eds. Ruth Hubbard et al. (Boston, 1979) 127–33; and Marion Woodman, *The Owl Was a Baker's Daughter* (Toronto, 1980) esp. 23. On anorexia and birth weight, see A. H. Crisp, "Reported birth weights and growth rates in a group of patients with primary anorexia nervosa," *J of Psychosomatic Research* 14 (1970) 23–50.

69. See, e.g., Helen Smiciklas-Wright and Anthony R. D'Augelli, "Primary prevention for overweight: Preschool Eating Patterns (PEP) program," *JADA* 72 (1978) 626–29; "Successful weight loss techniques with mentally retarded children and youth," *Exceptional Children* 49 (1982) 238–44; "American kids: more fat, less fit," *McCall's* 112 (May 1985) 70 on triathlons for kids; R. Wisdom, "Think thin, teach thin," *School and Community* 67 (Feb 1981) 18–19; Senate Select Committee on Nutrition and Human Needs, *Nutrition Education—1972* (Washington, D.C., 1973) 231–37; Tamara J. Keyser and Randall J. Souviney, *Measurement and the Child's Environment* (Santa Monica, Calif., 1980) 19, 30, 39–40; and Henrietta Fleck, *Introduction to Nutrition*, 2d ed. (London, 1971) 292, text used by San Dieguito High School in Encinitas, Calif. See also Mary Jane German et al., "Assessing nutrition education practices in the high school health curriculum," *J of School Health* 51 (1981) 405–7 revealing that weight control is taught even more frequently than the Basic Four food groups. On teachers' prejudices against fat children, see Richard N. Walker, "Body build and nursery school teachers' ratings," *Monographs of the Soc for Research in Child Development* 27,3 (1962), and David Brooks, "Fat 'n happy? not likely," *Thrust* 10 (March 1981) 32–31 (*sic*). Final quote from J. Robert McClintic, *Basic Anatomy and Physiology of the Human Body*, 2d ed. (NY, 1980) 606.

70. Jules Hirsch and B. Batchelor, "Adipose tissue cellularity in human obesity," *Clinical Endocrinology and Metabolism* 5 (1976) 299–311; Irving M. Faust, "Nutrition and the fat cell," *IJO* 4 (1980) 314–21; Ottavio Bosello et al., "Adipose tissue cellularity and weight reduction forecasting," *AJCN* 33 (1980) 776–82; and J. R. Bierich, "Therapeutic treatment in childhood obesity," in Cacciari, ed., *Obesity in Childhood*, 229 (quote).

71. Stanley M. Garn and Diane C. Clark, "Trends in fatness and the origins of obesity," *Pediatrics* 57 (1976) 443–56; Ross G. Mitchell, ed., *Child Health in the Community* (Edinburgh, 1977) 79, citing Mayer;

and Stanley M. Garn et al., "Effect of remaining family members on fatness prediction," *AJCN* 34 (Feb 1981) 148–53, giving a child a 40 percent chance of being obese if the other three members of the family are also obese. A recent study highlights the inheritability of obesity: Albert J. Stunkard et al., "An adoption study of human obesity," *NEJM* 314 (Jan 23, 1986) 193–97. Obesity is statistically associated with children of single-parent households; since the number of such households is growing and since nearly half of all children born in 1970 could expect to live in such a household before they were eighteen, the national proportion of obese children may well increase: J. Lawrence Angel, "Constitution in female obesity," *AJPA* ser. 2, 7 (1949) 437–38; "Infant feeding, somatic growth, and obesity," *Nutrition R* 35 (Sept 1977) 235–36; and Carl Degler, *At Odds* (NY, 1980) 456.

72. Isabelle Holland, *Heads You Win, Tails I Lose* (Philadelphia, 1973); Doris B. Smith, *Last Was Lloyd* (NY, 1981); Jan Greenberg, *The Pigout Blues* (NY, 1982); Robert K. Smith, *Jelly Belly* (NY, 1981); Ann Irwin, *One Bite at a Time* (NY, 1973); Judy Blume, *Blubber* (NY, 1974); Barbara Bottner, *Dumb Old Casey Is a Fat Tree* (NY, 1979); Ann Eve Bunting, *Oh, Rick* (Mankato, Minn., 1978); Barthe DeClementis, *Nothing's Fair in Fifth Grade* (NY, 1981); Doris Orgel, *Next Door to Xanadu* (NY, 1969); Robert Lipsyte, *One Fat Summer* (NY, 1977); Isabelle Holland, *Dinah and the Green Fat Kingdom* (Philadelphia, 1978); Daniel Manus Pinkwater, *Fat Elliot and the Gorilla* (NY, 1974); Mary Oldham, *White Pony* (NY, 1981); Nancy Saxon, *Panky and William* (NY, 1983); Molly Cone, *Mishmash and the Big Fat Problem* (Boston, 1982); R. Rozanne Knudson, *Rinehart Lifts* (NY, 1980); Lila Perl, *Hey, Remember Fat Glenda?* (NY, 1981), a sequel to her *Me and Fat Glenda* (NY, 1972); and Virginia Hamilton, *The Planet of Junior Brown* (NY, 1971).

73. Only Mary Oldham's *White Pony* argues firmly against the thinness mania. An earlier classic also does so: André Maurois, *Fattypuffs and Thinifers*, trans. Norman Penny (London, 1941 [1930]).

74. Michael T. Pugliese et al., "Fear of obesity," *NEJM* 309 (1983) 513–17, and cf. Joel D. Killen et al., "Self-induced vomiting and laxative and diuretic use among teenagers," *JAMA* 255 (March 21, 1986) 1447–49. Even in the 1970s, the weighing of children was often accomplished on scales not designed to accommodate squirming youngsters, and the frequent undermeasurement of height led to a common picture of short, stocky children: CDC, Bureau of Smallpox Eradication, Bureau of Training, *Identification and Quantification of Sources of Error in Weighing and Measuring Children* (Washington, D.C., 1976) 7–8, 15–16, and Patricia Freeman, "Obesity tipping the scales against an alarming number of children," *Los Angeles Herald Examiner* (Dec 1, 1985) A-1.

CHAPTER TEN
The Weightless Body

1. Joe B. Frantz, *Gail Borden* (Norman, Okla., 1951) 227–28; *NYT* (July 4, 1880) 5:5; Jack C. Drummond and Anne Wilbraham, *The Englishman's Food*, rev ed. (London, 1958) 352; and Elmer V. McCollum, *A History of Nutrition* (Boston, 1957) 94.

2. George W. Bo-Linn et al., "Starch blockers," *NEJM* 307 (1982) 1413–16; Frederick J. Stare, "Nutritional quackery," *Fourth National Congress on Health Quackery* (Chicago, 1968) 1–7, on Dr. Heinz Humplik's theory of minus-calorie foods, but cf. Mildred Klingman, *Secret Lives of Fat People* (Boston, 1981) 9–11 on popular beliefs about what is not fattening; John J. Beereboom, "Low calorie bulking agents," in *Low Calorie and Special Dietary Foods*, ed. Dasant K. Dwivedi (West Palm Beach, Fla., 1978) 40; "Toward a slimming pill," *New Scientist* 76 (Nov 24, 1977) 493; "A dieter's dream," *NYT* (Aug 30, 1977) 25; and M. Hussain et al., "Perfluoroctyl bromide," *J of Pharmaceutical Sciences* 66 (1977) 907.

3. I rely here on William Leiss, *The Limits of Satisfaction: An Essay on the Problem of Needs and Commodities* (Toronto, 1976) esp. 10, 27, 81.

4. Cf. Susan Stewart, *On Longing: Narratives of the Miniature, the Gigantic, the Souvenir, the Collection* (Baltimore, 1984).

5. See esp. L. H. Newburgh and Margaret W. Johnston, "Obesity," *MCNA* 27 (1943) 339, a summary of work since 1917.

6. William R. Mueller, "Of obesity and election," *Christian Century* 75 (Nov 26, 1958) 1366, quoting Donne; C. S. Lovett, "God's help for overweight Christians," *Personal Christianity* 19 (Jan 1979) 5; Deborah Pierce, *I Prayed Myself Slim* (NY, 1960) 15–16, 42, 76, 124; and Ellen Goodman, "The perils of paunches and pounds," *Washington Post* (Dec 12, 1977) A23.

7. Rosenteur, *Affair of the Flesh*, 218; Metropolitan Life, "Losing to Win" (16 mm., 11 mins., color, the "Cheers for Chubby" cartoon encapsulated within); Gerald Weales, "A family that prays together weighs together," *New Republic* 136 (March 25, 1957) 19–20; "Prayer and fasting," *Time* (March 4, 1957) 78; Mueller, "Of obesity and election," 1367–68; and Charlie W. Shedd, *The Fat Is in Your Head* (Waco, Tex., 1972) 13, 18, 39, 47, 87–89.

8. Kane, *Devotions*, 10, 91 (quote); Carol Showalter, *3D* (Orleans, Mass., 1977) 19, 53, 141; and Ron Enroth, "All isn't well in a popular Christian diet program," *Christianity Today* 26 (April 9, 1982) 54–58.

9. Evelyn Kliewer, *Freedom from Fat* (Old Tappan, N.J., 1977) 21, 38, 45, 55, 67–68.

10. Chapian, *Free to Be Thin* (Minneapolis, 1979) 14, 42, 86, 125; Hunter, *God's Answer to Fat—Lose It* (Houston, 1976) 44, 85; Cook, *Diary of a Fat Housewife* (Denver, 1977) 83–84; and Totie Fields, *I Think I'll Start on Monday* (NY, 1972) 61. See also Ann Thomas, *God's Answer to Overeating* (Washington, D.C., 1975); Jim Tear and Jan Houghton, *Fed Up with Fat* (Old Tappan, N.J., 1978); and Karen Wise, *God Knows I Won't Be Fat Again* (Nashville, 1978).

11. Shedd, *Fat Is in Your Head*, 21; Antonio S. Marotta and Lorraine F. Wurtzel, *Diet Cybernetics for Lean Lines* (NY, 1973); Richard B. Stuart, "Weight loss and beyond," in *Behavioral Medicine*, eds. Park O. Davidson and Shenna M. Davidson (NY, 1980) 188; and Theodore Rubin, *The Thin Book by a Formerly Fat Psychiatrist* (NY, 1966) 107. Cf. Peter M. Stalonas et al., "Do behavioral treatments of obesity last?" *Addictive Behaviors* 9,2 (1984) 175–83.

12. Vincent W. Antonetti, *The Computer Diet* (NY, 1973), and Walter H. Fanburg and Bernard M. Snyder, *How to Be a Winner at the Weight Loss Game* (NY, 1975).

13. Dannon Milk Products, *The Psychology of Dieting*, 12th ed. (Long Island City, N.Y., 1973) quote on 8. Martin Lederman, *The Slim Gourmet* (NY, 1955) 76 has perhaps the earliest food inventory chart. For behaviorist rules and ploys, see esp. James M. Ferguson, *Learning to Eat* (Palo Alto, Calif., 1975), and Alan Dolit, *Fat Liberation* (Millbrae, Calif., 1975). I have also used Richard B. Stuart and Barbara Davis, *Slim Chance in a Fat World*, condensed ed., rev. (Champaign, Ill., 1978 [1972]); C. Young, *Behavioral Modification Treatment of Obesity*, audiocassette (Chicago, 1974); Henry A. Jordan et al., *Eating is Okay!* (NY, 1976); Scene Two Productions, *Moods and Reactions* and *Binges and Snacking*, videocassette series (Detroit, 1979); and Lorraine Dusky and J. J. Leedy, *How to Eat Like a Thin Person* (NY, 1982). I have also benefited from conversations with James M. Ferguson, Sept 10, 1984; with Anne Seifert, author of *The Intelligent Woman's Diet* (La Jolla, Calif., 1982), Aug 16, 1984; and with Guy C. Qvistgaard of the Health-Wise Weight Control Program, Kaiser Permanente Hospital, La Mesa, Calif., Aug 21, 1984.

14. Edward M. Marshall, *The Marshall Plan for Lifelong Weight Control* (Boston, 1981) 110–11.

15. Annie Dillard, *Pilgrim at Tinker Creek* (NY, 1979) 91, 163–64, 232, 248, and Garrett Hardin, *Stalking the Wild Taboo*, 2d ed. (Los Altos, 1978) 221–44, essay dating from 1974.

16. Jean Anthelme. Brillat-Savarin, *The Physiology of Taste*, introduction (and trans.?) by Arthur Machen (NY, 1960), and cf. *The Philosopher in the Kitchen*, trans. Anne Drayton (London, 1970) 130–36.

17. Hal Lindsey, *The Late Great Planet Earth* (Grand Rapids, Mich., 1970) 124–34, quote on 130, and "Hal Lindsey's prophetic jigsaw puzzle," *Liberty* 80,6 (1985) 5.

18. Lindsey, *Late Great Planet Earth*, 124, 126.

19. Otto H. Gauer, "Historical aspects of gravitational stress," in *Gravitational Stress in Aerospace Medicine*, eds. Gauer and George O. Zuidema (Boston, 1961) 7–9; E. C. Dodds, commenting in A. W. Spence, "Discussion on obesity," *Royal Soc of Med Proc* 43 (1950) 344; "How zero gravity feels," *Time* 68 (Oct 8, 1956) 91–92; David Bushnell, *History of Research in Subgravity and Zero-G 1948–58* (Halloman Air Force Base, N.M., 1958); Charles C. Wunder et al., "Gravity as a biological determinant," in *Hypodynamics and Hypogravics*, ed. Michael McCally (NY, 1968) quote on 3; Theodore B. Van Italie, "Discussion: caloric requirements of long flights," in *Conference on Nutrition in Space and Related Waste Problems* (Washington, D.C., 1964) 131–33; and Theodore Berland, *Rating the Diets* (NY, 1979) 55–56 on the Astronaut's Diet. Cf. Mario Iona, "The meaning of weight," *Physics Teacher* 13,5 (1975) 263–74, esp. 264.

20. Shedd, *Fat Is in Your Head*, 35–37; Robert F. Capon, *The Supper of the Lamb* (Garden City, N.Y., 1969) 7 (quote), 114; Optifast weight-reducing program as described to me by Guy C. Qvistgaard of Kaiser Permanente Hospital, La Mesa, Calif.; Shana Alexander, "The Zero Calorie diet," *Life* (Oct 11, 1963) 3, 105–11; Robert Linn, *The Last Chance Diet* (NY, 1976); Alan Cott, *Fasting: The Ultimate Diet* (NY, 1975); Joy Gross, *The 30–Day Way to a Born–Again Body* (NY, 1978); and Eugene Garfield, "To fast or not too much fast," *Current Contents* 46 (Nov 16, 1981) 5–11 and 47 (Nov 23, 1981) 5–11 for a fine summary of the literature and the controversy over acidosis. During a low-carbohydrate, a very-low-calorie or a complete fasting diet, fat deposits are broken down faster than the body can use them. Acidic ketone bodies appear during the incomplete metabolism of fatty acids by the liver. The pH level of the blood may be upset. Whether this is unhealthy or healthy depends upon one's physiological disposition to diabetes or coronary thrombosis and upon one's philosophical disposition toward acids. Warnings and worries concerning acidosis date back at least eighty years. See Otto Folin and W. Denis, "On starvation and obesity, with special reference to acidosis," *J of Biological Chemistry* 21 (1915) 183–92; H. O. Beeson, "Obesity and starvation," *Western Med Times* 35 (1916) 422–25; Ronald M. Deutsch, *The Nuts Among the Berries*, rev. ed. (NY, 1967) 162–74; Jennie L. Rowntree, "Significance of studies of ketosis," *JADA* 8 (1932) 307–15; "Weight reduction: fasting vs. a ketogenic diet," *Nutrition R* 24 (May 1966) 133–34; Robert C. Atkins, *Dr.*

Atkins' Diet Revolution (NY, 1972) 13, "ketosis is a state devoutly to be desired"; and Edwin Bayrd, *The Thin Game* (NY, 1978) 21–22, 57–68.

21. Cott, *Fasting*, 3, 18 (quote), 68, 94, and Gross, *Born-Again Body*, 49 and flyleaf.

22. Cf. Ruth Gay, "Fear of food," *Amer Scholar* 45 (1976) 437–41. On skin treatments, see Jean Frumusan, *Cure of Obesity*, trans. Elaine A. Wood (London, 1924); Nicole Ronsard, *Cellulite* (NY, 1973); Denise Fortino, "Preventing cellulite," *Harper's Bazaar* 112 (March 1979) 126, 166–67; and Louise Fenner, "Cellulite," *FDA Consumer* (May 1980). On aerobics, Kenneth Cooper, *The New Aerobics* (NY, 1970). On surgery, Joachim Gabka and Ekkehard Vaubel, *Plastic Surgery Past and Present* (Basel, 1983); Edward E. Mason, *Surgical Treatment of Obesity* (Philadelphia, 1981); P. Castelnuovo-Tedesco, "Surgical treatment of obesity: psychiatric aspects," in *Eating, Sleeping and Sexuality*, ed. Michael R. Zales (NY, 1982) 84–101; W. O. Griffen, Jr., et al., "Decline and fall of the jejunoileal bypass," *Surgery, Gynecology and Obstetrics* 157 (1983) 301–8; and Frederick M. Grazer, "Suction-assisted lipectomy, suction lipectomy, lipolysis, and lipexeresis," *Plastic and Reconstructive Surgery* 72 (1983) 620–23. On abdominoplasty in particular, Frederick M. Grazer and Jerome R. Klingbeil, *Body Image* (St. Louis, 1980). On dietetic resurrections, Cott, *Fasting*, 82 (quote).

23. Mueller, "Of obesity and election," 1366, quoting St. Jerome; Lindsey, *Late Great Planet Earth*, 130.

24. Gail Sheehy, "Quest for the perfect body," *NY Daily News* (Aug 3, 1984); Judi Sheppard Missett, *Jazzercise* (NY, 1968) epigraph, 9; Cynthia Hall, "Jazzerbucks," *Executive* (May–June 1984), in Jazzercise press folder; Nietzsche, *Beyond Good and Evil*, trans. Marianne Cowan (Chicago, 1955) 15, and his "Why I am so clever," in *On the Genealogy of Morals and Ecce Homo*, trans. and ed. Walter Kaufman (NY, 1967) 237–40; George Sheehan, "From Sheehan," *Runner's World* 15 (Oct 1980) 25, cited by another runner, James C. Whorton, *Crusaders for Fitness* (Princeton, N.J., 1982) 249; Judi Sheppard Missett, *Student Guide to Jazzercise* (Carlsbad, Calif., 1985) 2; Louise Peterson quoted in Jazzercise invitational brochure, p. 5. Cf. critique in Rosalind Coward, *Female Desire* (London, 1984) 21–22.

25. See, e.g., Jonathan Wise and Susan K. Wise, *The Overeaters: Eating Styles and Personality* (NY, 1979) suggesting the use of dance therapy with the obese. On the energy crisis, see Martin V. Melosi, *Coping with Abundance* (Philadelphia, 1985) Part Four, esp. 295–96.

26. D. S. Miller and Pamela Mumford, "Gluttony," *AJCN* 20 (1967) 1212–22; D. S. Miller and Sally Parsonage, "Resistance to slimming, adaptation or illusion?" *Lancet* 1 (1975) 773–75; Ethan A. H. Sims,

"Experimental obesity, dietary-induced thermogenesis, and their clinical implications," *Clinics in Endocrinology and Metabolism* 5 (1976) 377–95; A. E. Dugdale and P. R. Payne, "The pattern of lean and fat deposition in adults," *Nature* 266 (March 1977) 349–51; George F. Cahill, Jr., et al., "Metabolism in obesity and anorexia nervosa," in *Nutrition and the Brain, Vol. 3: Disorders of Eating,* . . . eds. Richard J. Wurtman and Judith J. Wurtman (NY, 1979) 1–70, with 600 references; and Judith Rodin, "Current status of the internal–external hypothesis for obesity: what went wrong?" *Amer Psychologist* 36,4 (1981) 361–72, reviewing the literature on food cues; "Refractory obesity and energy homeostasis," *Nutrition R* 41 (Nov 1983) 349–52. Susan C. Wooley et al., "Theoretical, practical and social issues in behavioral treatments of obesity," *J of Applied Behavior Analysis* 12 (1979) 3–29 provides a fine critique of behaviorist models.

27. A. T. Rasmussen, "The so-called hibernating gland," *J of Morphology* 38 (1923) 147–93 with full review of studies on brown adipose tissue; H. Gideon Wells, "Adipose tissue, a neglected subject," *JAMA* 114 (1940) 2180–81; R. T. Jung et al., "Reduced thermogenesis in obesity," *Nature* 279 (1979) 322–23; David Sherry, "Body weight in balance," *New Scientist* 88 (Dec 18/25, 1980) 796 (quote); and David G. Nichols and Rebecca M. Locke, "Thermogenic mechanisms in brown fat," *Physiological R* 64 (1984) 1–64.

28. E. Stellar, "The CNS and appetite: historical introduction," in *Appetite and Food Intake*, ed. Trevor Silverstone (Berlin, 1976) 15–20; "Language enricher: the appestat," *New Yorker* 28 (Aug 9, 1952) 18–20; Jean Mayer and Donald W. Thomas, "Regulation of food intake and obesity," *Science* 156 (April 21, 1967) 328–37, with historical survey; P. J. Morgane and H. L. Jacobs, "Hunger and satiety," *World R of Nutrition and Dietetics* 10 (1969) 100–213, with long bibliography; Richard E. Nisbet, "Hunger, obesity, and the ventromedial hypothalamus," *Psych R* 79 (1972) 433–54; R. M. Gold, "Hypothalamic obesity: the myth of the ventromedial nucleus," *Science* 182 (1973) 488–89; Steven M. Paul et al., "(+) – Amphetamine binding to rat hypothalamus," *Science* 218 (Oct 1982) 487–89; Thomas W. Castonguay et al., "Hunger and appetite: old concepts/new distinctions," in *Present Knowledge in Nutrition*, 5th ed. (Washington, D.C., 1984) 19–34; articles by Stellar, Grossman, and Hoebel in Albert J. Stunkard and Eliot Stellar, eds., *Eating and Its Disorders* (NY, 1984) 1–38; Edward M. Stricker, "Biological bases of hunger and satiety: therapeutic implications," *Nutrition R* 10 (1984) 333–40; and David L. Wolgin and Juanita J. Salisbury, "Amphetamine tolerance and body weight set point," *Behavioral Neuroscience* 99 (1985) 175–85, critical of set point theory.

29. See Milton V. Kline, "Hypnotherapy in the treatment of obesity," in *Psychological Aspects of Obesity*, ed. Benjamin B. Wolman (NY, 1982) 268–90, and listen to Robert Parrish, "Listen and Lose," audiocassette (Habit Control, Inc., 1972).

CHAPTER ELEVEN
Fat and Happy?

1. Marvin Grosswirth, *Fat Pride* (NY, 1971) 161, D-Zerta ad, and American Physical Fitness Research Institute poster, "Fit to Quote" (Santa Monica, Calif., 1969).

2. Louis I. Dublin believed that he had demonstrated that weight-reducing decreased mortality: "Overweight shortens life," *MLIC* 32 (Oct 1951) 1–4, and idem, "Relation of obesity to longevity," *NEJM* 248 (1953) 971–74. But see Public Health Service, *Obesity and Health* (Washington, D.C., 1966) 59; George V. Mann, "Obesity, the national spook," *AJPH* 61 (1971) 1491–98; idem, "Influence of obesity on health," *NEJM* 291 (1974) 178–85, 226–32; and William Bennett and Joel Gurin, *The Dieter's Dilemma* (NY, 1982) 134–35.

   On the absence of a causal relationship between fatness or overweight and increased mortality, see Ancel Keys et al., "Coronary heart disease: overweight and obesity as risk factors," *AIM* 77 (1972) 15–27; Tavia Gordon and William B. Kannel, "Obesity and cardiovascular disease: the Framingham study," *Clinics in Endocrinology and Metabolism* 5 (1976) 367–75; Susan C. Wooley et al., "Obesity and women—I. A closer look at the facts," *Women's Studies Int Q* 2 (1979) 74; Reubin Andres, "Effect of obesity on total mortality,' *IJO* 4 (1980) 381–86; Kelly D. Brownell, "Obesity," *J of Consulting and Clinical Psych* 50 (1982) 820; and Carol Sternhill, "We'll always be fat, but fat can be fit," *Ms.* (May 1985) 142.

   On the dangers of a weight-loss/weight-gain cycle, see Vinne Young, *It's Fun to Be Fat* (NY, 1953) 10, 26 and quote on 23; Nick Lyons, *Locked Jaws* (NY, 1979) 13 quote; and Sharon G. Patton, "Why dieting can make you fat," *New Woman* (Aug 1984) 34.

   On deaths from dieting, see Roland C. Curtin, "The heart and its danger in the treatment of obesity," *J of Balneology and Climatology* 12 (1908) 223 on pokeberry; Chapter Seven on dinitrophenol and amphetamines; House of Representatives Subcommittee on Health and the Environment, *Hearing . . . on the Most Popular Diet in America Today, Liquid Protein, Dec 28, 1977* (Washington, D.C., 1978) 3–7; Center for Disease Control, "Follow-up on deaths associated with liquid protein diets," *Morbidity and Mortality Weekly Report* 27 (1978) 223–24; Harold E. Sours et al., "Sudden death associated with very low calorie weight reduction regimens," *AJCN* 34 (1981) 453–61, and see also 1639–40, 2855–57.

3. Ann M. Lingg, "A plump girl talks back," *Amer Mercury* 78 (March 1954) 30, an early reference to minority status; Lew Louderback, "More people should be fat," *SEP* 240 (Nov 4, 1967) 10; Grosswirth, *Fat Pride*, 40; and Mildred Klingman, *Secret Lives of Fat People* (Boston, 1981) 72 on Diet Conscience. See also Lisa Schoenfielder and Barb Wieser, eds., *Shadow on a Tightrope: Writings by Women on Fat Oppression* (Iowa City, Ia., 1983).

4. Robert J. Homant and Daniel B. Kennedy, "Attitudes toward ex-offenders: a comparison of social stigmas," *J of Criminal Justice* 10 (1982) 383–91.

5. Peter L. Benson et al., "Social costs of obesity," *Social Behavior and Personality* 8 (1980) 91–96 on colleges; Llewellyn Louderback, *Fat Power* (NY, 1970) 47, 52, 53, 55; Chris Chase, *The Great American Waistline* (NY, 1981) 196 on stewardesses; *New Yorker* (Sept 29, 1980) 49; and "Better than prison," *Time* 97 (June 7, 1971) 39. Concerning weight discrimination at law, see David H. Tucker for the Maryland Commission on Human Relations, *Report on the Study of Weight and Size Discrimination*, typescript (Baltimore, 1980); Jane O. Baker, "The Rehabilitation Act of 1973: protection for victims of weight discrimination?" *UCLA Law R* 29 (April 1982) 947–71; David Berreby, "Is being fat a handicap? Courts differ," *National Law J* 4 (Aug 30, 1982) 3:1; Lynne Reaves, "Fat folks' rights: weight bias issues emerging," *Amer Bar Assoc J* 69 (1983) 878; and Lauren R. Reskin, "Employers must give obese job applicants a fat chance," *Amer Bar Assoc J* 71 (Sept 1985) 104.

6. George L. Maddox et al., "Overweight as a problem of medical management in a public outpatient clinic," *AJMS* 252 (Oct 1966) 394–402; Hilde Bruch, *The Importance of Overweight* (NY, 1957) 318–24; Howard D. Kurland, "Obesity: an unfashionable problem," *Psychiatric Opinion* 7,6 (1970) 20–24; and Alfred J. Cantor, *How to Lose Weight the Doctor's Way* (NY, 1959) quote on 40.

7. Ruth Adams, *Did You Ever See a Fat Squirrel?* (Emmaus, Pa., 1972) 197; Tillie Lewis Tasti Diet ad in *Supermarket News* (March 29, 1976) on "Where Do Diet Food Customers Get Their Information?"; Louis Harris and Associates, *Harris Survey Yearbook* (NY, 1971) 203, 213; Diana Trilling, *Mrs. Harris: The Death of the Scarsdale Diet Doctor* (NY, 1981) 85 and cf. Peter Wyden and Barbara Wyden, *How the Doctors Diet* (NY, 1968); interview with Dr. Frederick J. Stare, Sept 27, 1984, concerning physician education in nutrition; and Martin Lederman, *The Slim Gourmet* (NY, 1955) quote on 8.

8. Vinne Young, "Don't get ill getting thin," *Science Digest* 36 (Aug 1954) 1 (quote); Abigail van Buren (= Pauline Phillips), *Dear Abby*

(Englewood Cliffs, N.J., 1958) 121; Walter W. Hamburger, "Psychology of dietary change," *AJPH* 48 (1958) 1342–48; Robert M. Lindner, *The Fifty-Minute Hour* (NY, 1955) 133 (quote); Albert J. Stunkard and A. J. Rush, "Dieting and depression reexamined," *AIM* 81 (1974) 526–33; and Colleen S. W. Rand, "Treatment of obese patients in psychoanalysis," *Psychiatric Clinics of North Amer* 1 (1978) 661–72.

9. Aldebaran, "Fat liberation—a luxury?" *State and Mind* 5 (June–July 1977) 34; Stuart Byron, "The unmaking of a fattie," *Village Voice* (Dec 17, 1970) 10; and Mark Dintenfass, *The Case Against Org* (Boston, 1978) 5, 189, 246, quoted with permission from Little, Brown & Co.

10. *NYDT* (Sept 3, 1899) illus. supp. 20:3; Louderback, *Fat Power*, 167.

11. Irvin S. Cobb, *At His Best* (Garden City, N.Y., 1929) 244 on gelati noids, and Totie Fields, *I Think I'll Start on Monday: The Official 8½ Oz Mashed Potato Diet* (NY, 1972) 32 on cottage cheese. On conviviality and its suppression by dieters, see James A. Pike and Howard A. Johnson, *Man in the Middle* (Greenwich, Conn., 1956) 53; Robert Waithman, "Plea to the joyless eaters," *NYT Mag* (Feb 12, 1956) 19, 62; and Jean Kerr, *Please Don't Eat the Daisies* (NY, 1957) 172.

12. Cf. Margaret Atwood, *Lady Oracle* (NY, 1976) esp. 74, 321; Susan C. Wooley and Orland W. Wooley, "Should obesity be treated at all?" in *Eating and Its Disorders*, eds. A. J. Stunkard and E. Stellar (NY, 1984) 185–92.

13. Margaret Dana, *Behind the Label* (Boston, 1938) 117–20; Marya Mannes, "Juno in limbo: the trauma of size 16," *Harper's Mag* (July 1964) 37–40; Grosswirth, *Fat Pride*, 69; Susie Orbach, *Fat Is a Feminist Issue* (NY, 1979) 90–91; Jean DuCoffe and Sherry Suib Cohen, *Making It Big* (NY, 1980) 12, 22, 25–31; Evelyn Roaman and Dee Ratterree, *The Evelyn Roaman Book: An Expert Shows You How Heavy Can Be Happy* (NY, 1980); Dale Godey, *Your Guide to Dressing Thin* (NY, 1981) 12–27; Ann Harper and Glenn Lewis, *The Big Beauty Book* (NY, 1982) 104; and William Johnston, "The fun of being a fat man," *Amer Mag* 94 (July 1922) 54–55.

14. Lila Austin, "I'm fat, and I like it!" *GH* III (Sept 1940) 48; Nora S. Kinzer, *Put Down and Ripped Off* (NY, 1977) 34, 49–50; Marcia Millman, *Such a Pretty Face: Being Fat in America* (NY, 1980) 106, 162–63; Harper and Lewis, *Big Beauty Book*, quote on 3; DuCoffe and Cohen, *Making It Big*, 258 (quote), 260–63; David Newman and Robert Benton, "Fat power," *Esquire* 66 (Dec 1966) 212–15 on visual grandeur of fat men; Carol S. Smith, *Fat People* (NY, 1978); and see "Fatso" film (20th-Century Fox, 1980).

15. Charlotte C. Rowett, "Success, avoirdupois, and clothes," *Woman Beautiful* 4 (June 1910) 40–41; DuCoffe and Cohen, *Making It Big*,

334; Anne Scott Beller, *Fat and Thin* (NY, 1977) esp. ch. 7; Kim Chernin, *The Obsession: Reflections on the Tyranny of Slenderness* (NY, 1981) esp. 133, 139; Jean Stafford, "The echo and the nemesis," *Children Are Bored on Sunday* (NY, 1953) 10–39, a fantasy self; Ruthanne Olds, *Big and Beautiful: Overcoming Fat Phobia* (Washington, D.C., 1982) 13; Stella J. Reichman, *Great Big Beautiful Doll* (NY, 1977) 26–28; and Marion Woodman, *The Owl Was a Baker's Daughter* (Toronto, 1980) 10, 18.

16. See Donald B. Meyer, *The Positive Thinkers* (Garden City, N.Y., 1965) 120 on the "flight from feelings"; Véronique Nahoum, "La belle femme ou le stade du miroir en histoire," *Communications* 31 (1979) 22–32 on mirrors; and Susan Griffin, *Pornography and Silence* (NY, 1981) esp. 60–62.

17. Nina W. Putnam, *Tomorrow We Diet* (NY, 1922) 89; Phillip W. Haberman, Jr., "How to diet if you have no character at all," *Vogue* 135 (June 1960) 148; and Thyra S. Winslow, *Think Yourself Thin* (NY, 1951) 113. On tapeworms, Ronald L. Baker, *Hoosier Folk Legends* (Bloomington, Ind., 1982) 226, and Jane Fonda, *Workout Book* (NY, 1981) 10.

18. Christopher Lasch, *The Culture of Narcissism* (NY, 1978) xvi (quote); Peter Clecak, *America's Quest for the Ideal Self* (NY, 1983) ch. 12; Louderback, *Fat Power*, 25, 28; Mike Featherstone, "The body in consumer culture," *Theory, Culture & Society* 1,2 (1982) 18–33; Bryan S. Turner, *The Body and Society* (Oxford, 1984) 93; and "Fear of fat," Pacifica Radio Archive audiocassette (1980).

19. On the *crise pléthorique*, see Friedrich Engels, "Socialism: utopian and scientific" (1880) in *Marx & Engels*, ed. Lewis S. Feuer (Garden City, N.Y., 1959) 100–101. Cf. Anne M. Christner, "Scrutiny of the Bounty: The Poor Quality of the U.S. Diet Amidst Agricultural Plenty," Ph.D. thesis, Univ of Massachusetts, 1983.

20. Letita Brewster and Michael F. Jacobson, *The Changing American Diet* (Washington, D.C., 1978) 55 on cost of vitamins. Infant formulas and prepared foods, often concocted from industrial chaff, have long been suspected of promoting the unnatural fatness of American babies. Bottle-feeding, which is to the advantage of dairymen and food manufacturers, may also restrict or reduce the natural weight-loss by postpartum mothers who would otherwise be breastfeeding. Commerce and physicians linked to the industrial concerns of drug manufacturers have worked together to argue for the early use of solid foods in infant diets, and for earlier weaning. To follow the controversy over the role of capitalism in producing unhealthy babies, see esp. Ted Greiner, *The Promoting of Bottle Feeding By Multinational Corporations* Cornell International Nutrition Monograph Se-

ries, 2 (1975); "Sally turns ten—and strained baby foods become big business," *Sales Management* 42 (May 1, 1938) 21, 65; Belle Wood-Comstock, "Obesity in children," *Med Women's J* 50 (1943) 125; "An anaysis of the baby food market," *Glass Packer* 23 (1944) 823–25, 860; Marguerite Rittenhouse and Ruth Kamerman, "Overweight child," *Cosmopolitan* 149 (July 1960) 79; Derrick B. Jelliffe and E. F. Patrice Jelliffe, "Fat Babies," typescript, UCLA Biomedical Library, 1973, esp. 33–36; Donald Naismith, "Bottle feeding makes fat mamas—and fat babies too!" *Med Opinion* 3 (Nov 1974) 38–40; Barbara Hall, "Changing composition of human milk and early development of an appetite control," *Lancet* 1 (1975) 779–81; David L. Yeung et al., "Infant fatness and feeding practices," *JADA* 79 (1981) 531–35; Steve Wirtz, "Infant formula practices in the U.S.," *Science for the People* 16,2 (March–April 1984) 14–17, 30–31 and see entire issue. The very first complaint about artificial feeds leading to obese babies may have been Carl F. H. Immermann, "Corpulence," in *Cyclopaedia of the Practice of Medicine*, trans. E. B. Baxter (NY, 1877) 632–33.

21. Jantzen/Dexaspan ad reprinted in Richard Kunnes, "Double dealing in dope," *Human Behavior* 2 (Oct 1973) 24.

22. On set points, see Bennett and Gurin, *Dieter's Dilemma*, and contrast David Wirtshafter and John D. Davis, "Set points, settling points and the control of body weight," *Physiology and Behavior* 19 (1977) 75–78; on the profitability of diet foods, Andrew Christian, "Diet soft drinks promise continued growth and profit potential," *FPD* 11 (Feb 1977) 59, and Christine Van Lenten, "Serving up health," *National Restaurant Assoc News* (Aug 1983) 11–14. Corinne Le Bovit and Hazen Gales estimated in 1971 that if the entire population were to go on a low-fat, low-cholesterol diet, Americans would spend 10 percent more on food and eat 15 percent more pounds of food: "Potential effects of fat-controlled, low-cholesterol diet on U.S. food consumption," *Agricultural Economics Research* 23 (July 1971) 49.

23. On the rice diet, Burr Snider, "Fat city," *Esquire* 79 (March 1973) 112–14; on hunger and obesity, see Thomas C. Desmond, "Fat men can't win," *Science Illustrated* 4 (June 1949) quote on 47. Cf. Vivek Bammi, "Nutrition, the historian and public policy," *JSH* 14 (1981) 627–48; Barbara Ehrenreich, "The cult of food in a world of hunger," *NYT* (Jan 17, 1985) IV, 14:1–3; and Mary Douglas, "Standard social uses of food," in *Food in the Social Order*, ed. Douglas (NY, 1984) 36.

24. See esp. the title stories in Peter Carey, *The Fat Man in History* (St. Lucia, Queensland, 1974) 114–41, and in Frederik Pohl, *The Man Who Ate the World* (NY, 1960) 7–37.

25. Phyllis Rosenteur, *Affair of the Flesh* (NY, 1952) 44–45 on Redeucit; Bruce M. Hannon and Timothy G. Lohman, "The energy cost of overweight in the U.S.," *AJPH* 68 (1978) 765–67; Carol Lynn Tiegs, "Growth is sweet for dessert concepts," *Restaurant Business* 83 (May 1, 1984) 176–87; Jeannie Willis, "How to feed a hungry family," *Amer Home* 55 (May 1956) 78–79; and "How fat is a fat man?" *Life* 23 (Oct 6, 1947) 88, ad on 89. On taxing the obese, there have been sporadic allusions to a Swedish law of the 1920s which was eventually ruled unconstitutional, but Inger Konradsson of the Swedish Ministry of Justice has been unable to locate such a law (letter of Jan 21, 1985). For other proposals to tax the obese, see "A British view on over-eating: tax on fat people?" *U.S. News and World Report* (Jan 7, 1955) 58–60, and Klingman, *Secret Lives*, 42.

26. Cf. Jessica R. Johnston, "The Double Bind: 'Eat and Stay Thin.' Food as a Condensed Cultural Symbol in Advertising and the Overweight Stigma, 1890–1980," MA thesis, California State Univ at Fullerton, 1983, and a recent essay by Aristides, "A fat man struggles to get out," *Amer Scholar* 54 (1985) 303–12, on the desire "to live fat but be thin."

On class, obesity and dieting, see Phillip B. Goldblatt et al., "Social factors in obesity," *JAMA* 192 (1965) 1039–42, generally referred to as part of the Midtown Manhattan study; Public Health Service, *Obesity and Health*, 68; Harris and Associates, *Harris Survey Yearbook* (1971) April 1970 survey of doctors; Albert J. Stunkard et al., "Influence of social class on obesity and thinness in children" *JAMA* 221 (1972) 579–84, showing that obesity was more prevalent among lower-class than upper-class girls by age six, perhaps because thinness was an upper-class value, perhaps because of the kinds of foods available to the poor; Stanley M. Garn and Diane C. Clark, "Economics and fatness," *Ecology of Food and Nutrition* 3 (1974) 19–20, analyzing the Ten-State Nutrition Survey 1968–70, which showed that poverty-level women of all groups were fatter than women of median incomes; idem, "Trends in fatness and the origins of obesity," *Pediatrics* 57 (1976) 443–56; Albert J. Stunkard, *The Pain of Obesity* (Palo Alto, Calif., 1976) 146–48; Wooley et al., "Obesity and women—II. A neglected feminist topic," 81, 87; and April E. Fallon and Paul Rozin, "Sex differences in perceptions of desirable body shape," *J of Abnormal Psych* 94 (1985) 102–5, suggesting that women of all classes are highly conscious of an upper-class-male figure preference for thin women.

On blacks, and black women in particular, see George D. Maddox et al., "Overweight as social deviance and disability," *J of Health and Social Behavior* 9 (1968) 287–98; Sandra L. Benbrook, "Obesity in the U.S.—Stratifying Factors," Ph.D. thesis, Univ of Southern California, 1978; Sue R. Dyrenforth et al., "A women's body in a man's world: a review of findings on body image and weight control," in *A Woman's Conflict* ed. June R. Kaplan (Englewood Cliffs, N.J., 1980) esp. 42, and in the same volume, Marvalene H. Styles, "Soul, black women and food," 161–76.

27. Katherine M. H. Blackford and Arthur Newcomb, *Analyzing Character*, 4th ed. (NY, 1916) ch. 5; Woods Hutchinson, "A defense of fat men," *SEP* 196 (June 7, 1924) 62; Leonard H. Robbins, "Plea in defense of the fat man," *NYT Mag* (Jan 5, 1936) 14; and Les A. Murray, *The Vernacular Republic* (Edinburgh, 1982), "Quintets for Robert Morley," stanzas 2, 7, quoted with permission from Persea Books.

28. Du Coffe and Cohen, *Making It Big*, 234; Orbach, *Fat Is a Feminist Issue*, quote on 12; *NYT* (June 5, 1967) 54:1 on Fat-In; CBS-TV, "Fat . . . And Proud Of It," *Sixty Minutes*, Dec 10, 1978; and Paul Deutschman, *The Adipose Complex* (NY, 1972) 357–59. Cf. Michel Foucault, "Body/Power," in his *Power/Knowledge*, ed. and trans. Colin Gordon et al. (NY, 1980) 58.

29. Trilling, *Mrs. Harris*, 310–11.

30. Hilde Bruch, *The Golden Cage* (Cambridge, Mass., 1978); Emily E. Hudlow, *Alabaster Chambers* (NY, 1977); L. M. Vincent, *Competing with the Sylph* (Kansas City, Mo., 1979); Nu-Weigh Hospital Treatment Program ad in *Los Angeles Times* (Feb 12, 1985) V, 8; Craig Johnson et al., "Anorexia nervosa and obesity," in *Progress in Pediatric Psychology*, eds. W. J. Burns and J. V. Lavigne (Orlando, Fla., 1984) 193 on pessimistic outcome and cure rates; National Assoc of Anorexia Nervosa and Related Disorders, introductory brochure (Highland Park, Ill., 1984); Steven Levenkron, *Best Little Girl in the World* (Chicago, 1978); Richard Bachman, *Thinner* (NY, 1984); and Susan Squire, *The Slender Balance* (NY, 1983) esp. 106, 156.

31. Corey Ford, "Never say diet," *RD* 62 (May 1953) 95, 96; idem, *Never Say Diet: How to Live Older and Look Longer* (NY, 1954) 14; Fields, *I Think I'll Start on Monday*, quote on 41. Cf. Mark Twain, "At the Appetite-Cure," *Cosmopolitan* 25 (Aug 1898) 425–33.

32. Russell Baker, *So This Is Depravity* (NY, 1980) 103, and National Public Radio, "Prairie Home Companion," Oct 29, 1983. Joseph Bones of NY has recently formed an actual fat squad. Robert Pfeiffer, "Policing the pounds," *Washington Post* (May 2, 1986) D2.

33. "Handbook of diets," *Vogue* 121 (April 15, 1953) 76; Edward Sagarin, *Odd Man In: Societies of Deviants in America* (Chicago, 1969) 73; and interview with Richard Simmons, Feb 4, 1985.

34. Chernin, *The Obsession*, 100; Nicole Hollander, *More Sylvia* (NY, 1982) 23; Millman, *Such a Pretty Face*, 112–13; and Nicky Diamond, "Thin is the feminist issue," *Feminist R* 19 (Spring 1985) 45–65.

35. Fonda, *Workout Book*, 13–20, quote on 20.

36. *Ibid.*, 68, and *Jane Fonda's Workout Record* (Columbia Records, 1982) cover notes and side 4, cut 3.

37. Fonda, *Workout Book*, 33, 41 (quote), 71, 228 (quote), and Charles Krauthammer, "Stretch Marx: *Jane Fonda's Workout Book*," *New Republic* 187 (Aug 16–23, 1982) 30–31.

38. "Thin model ban," *AA* (Aug 3, 1981) 2, 63; "One voice does count," ANAD *Working Together* newsletter (March–April 1984) 2 on *Glamour Mag*'s "recent editorial decision to begin featuring fashion & beauty strategies for women who don't fall in that 'model perfect' category."

39. Public Health Service, *Obesity and Health*, 68; "Land of the fat," *Time* (Jan 2, 1978) 53; Craig Norback, ed., *Complete Book of American Surveys* (NY, 1980) 211–12; and Brewster and Jacobson, *Changing American Diet*, 56, 58 (quote). P. V. Sukhatme, "Trend of obesity in the U.S.A.," FAO Working Paper WS/77438, argues that the increase of weight is also an increase in obesity (fatness), but contrast Sidney Abraham, ed., "Obese and overweight adults in the U.S.," *Vital and Health Statistics* ser. 11, 230 (1983) arguing (p. 23) that far more people are overweight than obese.

40. Ann Blackman, "Sizing up today's woman," *NY Post* (Jan 7, 1971) 30; DuCoffe and Cohen, *Making It Big*, 47; Joseph M. Fee and Roger H. L. Wilson, "Obesity: a gross national product," in *Obesity*, ed. Nancy L. Wilson (Philadelphia, 1969) 244; and letter from Fred Rose, Director of Products, American Seating Company, Dec 27, 1984.

41. Letter from Frederic Seltzer, Asst. Actuary for Metropolitan Life, Dec 5, 1984, with enclosed paper, "Construction of weight tables based on lowest mortality."

42. "Ideal weight rises," *RD* 123 (July 1983) 18; interviews with Lois Lindauer, International Director of Diet Workshop, Inc., Nov 15, 1984, and Linda Konner, editor of *WW*, Oct 12, 1984; and Pat McManus, "Yes, you can be too thin," *NY Mag* 14 (June 22, 1981) 43–45.

43. "Why weight tables don't work," *Vogue* (Dec 1984) 371, and "Health benefits of lifelong leanness are challenged by new weight tables," *NYT* (Aug 6, 1985) Section C, pp. 1, 7.

44. Richard Smith, *The Bronx Diet* (NY, 1981) 141.

45. On climate, see entire issue of *JIH* 10,4 (1980), and Hubert H. Lamb, *Climate, History and the Modern World* (London, 1982) 253–71. On obesity in the Northern Hemisphere, see P. V. Sukhatme, "On the trend of obesity in the advanced countries," FAO Working Paper, ST: Misc/68; Kateřina Ošancová and Stanislav Hejda, "Epidemiol-

ogy of obesity," in *Obesity: Its Pathogenesis and Management*, ed. Trevor Silverstone (Acton, Mass., 1975) 57–91.

46. Kenneth Clark, *The Nude* (NY, 1956) ch. 8; Walter C. Curry, *The Middle English Ideal of Personal Beauty* (Baltimore, 1970) 3, 102–3, 107, 110–11, 115–16; and William A. Shack, "Hunger, anxiety and ritual: deprivation and spirit possession among the Gurage of Ethiopia," *Man* 6 (1971) 30–43.

47. Cf. Melvin Cherno, "Feuerbach's 'Man Is What He Eats': a rectification," *J of the History of Ideas* 24 (1963) 397–406; Gillian Gillison, "Images of nature in Gimi thought," in *Nature, Culture and Gender*, eds. Carol P. MacCormack and Marilyn Strathern (Cambridge, 1980) 143–73.

48. Kerr, *Please Don't Eat the Daisies*, 172.

Index

Note: Due to considerations of weight and economy, this index is leaner than it might be. Place names, passing references, incidental proper names, cartoon characters, book and magazine titles have been omitted. Reducing aids are indexed separately at the end, alphabetically by trade name.

Watkins, Henry, 273
Watling Mfg Co, 165
Weber, Mathias C., 169
weighing: of babies, 4, 271–80; of
children, 271, 280–86, 437; of
criminals, 153; of excrement, 12,
127; of food, 13–14, 27, 83, 171–76;
of patients, 152–53, 393; of the
soul, 11, 13, 50, 155, 308
—frequency of, 17, 27, 39, 57, 120–
21, 155, 282
—popularity of, 4, 5, 17, 57–58, 147,
164–75, 271
"Weighing the Baby," 270, 272
weight: "dead," 75, 103, 105, 111,
132, 216, 220; ideal, 153, 157, 159,
164, 166, 177, 201, 334, 336–38;
sensation of, 3, 10, 14, 19, 51, 58–
59, 67–68, 73, 109, 128, 145, 147,
151–53
Weight Watchers, 204, 208–11, 220,
225, 242, 244, 246, 247, 255, 309,
337
weight-watching: origins of, 10, 26,
46, 147, 214, 239, 271, 279–80,
285 86, 320; prevalence of, 5, 57,
145, 246–51, 325
Weight Worthy, 331
weightlessness, 8, 54, 301, 303,
314–15
weights, 17, 27, 40, 68, 157, 336–37
Weld, Theodore D., 65, 67
Wells, David A., 85
Wheeler, Elmer, 211–13, 220
White, Barry, 249
White, Ellen G., 64, 184
White, Paul Dudley, 234
White House Conference on Food,
Nutrition and Health, 295
Whiteman, Margaret, 183
Whiteman, Paul, 183
Wilder, Russell M., 193
Wiley, Harvey W., 264
Wilkinson, William S., 122
Williams-Heller, Annie W., 242
will power, 17–18, 31, 72, 98, 103,
107, 119, 140, 228, 308–9, 316–17
Wilson, William G., 204

Windom, William, 91
Winslow, Rose, 123–24
Winslow, Sam, 179–80
Winthrop, Alice W., 99
Wollheim, Louis, 183
women: their bodies, 46, 136–37,
325–26; as dieters, 16–18, 38, 136–
37, 140, 158–59, 196–97, 209–11,
246–51, 254, 330, 398–99; as
fasters, 123–24; as gatekeepers,
194–95; in groups, 59, 61–64, 204–
11, 309; as mothers, 23–26, 32, 70,
194–96, 201–4, 248–49, 254, 275,
286, 291–92, 301, 330; as suffrag-
ists, 123–24
Wood, Thomas, 239–45, 268
Workshop in Lenten Living, 309
World War I, 140–45, 157–58, 174,
191, 194, 204, 230
World War II, 157–59, 195, 231–32,
262, 263, 280, 286, 294
Wright brothers, 78–79, 102
Wrigley, William, Jr., 182
Wurtman, Richard, 266
Wyden, Barbara, 248
Wyden, Peter, 248

Yorke-Davies, N. E., 111

Zachar, John, 123
Zander, Gustaf, 185
zippers, 178, 288

REDUCING AIDS
(alphabetical by trade name)

Absorbit, 110; Allan's Anti-Fat, 114,
139; Anorexine, 7; Appedrine, 7, 245;
Appetrol, 197, 403; Aunt Leah's diet
borscht, 241; Ayds, 7; Basy Bread,
241; Battle Creek Health Builder,
182; Berledets, 97; Bertha C. Day's
prescriptions, 139; Biphetamine, 197;
Body Taper-Trim Shirt, 249; Carnation Slender, 199; Cellu wafers, 241;
Chichester's Corpus Lean, 98; Coffee,
Tea & A New Me, 7; Control, 245;
Corpu-Lean, 191; Corpulin, 139;